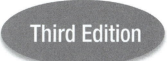
Third Edition

Understanding and Managing
VISION DEFICITS

A Guide for Occupational Therapists

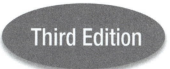

Third Edition

Understanding and Managing
VISION DEFICITS
A Guide for Occupational Therapists

Mitchell Scheiman, OD, FCOVD, FAAO
Professor
Chief, Pediatric/Binocular Vision Service
Pennsylvania College of Optometry at Salus University
Philadelphia, Pennsylvania

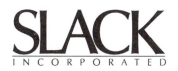

www.slackbooks.com

ISBN: 978-1-55642-937-8

Copyright © 2011 by SLACK Incorporated

SLACK Incorporated uses a review process to evaluate submitted material. Prior to publication, educators or clinicians provide important feedback on the content that we publish. We welcome feedback on this work.

Published by: SLACK Incorporated
                       6900 Grove Road
                       Thorofare, NJ 08086 USA
                       Telephone: 856-848-1000
                       Fax: 856-848-6091
                       www.slackbooks.com

Contact SLACK Incorporated for more information about other books in this field or about the availability of our books from distributors outside the United States.

Library of Congress Cataloging-in-Publication Data

Scheiman, Mitchell.
  Understanding and managing vision deficits : a guide for occupational therapists / Mitchell Scheiman.
-- 3rd ed.
      p. ; cm.
  Includes bibliographical references and index.
  ISBN 978-1-55642-937-8 (alk. paper)
  1. Vision disorders. 2. Ocular manifestations of general diseases. 3. Occupational therapy. I. Title.
  [DNLM: 1. Vision Disorders--diagnosis. 2. Occupational Therapy--methods. 3. Vision Disorders--reha-
bilitation. 4. Vision, Ocular--physiology. WW 141]
  RE91.U53 2011
  617.7'0024615--dc22
                              2010041846

Printed in the United States of America.

Contents

About the Author

Mitchell Scheiman, OD, FCOVD, FAAO, is a nationally known optometric educator, lecturer, author, and private practitioner. He graduated from the New England College of Optometry, Boston, MA, in 1975 and completed a residency in vision therapy at the State University of New York College of Optometry in 1976. He has specialized in vision therapy for the past 35 years. Dr. Scheiman is currently director of Pediatric and Binocular Vision Programs at The Eye Institute and professor of optometry at the Pennsylvania College of Optometry. He has written three books for optometrists, covering the topics of binocular vision and vision therapy, pediatric optometry, and learning-related vision problems, and he has published more than 140 articles in the professional literature. He is a Diplomate in Binocular Vision and Perception and a Fellow in the College of Optometrists in Vision Development. Dr. Scheiman maintains a private practice in the Philadelphia suburbs where he specializes in vision therapy.

Dr. Scheiman has a long and close relationship with occupational therapists. He is the founder of Vision Education Seminars, a company that develops and provides continuing education programs about vision to occupational therapists. In the past 15 years he has lectured to more than 7000 occupational therapists. He co-manages patients with occupational and physical therapists in his practice, and his wife, Maxine Scheiman, has been an occupational therapist for more than 20 years.

Contributing Authors

Sarah D. Appel, OD, FAAO (Chapters Eleven and Twelve)
Associate Professor of Optometry
Diplomate in Low Vision Rehabilitation (American Academy of Optometry)
Co-Director, Special Populations Assessment and Rehabilitation Clinic
Pennsylvania College of Optometry at Salus University
Elkins Park, Pennsylvania

Elise B. Ciner, OD, FAAO (Chapters Eleven and Twelve)
Associate Professor of Optometry
Director, Infant Vision Care
Co-Director, Special Populations Assessment and Rehabilitation Clinic
Pennsylvania College of Optometry at Salus University
Elkins Park, Pennsylvania

Maureen A. Duffy, MS, CVRT (Chapter Fourteen)
Editorial Director
Associates for World Action in Rehabilitation & Education (AWARE)
Associate Editor
Journal of Visual Impairment and Blindness

Beth I. Fishman, OTR, COVT (Chapter Ten)
Private Practice
Centennial, Colorado

Lynn Fishman Hellerstein, OD, FCOVD, FAAO (Chapters Nine and Ten)
Adjunct Professor
Pacific University College of Optometry
Illinois College of Optometry
Southern College of Optometry
Private Practice
Centennial, Colorado

Paul B. Freeman, OD, FAAO, FCOVD (Chapter Thirteen)
Diplomate Low Vision
Chief of Low Vision Services
Allegheny General Hospital
Pittsburgh, Pennsylvania

Marcy Graboyes, ACSW, LSW (Chapter Twelve)
Associate Professor
College of Education and Rehabilitation
Coordinator of Social Services
William Feinbloom Vision Rehabilitation Center
Pennsylvania College of Optometry at Salus University
Elkins Park, Pennsylvania

Kathleen Mary Huebner, PhD, COMS (Chapter Fourteen)
Professor and Associate Dean
College of Education and Rehabilitation
Director, National Leadership Consortium for Sensory Disabilities
Salus University
Elkins Park, Pennsylvania

Maxine Scheiman, MEd, OTR/L, CLVT (Chapters Fifteen and Sixteen)
Low Vision Occupational Therapist
Thomas Jefferson University
Philadelphia, Pennsylvania

Valorie Todd, OTR (Chapter Seventeen)
Occupational Therapist
Kingston City Schools
Lecturer
Rutgers University
Stone Ridge, New York

Kathleen Tsurumi, OTR (Chapter Seventeen)
Private Practice
Pediatric Occupational Therapy
Highland Park, New Jersey

Stephen G. Whittaker, OTR, PhD, CLVT (Chapter Ten)
Vision Rehabilitation Consulting
Southampton, Pennsylvania

Diane P. Wormsley, PhD (Chapter Fourteen)
Brenda Brodie Endowed Chair
Professor of Special Education in Visual Impairment
North Carolina Central University
Durham, North Carolina

Preface to the Third Edition

The primary goal of this new edition is to ensure that this book continues to be an up-to-date resource for occupational therapists about vision, enabling them to develop a comprehensive understanding of vision, to appreciate the various effects vision problems can have on the practice of occupational therapy, and to more effectively manage patients with vision disorders. Eight years have passed since the publication of the Second Edition and, as can be expected, there have been many new developments in vision care.

Some of the general changes in each chapter include updated figures, incorporation of new research, and updated references. Several areas required more extensive updates. For example, there have been very important developments in vision therapy research over the past 8 years with a number of randomized clinical trials published since 2005. Another area of significant change is in traumatic brain injury. As a result of the wars in Iraq and Afghanistan, more than 30,000 soldiers have returned to the United States with injuries requiring rehabilitation. Over 50% of those returning with injuries due to traumatic brain injury have significant vision problems. Studies have shown that binocular vision, accommodation, eye movements, and visual field disorders are prevalent in this population. If left undetected and uncorrected these problems can interfere with the patient's ability to regain independence in activities of daily living. We have incorporated updated information about research and treatment of the vision conditions that are prevalent after traumatic brain injury.

Finally, occupational therapy continues to emerge as one of the important professions involved in the care of patients with visual impairment. Legislative changes in the past decade have created an atmosphere in which occupational therapists can be more easily reimbursed for low vision rehabilitation. These factors combined with the aging of the population and an increase in the prevalence of visual impairment have created a very strong interest from occupational therapists in topics such as the low vision evaluation, low vision aids, and low vision rehabilitation. As a result, we have updated the three chapters related to low vision in this Third Edition.

My hope is this book will continue to bring the professions of occupational therapy and optometry closer together, which will ultimately lead to the best possible care for patients being treated by both professions.

Preface to the Second Edition

The first edition of this book was written to meet a perceived demand for information about vision by occupational therapists. The response to this book during the past 4 years has been outstanding and demonstrates that there is indeed very strong interest from occupational therapy about vision problems and intervention strategies for these problems.

The need for a second edition became apparent shortly after completion of the first edition. In the past few years, occupational therapy has emerged as one of the professions involved in the care of patients with visual impairment. This emergence has been a gradual process and has evolved for at least two reasons. First, occupational therapists are uniquely trained to care for patients with low vision. Low vision problems significantly affect an individual's ability to perform activities of daily living. Helping individuals regain independence in activities of daily living is the distinctive skill of occupational therapists. In addition, legislative changes in the past few years have created an atmosphere in which occupational therapists can be more easily reimbursed for low vision rehabilitation. These factors combined with the aging of the population and an increase in the prevalence of visual impairment have created a very strong interest from occupational therapists in topics such as low vision evaluation, low vision aids, and low vision rehabilitation.

To meet this need, I have added three new chapters that specifically address the area of low vision. These chapters are written by experienced clinicians from optometry, occupational therapy, and the three other important low vision professions: rehabilitation teachers, orientation and mobility instructors, and teachers of the visually impaired.

Chapter Fourteen is an introductory chapter and provides an overview of the low vision evaluation, low vision aids, and low vision rehabilitation from an optometric viewpoint. Chapter Fifteen describes the various professional disciplines involved in low vision rehabilitation and how occupational therapy fits into the team of rehabilitation professionals. This chapter also provides detailed information about environmental assessment and modification for individuals with low vision. The final chapter on low vision is written by an occupational therapist who has developed a low vision rehabilitation program in her rehabilitation facility. It is a practical presentation of how an occupational therapist can develop a low vision specialty. It includes information about necessary competencies for treating low vision patients, educational opportunities for occupational therapists to gain these competencies, becoming certified in low vision, generating patient referrals, marketing low vision rehabilitation services, documentation, reimbursement issues, and billing.

The original 15 chapters have all been revised and updated based on recommendations from reviewers and changes that have occurred in theory, diagnosis, and treatment over the past 4 years.

Preface to the First Edition

My primary goal for writing this book is to create a resource for occupational therapists about vision, enabling them to develop a comprehensive understanding of vision, to appreciate the various effects vision problems can have on the practice of occupational therapy, and to manage patients with vision disorders more effectively. There can be little argument that occupational therapists evaluate and treat patients with a high prevalence of vision disorders. For example, adults with traumatic brain injury and cerebrovascular accident and children with pervasive developmental disabilities, cerebral palsy, mental retardation, learning disorders, and traumatic brain injury are all commonly seen by occupational therapists. One of the major health concerns present in all of these patients is vision problems.

In some instances, these vision problems may be primary and may prevent any meaningful progress. In other cases, the vision problem is not the key factor but, if left untreated, may interfere with the occupational therapy care process, leading to less than optimal treatment outcomes.

A second motive for writing this book is to develop a text that will help the professions of optometry and occupational therapy relate to and understand each other more effectively. In recent years, a number of authors have described several striking similarities between optometry and occupational therapy. These include a strong emphasis on investigating the relationship between physical and cognitive deficiencies and performance on activities of daily living, the importance of therapeutic intervention, and the importance of eliminating underlying skills problems. At the same time, the differences between the professions are also obvious, each having its own unique perspectives and strengths. These similarities and differences have led many individual professionals from optometry and occupational therapy to realize that, in some instances, optimal care for patients requires a joint effort between the two professions.

Although optometry and occupational therapy have traditionally not worked in the same clinical settings, this is occurring more often. Optometrists are becoming part of the health care team in rehabilitation settings, providing both direct care and, in some cases, consultative services. In the private sector, more and more optometrists and occupational therapists are working together in practices to meet the needs of their patients. Continuing education courses for occupational therapists about vision, visual perception, and vision therapy are becoming commonplace.

From my own personal experience being married to a pediatric occupational therapist and having interacted with many therapists in early intervention programs, rehabilitation hospitals, and school-based programs, I know that in many cases occupational therapists are anxious to acquire as much knowledge as possible about vision and that they recognize its importance in the care of their patients. I have often been asked to lecture about vision problems, screening procedures to help determine if such problems exist, and even information on intervention when these problems are present.

The objectives of this book are to meet these needs. The first five chapters of the book are designed to provide background information about vision. After the introductory chapters, Chapters Three through Five develop an understanding of the complexity of vision and present a three-component model, including acuity, refraction, eye health, visual efficiency disorders, and visual processing problems. Chapter Six describes a screening battery that can be used in a variety of settings by occupational therapists to screen for visual acuity, refractive, visual efficiency, and visual information processing problems. The screening procedures described can generally be done in a short period of time and without an investment in expensive instrumentation.

Chapter Seven reviews the management of refractive, visual efficiency, and visual information processing problems. This chapter is not designed to teach occupational therapists to perform optometric vision therapy. The optometric viewpoint is that vision therapy should be performed by optometrists or under the supervision of optometrists. However, there are several ways in which the occupational therapist can help in the management of patients with vision disorders. This chapter is designed to accomplish several objectives regarding intervention. The first goal is to provide information about how optometrists treat various vision disorders using lenses, prism, and vision therapy. The second objective is to provide detailed suggestions about how the occupational therapist can work along with the optometrist when treating children who are also being treated for a vision disorder. The final goal is to provide several treatment sequences that can be used by occupational therapists to supplement the vision therapy being performed by an optometrist in the areas of eye movements and visual information processing skills.

Chapters Eight through Twelve provide detailed information about common vision problems in three very important populations: those with developmental disabilities, children and adults who have experienced traumatic brain injury, and children with learning disabilities. Chapter Thirteen provides details about visual field deficits and neglect, two of the more common and enigmatic vision disorders occurring after cerebrovascular accident and traumatic brain injury. Chapter Fourteen presents a four-step inter-relationship model for optometrists and occupational therapists.

The final chapter, written by two experienced pediatric occupational therapists, provides a frame of reference for occupational therapists interested in managing patients with vision problems. The entire text has been reviewed by occupational therapist Maxine Scheiman to ensure accuracy and relevance for occupational therapists. In addition, it has been peer reviewed by occupational therapists.

My hope is that, by developing a better understanding of vision, this book will serve to bring the two professions closer together, which will ultimately lead to the best possible care for patients being treated by both professions.

Chapter One

Background Information

Mitchell Scheiman, OD, FCOVD, FAAO

The Importance of Vision for Occupational Therapists

Occupational therapy is concerned with a person's ability to participate in desired life tasks, including caring for one's self, working, going to school, playing, and living independently. If a person's ability to perform these tasks is affected by an illness, disease, or disability, occupational therapy can be important in improving the individual's quality of life.[1] The premise of this book is that, given the high prevalence of vision disorders in the patients they serve, occupational therapists must understand the complexity and importance of vision and how visual deficits can interfere with occupational therapy, to be maximally effective in achieving these goals.

Reading, writing, and driving, for example, are three important functional skills that are very dependent on normal visual function.[2,3] There is a strong overflow to most other daily tasks. Vision problems may interfere with mobility, filling out forms, dressing, eating, locating objects, shopping, cooking, grooming, and managing finances. Hemiplegic patients with visual field deficits and/or visual neglect have also been shown to be accident prone.[4] This type of behavior may prolong treatment programs and may affect how the therapist grades the patient's level of competence in various activities of daily living. Visual scanning disorders may be one of the key factors causing the accident prone behavior.[5] In children, vision problems may interfere with learning to read, write, and play. Studies have also looked at the importance of vision for normal social interaction and found that a significant amount of social interaction involves nonverbal communication, which is often based on recognition of facial cues during conversation. Vision problems can, therefore, interfere with conversation and can cause social interaction problems for both adults and children. Recognizing faces and facial expressions is a common problem after traumatic brain injury or cerebrovascular accident.[6] It is not unusual for brain injury patients to miss important social cues, become more passive during conversation, and retreat from normal social interaction. Clearly, a change in visual processing can affect all aspects of a person's functioning.

Pediatric occupational therapists care for children with a wide variety of problems, including cerebral palsy, Down syndrome, other types of mental retardation, spina bifida, low birth weight syndrome, pervasive developmental delay, sensory integrative dysfunction, and child abuse and neglect. Studies have shown that most of these patients have a high prevalence of vision disorders, which creates a need for a comprehensive understanding of vision.[7-18] The most common conditions found in these children include optical problems such as hyperopia, myopia, and astigmatism; strabismus; amblyopia; nystagmus; optic atrophy; and visual processing problems.[7] Ciner et al[17] performed a comprehensive visual examination on 135 preschool children at an early intervention program in Philadelphia. These children had various mentally and physically handicapping conditions, including Down syndrome, cerebral palsy, history of parental substance abuse, failure to thrive, and unlabeled developmental delays. They found that 60% of this population had significant vision problems. Strabismus was the most common condition, followed by refractive conditions such as hyperopia, myopia, and astigmatism.

For occupational therapists working with adults, the most common patients seen are those who have experienced cerebrovascular accidents, head trauma, and spinal cord injuries. Gianutsos reported that nearly half of the people admitted to a long-term rehabilitation facility after brain injury had visual system deficits, primarily in the area of binocular vision and accommodation.[19,20] Suchoff et al[21] evaluated 62 consecutive patients entering a rehabilitation hospital with acquired brain injury (mean age: 49, range: 19 to 70). They found a high prevalence of vision disorders including problems with eye teaming (42%), eye movement (40%), focusing (10%), external eye disease (23%), glaucoma (19%), and visual field defects (32%). Ciuffreda et al[22] reported on a retrospective study of 220 patients with traumatic brain injury or stroke and found that 90% of the individuals with traumatic brain injury and 86.7% with stoke had ocular motor dysfunction. Accommodative and binocular vision problems were most common in the traumatic brain injury group while cranial nerve palsy and strabismus were most common in the stroke population. Most recently several authors[23-25] reported on the frequency of vision problems in combat-injured inpatient and outpatient military personnel. Convergence, accommodative, and eye movement dysfunction were common in both populations. In these studies the most common vision problem found in both populations was a binocular vision problem called convergence insufficiency. Other commonly reported vision problems include reduced visual acuity, decreased contrast sensitivity, visual field deficits and neglect, strabismus, ocular motor dysfunction, accommodative dysfunction, and reduced stereopsis.[26-40]

Whether working with children or adults, occupational therapists often manage patients who have vision disorders. Unfortunately, visual deficits are not always recognized in the evaluation process or taken into consideration in therapy. Warren,[41] Bouska et al,[42,43] and Gianutsos[44] have all expressed concern that there appears to be little systematic consideration of a patient's visual profile in occupational therapy. Gianutsos[44] suggests that there "is a real delivery system vacuum." After brain injury, patients generally fail to articulate complaints due to impaired subjective experience or reduced cognition.[44] Bouska et al[42] also suggest that vision problems are not routinely detected in rehabilitation settings. They describe the patient who is labeled confused, clumsy, anxious, uncooperative, or unmotivated by professionals who are unaware that vision deficits may be the cause of the patient's behavior. When vision is addressed, it is usually from a strictly medical perspective, with attention given only to visual acuity and eye health. Chapters Three through Five will fully develop the concept that vision is more than good visual acuity and eye health.

Because visual function is dynamically interwoven within functional task performance,[44] ignoring visual deficits is likely to result in invalid assessment, faulty clinical reasoning, and, ultimately, ineffective treatment. The following are examples of how a visual deficit can interfere with occupational therapy and why a comprehensive vision examination is important before beginning occupational therapy:

- A 3-year-old child was referred for occupational therapy because she could not maintain eye contact, had poor fine motor skills, could not follow directions, could not sit still, and feared movement-based activities. The occupational therapy evaluation revealed low tone, tactile hyposensitivity, postural insecurity, and poor fine motor skills. A treatment plan was designed to deal with each of these problems. Although some progress was noticed, the therapist felt that the child still had great difficulty maintaining eye contact and concentrating on tasks, particularly if the task involved small objects. Finally, a vision evaluation was performed, and a very high degree of hyperopia (farsightedness) was found. The presence of high hyperopia would be expected to cause blurred vision and an inability to remain focused on a near activity for even short periods of time. Eyeglasses were prescribed, and occupational therapy proceeded much more effectively.

- A learning disabled, 7-year-old second grader was referred for a school occupational therapy consultation because the child frequently lost his place when reading, reread the same line, and showed a lack of interest in reading. The occupational therapist performed an evaluation and found normal sensory motor integration skills and visual processing. Tests to probe the area of scanning and tracking revealed mild problems, and treatment was designed to improve these skills. Little progress was achieved after 6 months of intervention. A visual evaluation revealed a significant binocular vision disorder called convergence insufficiency. What was overlooked in this case was that the child's behavior was characteristic of a child with a binocular vision (eye teaming) disorder. Inefficient use of the two eyes together as a team can mimic the symptoms and signs of a tracking or scanning problem. This child required a program of optometric vision therapy to improve binocular vision.

- An occupational therapist was treating a 74-year-old woman after a cerebrovascular accident. The therapist was struggling to help this patient regain independence in daily activities. She appeared fearful of walking in new environments and also had great difficulty localizing objects and reaching for things. An optometric evaluation revealed the presence of an inferior visual field deficit along with intermittent double vision. This patient required prism in her glasses to treat the double vision and occupational therapy to teach her how to compensate for the visual field deficit.

In each of these three cases, the vision problem may have been the primary factor interfering with progress for the patient. An attempt to continue occupational therapy without an evaluation and appropriate treatment of the vision problem would lead to frustration for both the therapist and the patient and less than optimal progress. In other cases, the vision problem may not be the key factor, but if left untreated, may interfere with the occupational therapy care process and lead to less than optimal treatment outcomes.

Vision is our most far-reaching sense, and it is clear that vision is critical for most activities of daily living. It is evident that for an occupational therapist to be maximally effective, a comprehensive understanding of vision is important.

Optometry and Occupational Therapy

The Eye Care Professions

There are two primary providers in the eye care profession. The differences between the two professions are significant and are related to the respective educational and clinical training programs for each profession. An *ophthalmologist* is a medical doctor who specializes in diseases of the eye and eye surgery. The initial training for an ophthalmologist is similar to any other medical doctor and has a heavy emphasis on disease. Following completion of medical school and an internship, the physician enters a residency and fellowship training program to specialize in ophthalmology. This period of training can last another 3 to 8 years, with a continuing focus on disease. The treatment approaches that are emphasized are medication and surgery. Rehabilitation of the visual system using vision therapy, lenses, low vision devices, or prism is not an important part of training. In fact, in many instances, negative opinions about visual rehabilitation are developed during this period of specialization.[45]

An *optometrist* is a primary health care provider who specializes in the examination, diagnosis, treatment, and management of diseases and disorders of the visual system, the eye, and associated structures, as well as the diagnosis of related systemic conditions.[46] To become an optometrist, an individual must graduate from a 4-year college program and then enter a 4-year program in a college of optometry. The emphasis in both didactic and clinical education is different from the ophthalmological residency programs. Although optometrists are also educated to diagnose and treat eye disease, a significant portion of the educational program deals with the concept of vision and its relationship to performance in play, school, work, and sports.

The optometrist is taught to evaluate the visual system in a manner that allows diagnosis of visual conditions that can interfere with performance and affect the quality of life. An integral concept in the optometric curriculum that is absent in ophthalmological training is that the status of the visual system is directly related to the environment and to how the individual uses his or her eyes. With increased close work such as reading and computer work, the visual system becomes more susceptible to disorders of accommodation, binocular vision, and refractive error. In fact, optometric theory suggests that many of the common vision problems that are prevalent in society are actually caused by the excessive close work that all of us experience in modern society.[47] Finally, optometrists are taught that rehabilitation using lenses, prism, low vision devices, and vision therapy is indeed an effective alternative to help patients become more comfortable and productive in school and work.[48] Many hours in the typical optometric curriculum are devoted to the study of the use of vision therapy to rehabilitate a wide variety of vision disorders.

Although all optometrists receive this training, only a percentage choose to offer this service in practice. Optometrists who offer vision therapy and vision rehabilitation in practice often have completed additional residency training or have passed comprehensive examinations designed to assess their level of expertise in these areas. The two organizations that administer such examinations are the American Academy of Optometry (Binocular Vision, Perception, and Pediatric Optometry Section) and the College of Optometrists in Vision Development (COVD). Optometrists successfully completing the examination process for the American Academy of Optometry are called Diplomates in Binocular Vision, Perception, and Pediatric Optometry. Approximately 50 optometrists in the United States have achieved this status. Optometrists successfully completing the examination process for COVD are called Fellows of COVD (FCOVD). Approximately 500 optometrists in the United States are FCOVDs, and about another 700 optometrists are associate members of COVD. Another organization that has established a certification process is the Neuro-Optometric Rehabilitation Association International (NORA). This organization is focused on advancing the art and science of the rehabilitation of the neurologically challenge individual and has a membership list of optometrists with an interest in vision therapy and vision rehabilitation after acquired brain injury.

There are also other optometrists who have expertise in the area of vision therapy but have not passed the examinations administered by these three organizations. My advice is to first look for an optometrist with at least one of the credentials described above to help you manage your patients. All three organizations maintain lists of these optometrists, and their addresses and phone numbers of the organizations are included at the end of this chapter. You can also access these membership directories at the Web sites of these organizations. If you are unable to find a local optometrist who has been certified by one of these three organizations, there is an additional organization—the Optometric Extension Program—that has a membership list of optometrists with an interest in vision therapy and vision rehabilitation. While members of this organization have a strong interest in these areas, they may not have passed any additional testing to certify their competence.

These differences in educational experience and clinical training explain the experiences of many therapists relative to the eye care professions. I have often heard occupational therapists comment about the frustration they experience when attempting to help a patient who they suspect may have a vision problem. For example, a therapist may refer a child for an eye examination because of concern about tracking or focusing skills. Depending on the doctor to whom the child is referred, it would not be unusual for the child to be sent back with completely contradictory reports. One doctor might suggest that there is no vision problem, that visual acuity is 20/20, that glasses are unnecessary, and that the eyes are healthy. The other doctor agrees that acuity is normal, glasses are not required, and the eyes are healthy, but reports the presence of a significant binocular vision problem that can explain the therapist's observations.

This lack of uniformity in vision care is confusing to therapists and to the public and may lead to lack of identification and treatment of vision disorders that can interfere with occupational therapy. The differences in approach between optometry and ophthalmology are important, and even within the optometric profession, philosophical differences may be significant. It is critical, therefore, that therapists seeking meaningful information about a patient's or client's visual status make the referral to an eye care professional who has training and expertise in the areas of binocular vision, vision and learning, and vision therapy. This will most likely require a referral to an optometrist who is either a FCOVD or a Diplomate in Binocular Vision, Perception, and Pediatric Optometry. Another acceptable credential is completion of a residency in pediatric optometry or vision therapy.

Optometry and Occupational Therapy Similarities and Differences

In recent years, a number of authors have described several striking similarities between optometry and occupational therapy.[49-51] These include a strong emphasis on the relationship between physical and cognitive deficiencies and performance in activities of daily living; the importance of therapeutic intervention, including both remedial and adaptive approaches; and the importance of eliminating underlying skills problems.

Optometrists routinely try to find relationships between vision disorders and problems with learning, work, and play. This is remarkably similar to occupational therapy's consistent concern about the effects of dysfunction on activities of daily living. Occupational therapy is the art and science of directing man's participation in selected tasks to restore, reinforce, and enhance performance.[52] The goals of optometric intervention are similar and revolve around restoring normal visual function to enhance performance in everyday tasks. When it is clear that there is a relationship between a diagnosed condition and performance, both occupational therapists and optometrists use all available treatment options to try to eliminate the interference or to teach the patient how to compensate for the problem. In some cases, this involves an adaptive approach to capitalize on the patient's remaining strengths and, in other cases, a remedial approach to restore normal function. The goal of treatment for both professions is ultimately to improve the patient's quality of life. As an optometrist, I was elated when I discovered another profession with such a strong commitment to the restoration and enhancement of function and performance.

At the same time, differences between the professions are also apparent, with each having its own unique perspectives and strengths. Occupational therapists generally use activities of daily living to improve function, while optometrists work directly with the affected function. Optometrists test and treat disorders of the peripheral visual system, such as eye movements, accommodation, and binocular vision. Occupational therapists may screen for these disorders but do not generally treat them, with the exception of some work with eye movements. Optometric testing tends to concentrate primarily on higher level functioning at the level of the cerebral cortex, while occupational therapists may focus more on lower level brainstem functions of the vestibular and proprioceptive system and how they are organized and processed.[51] Optometrists stress the predominance of the visual system in treatment, while occupational therapists stress the importance of the vestibular system and sensory motor integration. These similarities and differences have led many individual professionals from optometry and occupational therapy to realize that, in some instances, optimal care for patients requires a joint effort between the two professions.[49-51]

Optometry and occupational therapy have traditionally not worked in the same clinical settings. This is occurring more often, however. Optometrists are becoming part of the health care team in rehabilitation settings, providing both direct care and, in some cases, consultative services.[53-56]

In the private sector, more and more optometrists and occupational therapists are working together in practices to meet the needs of their patients. Continuing education courses for occupational therapists about vision, visual perception, and vision therapy are becoming commonplace.

Understanding Vision

Optometric Model of Vision

When people are asked to define good vision, they generally respond with one of the following three answers:

1. Good vision is the ability to see 20/20 or to see clearly.

2. Good vision means having healthy eyes and not needing glasses.

3. Good vision means that I am able to pass the school vision screening or the eye test at my doctor's office.

While an individual with "good vision" would certainly see clearly, have 20/20 vision, have healthy eyes, and pass a vision screening, there is much more that must be considered when answering this question. In addition to clear vision, an individual must have the ability to use his or her eyes for extended periods of time without discomfort, be able to analyze and interpret the incoming information, and be able to respond to what is being seen.

Optometric authors have developed models of vision that tend to emphasize that vision is a learned process dependent upon how the child interacts with his or her environment and that, in particular, it is related to a child's motor development. Hendrickson stressed that instead of asking what vision is, we should be asking what vision is for.[57] Suchoff[58] proposed an answer to this question, stating that "A primary mission of vision in the human organism is the organization and manipulation of space." This concept that vision is used to interact with and not just receive information is central to the optometric concept of vision. Getman[59] described vision as "The learned ability to see for information and performance. Vision is the ability to understand the things we cannot touch, taste, smell, or hear. Vision is the process whereby we perceive space as a whole." Another emphasis in optometric models of vision has been the important role of movement. Movement has been called the key to learning, thinking, and vision.[57] Skeffington said, "Thinking is a movement pattern. Vision is a movement pattern."[60] This emphasis on movement and motor skills is one of several key similarities in the philosophy that links optometry and occupational therapy.

One of my key objectives in writing this book is to demonstrate to the reader the complexity of vision and how vision disorders can impact on the occupational therapy process. To accomplish this, I will present the Three Component Model of Vision, which goes beyond 20/20 visual acuity, good optics, and normal eye health. The individual must also have normal binocular vision, accommodation, ocular motility, and visual information processing skills and be able to respond to the environment. The Three Component Model of Vision presented in Chapters Three through Five, therefore, consists of three distinct but interrelated components, which are visual integrity (acuity, refraction, and eye health); visual efficiency (accommodation, binocular vision, and eye movements); and visual information processing (visual spatial, visual analysis, and visual motor integration skills).

Although I will present these three components separately, they are closely related and interdependent. Disorders and delayed development in one component invariably will affect function in the other areas. Once the reader understands the complexity of vision, it should be apparent why occupational therapy and optometry should work closely together.

Directory of Optometrists With Expertise in Vision Therapy and Vision Rehabilitation

American Academy of Optometry, Diplomates in Binocular Vision, Perception, and Pediatric Optometry
http://aaopt.org/section/bv/diplomates/index.asp

College of Optometrists in Vision Development
www.covd.org

Neuro-Optometric Rehabilitation Association, International
http://nora.cc/

References

1. American Occupational Therapy Association. *Occupational Therapy Services for Children With Visual Dysfunction.* Bethesda, MD: Author; 1994.
2. Lorenze EJ, Cancro R. Dysfunction in visual perception with hemiplegia: its relation to activities of daily living. *Arch Phys Med Rehabil.* 1962;43:514-517.
3. Weinberg J, Diller L. On reading newspapers by hemiplegics—denial of visual disability. *Proc 76th Ann Con Am Psychol Assoc.* 1968;3:655-656.
4. Diller L, Weinberg J. Evidence for accident prone behavior in hemiplegic patients. *Arch Phys Med Rehabil.* 1970;51:358-363.
5. Diller L, Weinberg J. Attention in brain damaged people. *J Educ.* 1968;150:20-27.
6. Hier DB, Mondlock J, Caplan LR. Behavioral abnormalities after right hemisphere stroke. *Neurol.* 1983;33:337-344.
7. Scheiman M. Assessment and management of the exceptional child. In: Rosenbloom AA, Morgan MW, eds. *Pediatric Optometry.* Philadelphia, PA: JB Lippincott; 1990:388-419.
8. Kirschen M. A study of visual performance of mentally retarded children. *American Journal of Optometry and Archives of the American Academy of Optometry.* 1954;31:282-286.
9. LoCascio GP. A study of vision in cerebral palsy. *Am J Optom Physiol Opt.* 1977;54:332-335.
10. LoCascio GP. A longitudinal study of vision in cerebral palsy. *Am J Optom Physiol Opt.* 1984;61:689-674.
11. Scheiman M. Optometric findings in children with cerebral palsy. *Am J Optom Physiol Opt.* 1984;61:321-327.
12. Lyle WM, Woodruff ME, Zuccaro VS. A review of the literature on Down syndrome and an optometrical survey of 44 patients with the syndrome. *Am J Optom Physiol Opt.* 1972;49:715-721.
13. Pesch RS, Nagy DK, Caden B. A survey of the visual and developmental abilities of the Down syndrome child. *J Am Optom Assoc.* 1978;49:1031-1036.
14. Shapiro MB, France TD. The ocular features of Down syndrome. *Am J Ophthalmol.* 1985;99:659-665.
15. Clements DB, Kausal K. A study of the ocular complications of hydrocephalus and meningomyelocele. *Trans Ophthalmol Soc UK.* 1970;40:383-394.
16. Gottlieb DD, Allen WA. Incidence of visual disorders in a selected population of hearing impaired students. *J Am Optom Assoc.* 1985;56:292-297.
17. Ciner EB, Macks B, Schanel-Klitsch E. A cooperative demonstration project for early intervention vision services. *Occup Ther Pract.* 1991;3:42-56.
18. Akinci A, Oner O, Bozkurt OH, et al. Refractive errors and ocular findings in children with intellectual disability: a controlled study. *Journal of AAPOS.* 2008;12:477-481.
19. Gianutsos R, Ramsey G. Enabling survivors of brain injury to receive rehabilitative optometric services. *J Vis Rehab.* 1988;2:37-58.
20. Gianutsos R, Ramsey G, Perlin R. Rehabilitative optometric services for survivors of brain injury. *Arch Phys Med Rehabil.* 1988;69:573-578.
21. Suchoff IB, Kapoor N, Waxman R, Ference W. The occurrence of ocular and visual dysfunctions in an acquired brain-injured patient sample. *J Am Optom Assoc.* 1999;70:301-308.
22. Ciuffreda KJ, Kapoor N, Rutner D, et al. Occurrence of oculomotor dysfunctions in acquired brain injury: a retrospective analysis. *Optometry.* 2007;78:155-161.
23. Goodrich L, Kirby J, Cockerham G, Ingalla SP, Lew HL. Visual function in patients of a polytrauma rehabilitation center: a descriptive study. *J Rehabil Res Dev.* 2007;44:929-936.
24. Brahm KD, Wilgenburg HM, Kirby J, Ingalla S, Chang CY, Goodrich GK. Visual impairment and dysfunction in servicemembers with TBI. *Opt Vis Sci.* 2009;86:817-825.

25. Stelmack JA, Frith T, Van Koevering D, Stelmack TR. Visual function in patients followed at a Veterans Affairs poly-trauma network site: an electronic medical record review. *Optometry.* 2009;80:419-424.
26. Kwatny E, Bouska MJ. *Visual System Disorders and Functional Correlates: Final Report.* Philadelphia, PA: Temple University Rehabilitation Research and Training Center #8; 1980.
27. Mitchell R, MacFarlane A, Cornell E. Ocular motility disorders following head injury. *Aust Orthop J.* 1983;20:31-36.
28. Cohen M, Groswasser Z, Barchadski R, Appel A. Convergence insufficiency in brain-injured patients. *Brain Inj.* 1989;3:187-191.
29. Schlageter Gray B, Hall K, Shaw R, Sammet R. Incidence and treatment of visual dysfunction in traumatic brain injury. *Brain Inj.* 1993;7:439-448.
30. Elisevich KV, Ford RM, Anderson DP, et al. Visual abnormalities with multiple trauma. *Surg Neurol.* 1984;22:565-575.
31. Tierney DW. Visual dysfunction in closed head injury. *J Am Opt Assoc.* 1988;59:614-622.
32. Padula WV. Head injury causing post trauma vision syndrome. *N Engl J Optom.* 1988;Dec:16-21.
33. Krohel GB, Kristan RW, Simon JW, et al. Post-traumatic convergence insufficiency. *Ann Ophthalmol.* 1986;18:101-104.
34. Roca PD. Ocular manifestations of whiplash injuries. *Ann Ophthalmol.* 1972;4:63-73.
35. Uzzell BP, Dolinskas CA, Langfitt TW. Visual field defects in relation to head injury severity. *Arch Neurol.* 1988;45:420-424.
36. Rutner D, Kapoor N, Ciuffreda KJ, et al. Occurrence of ocular disease in traumatic brain injury in a selected sample: a retrospective analysis *Brain Inj.* 2006;20(10):1079-1086.
37. Jones, SA, Shinton, RS. Improving outcome in stroke patients with visual problems. *Age Ageing.* 2006;35:560-565.
38. McKenna K, Cooke, DM, Fleming J, et al. The incidence of visual perceptual impairment in patients with severe traumatic brain injury. *Brain Inj.* 2006;20(5):507-518.
39. Suchoff, IB, Kapoor, N, Ciuffreda KJ, et al. The frequency of occurrence, types, and characteristics of visual field defects in acquired brain injury: a retrospective analysis. *Optometry.* 2008;79:259-265.
40. Rowe F. Visual perceptual consequences of stroke. *Strabismus.* 2009;17:24-28.
41. Warren M. Identification of visual scanning deficits in adults after cerebrovascular accident. *Am J Occup Ther.* 1990;44:391-399.
42. Bouska MJ, Kauffman NA, Marcus SE. Disorders of the visual perceptual system. In: Umphred DA, Jewell MJ, eds. *Neurological Rehabilitation.* St. Louis, MO: CV Mosby Co; 1985:552-585.
43. Bouska MJ, Gallaway M. Primary visual field deficits in adults with brain damage: management in occupational therapy. *Occup Ther Pract.* 1991;3:1-11.
44. Gianutsos R. Working relationships between psychology and optometry. *J Beh Optom.* 1991;2:30-36.
45. American Academy of Ophthalmology. *Policy Statement: Learning Disabilities, Dyslexia, and Vision.* San Francisco, CA: American Academy of Ophthalmology; Revised 2009.
46. American Optometric Association. *Position Statement on Vision Therapy.* St. Louis, MO; 1999.
47. Skeffington AM. *Introduction to Clinical Optometry.* Santa Ana, CA: Optometric Extension Program Foundation, Optometric Extension Program Postgraduate Courses. Vol 37, Oct. 1964-Sept 1965.
48. Scheiman M, Wick B. *Clinical Management of Binocular Vision.* 3rd ed. Philadelphia, PA: JB Lippincott; 2008.
49. Cool SJ. Occupational therapy and functional optometry: an interaction whose time has come? *Sensory Integration Special Interest Newsletter.* 1987;10:1-6.
50. Appelbaum SA. Sensory integration: optometric and occupational therapy perspectives. *Optom Ext Program Curriculum II.* 1988;61(1-12).
51. Hellerstein LF, Fishman B. Vision therapy and occupational therapy: an integrated approach. *Sensory Integration Special Interest Newsletter.* 1987;10:4-5.
52. Hopkins HL, Smith HD. *Occupational Therapy.* 6th ed. Philadelphia, PA: JB Lippincott; 1983:27.
53. Mastrangelo R. Visionary effort: OT and optometry join hands. *OT Week.* 1990;6(28):1-2.
54. Breske S. Opening eyes to vision deficits in rehab. *Advance for Occupational Therapists*; 1995.
55. Schlageter K, Shaw R. Vision therapy. *OT Week.* 1991;5(31):12-13.
56. Scheiman M. The eyes have it. *Advance for Physical Therapists and Rehab Medicine.* 2000;October 1:61-62.
57. Hendrickson H. *Vision Development in Man—A Review. Vision and Learning.* St. Louis, MO: American Optometric Association; 1976:21-45.
58. Suchoff I. *Visuo-Spatial Development in the Child: An Optometric Theoretical and Clinical Approach.* New York, NY: State University of New York; 1981.
59. Getman GN, Hendrickson H. The needs of teachers for specialized information on the development of visuomotor skills in relation to academic performance. In: Cruickshank WM, ed. *The Teacher of Brain Injured Children.* New York, NY: Syracuse University Press; 1966:156-157.
60. Skeffington AM. *The Low Acuity Emmetrope Who Constricted Her Visual System.* Duncan, OK: Clinical Optometry, Optometric Extension Program; 1972:45(1,3).

Chapter Two

Review of Basic Anatomy, Physiology, and Development of the Visual System

Mitchell Scheiman, OD, FCOVD, FAAO

Basic Anatomy and Physiology of the Visual System

This chapter is designed to provide a review of the basic anatomy and physiology of the visual system. Space limitations prevent a comprehensive discussion of this topic. Readers requiring more in-depth information about these topics should review the texts listed in the Bibliography of this chapter.

Orbit, Eyelids, Eyeball

A traditional method of describing the anatomy of the eye is to begin with the outermost structures and move inward. The orbit of the eye, which is a bony recess in the skull, contains a number of major structures, including the eyeball, the optic nerve, the muscles of the eye, and their nerves and blood vessels. The eyeball, which is about 2.5 cm long, is suspended in the orbital cavity in such a way that the six ocular muscles can move it in all directions.

The eyelids protect the eyes from injury and excessive light and keep the cornea moist. As illustrated in Figure 2-1, the upper eyelid partially covers the iris, whereas the entire inferior half of the eye is normally uncovered. The eyelids are covered internally by the highly vascular palpebral conjunctiva. The palpebral conjunctiva continues onto the eyeball and is called the bulbar conjunctiva. Inflammation of either the bulbar or palpebral conjunctiva is referred to as conjunctivitis, commonly called pink eye. Conjunctivitis can be secondary to bacterial, viral, or allergic etiology. Infection of the conjunctiva is generally self-limiting, but occasionally conjunctivitis can lead to inflammation of the cornea as well.

The bulbar conjunctiva covers the white portion of the eye called the sclera. The sclera is the external coat of the eye and is a white tissue covering the posterior five-sixths of the eye. The anterior one-sixth of the outer coat of the eye is the transparent structure called the cornea (Figure 2-2). The cornea is an extremely important structure of the eye because it is the key optical component responsible for refraction of light that enters the eye. It is an unusual tissue because it is clear and

Figure 2-1. The upper eyelid partially covers the iris, whereas the entire inferior half of the eye is normally uncovered. (Reprinted with permission from Scheiman M, Scheiman M, Whittaker SG. *Low Vision Rehabilitation: A Practical Guide for Occupational Therapists*. Thorofare, NJ: SLACK Incorporated; 2007.)

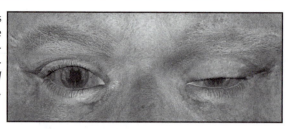

has no blood vessels. The cornea is susceptible to infection from bacterial, viral, fungal or allergic causes, and inflammation of the cornea is referred to as keratitis. Severe inflammation, a corneal burn due to exposure to toxic substances, or trauma to the cornea can all lead to scarring and loss of transparency of the cornea. This can then lead to a loss of vision if the scarring is located in the central portion of the cornea. Reduced visual acuity secondary to central corneal scarring is a disease condition that may be encountered by occupational therapists in clients who have experienced head trauma. Other common other age-related problems of the anterior part of the eye that affect vision and cause discomfort include blepharitis (chronic inflammation of the lids) and dry eye. These can be managed medically but with varying success.

Directly behind the cornea is a clear, watery fluid called the aqueous humor, which is produced in the posterior chamber and fills the anterior chamber of the eye (see Figure 2-2). The aqueous is continuously produced by the ciliary body and provides nutrients for the avascular cornea and lens. After passing through the pupil from the posterior chamber into the anterior chamber, the aqueous is drained off through the canal of Schlemm (see Figure 2-2).

Lens

The lens is a transparent, flexible structure that is held in position by zonular fibers (see Figure 2-2). It is located posterior to the iris and anterior to the vitreous humor. Like the cornea, the lens is both transparent and avascular and is another key part of the refractive system of the eye. To accommodate or focus on objects, the lens must change shape. The ciliary muscle contracts, and this allows the lens to thicken, enabling the individual to focus. As an object moves away, the ciliary muscle relaxes, the lens becomes thinner, and the focusing system relaxes. The lens of the eye is the structure that gradually loses its transparency as a person ages. This loss of transparency and development of opacities is referred to as cataracts.

Vitreous

The vitreous body is located behind the lens (Figure 2-3). It consists of a jelly-like substance called vitreous humor, in which there is a meshwork of collagen fibrils. Vitreous humor is a colorless, transparent gel. It consists of 99% water and forms four-fifths of the eyeball. In addition to transmitting light, it holds the retina in place and provides support for the lens. In contrast to the aqueous humor, it is not continuously replaced.

Choroid

The eyeball has three concentric coats. The first or outermost coat, the sclera, was described above. The middle coat is a heavily pigmented, vascular layer consisting of the iris, ciliary body, and the choroid. The iris, which is the colored portion of the eye, is located between the cornea and the lens. The eye color depends on the amount and distribution of pigment in the iris. The iris is a contractile diaphragm that has a central, circular aperture for transmitting light, which is called the pupil. The size of the iris continually varies to regulate the amount of light entering the eye through the pupil. The ciliary body lies between the iris and the choroid. This structure secretes

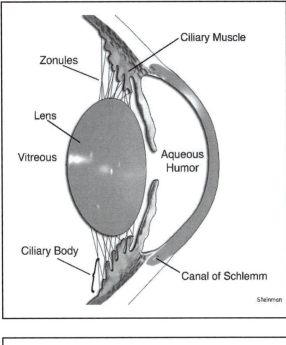

Figure 2-2. The anterior one-sixth of the outer coat of the eye is the transparent structure called the cornea. (Reprinted with permission from Scheiman M, Scheiman M, Whittaker SG. *Low Vision Rehabilitation: A Practical Guide for Occupational Therapists*. Thorofare, NJ: SLACK Incorporated; 2007.)

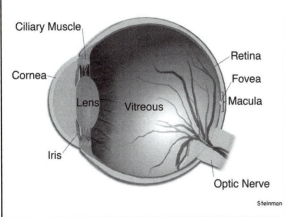

Figure 2-3. Cross-section of the eye. (Reprinted with permission from Scheiman M, Scheiman M, Whittaker SG. *Low Vision Rehabilitation: A Practical Guide for Occupational Therapists*. Thorofare, NJ: SLACK Incorporated; 2007.)

aqueous humor. The ciliary body also contains the ciliary muscle, which can contract or relax to permit accommodation or focusing of the eye. The choroid is a dark brown membrane and is also part of this middle coat of the eye. It continues from the ciliary body and covers the entire posterior portion of the eye. The choroid attaches firmly to the retina and contains the venous plexus and layers of capillaries that are responsible for nutrition of the retina.

Retina

The most internal coat of the eye is the retina, which is a thin, delicate membrane. The retina is the posterior portion of the eye and there is a circular depressed area called the optic nerve (see Figure 2-3). This is where the optic nerve enters the eye and its fibers spread out in the neural layer of the retina. Because it contains nerve fibers and no photoreceptor cells, the optic disc is insensitive to light. For this reason it is sometimes referred to as the blind spot. Another very important

Figure 2-4. The fovea is the part of the eye that contains the area of most acute vision. (Reprinted with permission from Scheiman M, Scheiman M, Whittaker SG. *Low Vision Rehabilitation: A Practical Guide for Occupational Therapists.* Thorofare, NJ: SLACK Incorporated; 2007.)

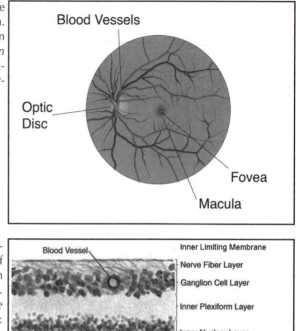

Figure 2-5. Beneath the pigmented epithelium of the retina are the 10 layers of the retina. (Reprinted with permission from Scheiman M, Scheiman M, Whittaker SG. *Low Vision Rehabilitation: A Practical Guide for Occupational Therapists.* Thorofare, NJ: SLACK Incorporated; 2007.)

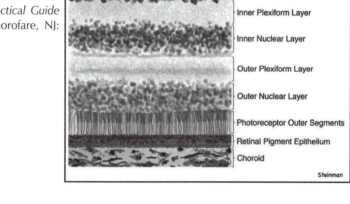

structure just lateral to the optic disc is the fovea (Figure 2-4). The fovea is the part of the eye that contains the area of most acute vision. Whenever we look at an object we must aim the eye so that the image of the object is focused on the fovea. Smooth eye movements, called pursuits, and jump eye movements, called saccades, are both designed to allow the individual to use the fovea.

The retina is composed of 10 layers including the pigment epithelium, which is closest to the choroid and the photoreceptors (cones and rod photoreceptors). Beneath the pigment epithelium of the retina are the 10 layers of the retina (Figure 2-5) from the outside (furthest from the retina) to the inside (closest to the retina):

- Sclera (white part of the eye)
- Large choroidal blood vessels
- Choriocapilaris
- Bruch's membrane (separates the pigment epithelium of the retina from the choroid)

Note that light must pass through all layers of the retina to reach the photoreceptors where the visual process begins. Diseases such as macular degeneration or diabetic retinopathy that affect the clarity of retina or swelling that affects the shape of the retina will have a profound effect on vision.

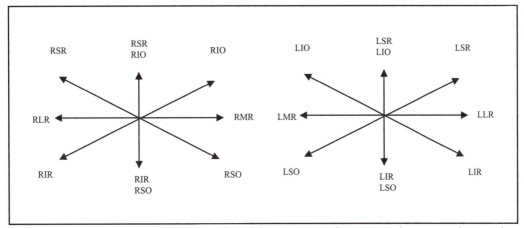

Figure 2-6. Positions of gaze that are evaluated by clinicians when testing the extraocular muscles. (RSR=right superior rectus, RLR=right lateral rectus, RIR=right inferior rectus, RSO=right superior oblique, RMR=right medial rectus, RIO=right inferior oblique, LSR=left superior rectus, LLR=left lateral rectus, LIR=left inferior rectus, LSO=left superior oblique, LMR=left medial rectus, LIO=left inferior oblique.)

Photoreceptors (Cones and Rods)

Light causes a chemical reaction in cones and in rods, beginning the visual process. Activated photoreceptors stimulate bipolar cells, which in turn stimulate ganglion cells. The impulses continue into the axons of the ganglion cells, through the optic nerve, and to the visual cortex at the occipital lobe of the brain.

There are about 6.5 to 7 million cones in each eye, and they are sensitive to bright light and to color. The highest concentration of cones is in the macula. The center of the macula contains only cones and no rods. The highest concentration of rods is in the peripheral retina, decreasing in density up to the macula. Rods do not detect color, which is the main reason it is difficult to tell the color of an object at night or in the dark. Defective or damaged cones results in color deficiency, whereas, defective or damaged rods result in problems seeing in the dark and at night.

Muscles of the Orbit and Their Innervation

Six extraocular muscles attach to each eye and allow movement in all directions of gaze. There are four rectus muscles—the superior, inferior, lateral, and medial recti muscles—and two oblique muscles—the inferior and superior oblique muscles.

Each of the six muscles has one position of gaze in which it exerts the main influence on eye position. Figure 2-6 illustrates the various positions of gaze that are evaluated clinically. The diagram also displays the muscle that is primarily responsible for movement into each position of gaze. This diagram is the basis for the clinical evaluation of eye muscle problems. For example, if a client has difficulty moving his or her eyes down and to the right, the two possible muscles involved would be the right inferior rectus and the left superior oblique. The left superior oblique moves the left eye down and to the right and the right inferior rectus moves the right eye down and to the right. To determine which of the two remaining muscles is at fault requires additional clinical testing.

Three cranial nerves supply innervation to the six extraocular muscles. The third cranial nerve innervates the superior, inferior, medial recti, and the inferior oblique muscle. The fourth cranial nerve supplies innervation to the superior oblique, and the sixth cranial nerve innervates the lateral rectus.

Diplopia, or double vision, is a very common symptom of clients treated by occupational therapists, particularly after cerebrovascular accident or head trauma. Diplopia occurs when the object at which the individual is looking stimulates the fovea of one eye and a non-foveal part of the retina of the other eye. Thus, diplopia suggests misalignment of the eyes. There are a number of disorders that can lead to diplopia. Brain injury from stroke or trauma that affects the midbrain or cerebellum area often affects both balance and eye movements. Among the more common problems are cranial nerve palsies. The most common nerve palsies seen by occupational therapists are sixth and fourth nerve palsies.

The most common causes of fourth nerve palsy are head trauma and vascular problems. Fourth cranial nerve palsy can be unilateral or bilateral and can affect the superior oblique muscle. Bilateral fourth nerve palsy is often seen following vertex blows to the head, such as those that occur in motorcycle accidents. The presence of a fourth nerve palsy causes the eye with the affected muscle to drift upward. The client has difficulty looking down and to the right if it is a left superior oblique problem, and down and to the left if it is a right superior oblique problem.

Sixth cranial nerve palsies are the most frequently reported ocular motor nerve palsies. The nerve has the longest intracranial course of any nerve and is often subject to embarrassment with raised intracranial pressure. The causes include vascular disease, trauma, elevated intracranial pressure and neoplasm. The sixth nerve innervates the lateral rectus. A sixth nerve palsy will interfere with the client's ability to abduct the eye (move the eye away from the nose).

Visual Pathways

One of the most common vision problems occupational therapists encounter after acquired brain injury is visual field deficits. One of the most common is a right or left field loss referred to as an homonymous hemianopsia. To understand why a client would lose vision to just one side, it is necessary to understand how visual information travels from the retina to the visual cortex. Vision begins with the capture of images focused by the optical media on photoreceptors of the retina. The fibers from the upper half of each retina enter the optic nerve above the horizontal meridian, and those from the lower half enter below the horizontal meridian. Fibers from the periphery of the retina lie peripherally in the optic nerve, and fibers from the fovea lie centrally. This arrangement persists throughout the entire course of the visual pathways from the optic nerve through the chiasm, the optic tracts, and optic radiations.

Visual information from the right field strikes the nasal half of the retina of the right eye and the temporal half of the retina of the left eye. Similarly, visual information from the left field strikes the nasal half of the retina of the left eye and the temporal half of the retina of the right eye (Figure 2-7). When the fibers from each optic nerve reach the optic chiasm, a decussation takes place. The fibers from the temporal part of the retina remain on the temporal or outside aspect of the chiasm and are called uncrossed fibers (see Figure 2-7). The nasal fibers of the retina cross over in the chiasm and are called crossed fibers. After leaving the chiasm, the fibers form the optic tract. Thus, all visual information originating from the right field travels in the left optic tract, and all of the visual information originating from the left field travels in the right optic tract. The fibers in the upper half of the tract originate from the upper half of the two retinas, and the fibers from the lower half of the tract come from the lower half of the two retinas. The fibers from the optic tract synapse in the lateral geniculate body. The cells of the lateral geniculate body give rise to new fibers which form the optic radiation. These fibers then proceed to the cells of the visual cortex (see Figure 2-7). Any lesion that affects the visual pathway on only the right or left side after this decussation takes place will affect either the left visual field or right visual field.

Vision Areas of the Brain

The brain is divided into several different lobes. Starting anteriorly are the frontal lobes, which are responsible for decision making, planning ahead, emotional tone, abstract thinking, and

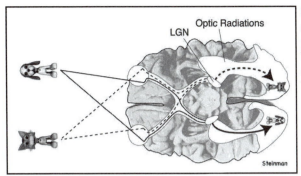

Figure 2-7. Visual pathway from the optic nerve to the visual cortex. (Reprinted with permission from Scheiman M, Scheiman M, Whittaker SG. *Low Vision Rehabilitation: A Practical Guide for Occupational Therapists.* Thorofare, NJ: SLACK Incorporated; 2007.)

carrying out intentions. Immediately behind them and in front of the motor area is the prefrontal cortex, which is involved in organizing and sequencing complex motor behavior. The temporal lobes are associated with hearing and also provide some contribution to vision. The parietal lobes are responsible for tactile recognition. Parietal lobe injury commonly results in perceptual deficits that disrupt ambulation and self-care activities. Hemisensory neglect is a common problem in clients with a lesion in the posterior parietal cortex.

The occipital lobe contains the visual cortex, with nerve pathways leading to higher centers in the parietal and temporal lobes, where visual sensations acquire meaning. Lesions in the visual cortex and in associated areas can produce visual and perceptual problems. The cerebellum integrates the smooth coordination of muscular activity. If it is damaged, general motor clumsiness occurs. This may interfere with manual dexterity and other forms of fine muscular performance, as well as eye movement control. Dysfunction within the cerebellum yields problems with equilibrium, motor control, body image, laterality, and sometimes with reading and speech.

All of the visual fibers end in the striate area of the cortex which is called area 17. Area 17 is considered to be the primary visuosensory area in man. Outside of area 17 and closely following its contours are two other areas that are concerned with visual reactions as well. These are called areas 18 and 19. Most physiologists agree that vision is a function of higher parts of the brain than just the visual cortex. The message relayed to area 17 enables a person to see. It does not enable a person to recognize what he or she sees or to recall things that have been seen. These functions are dependent on other parts of the brain. In order for a person to be able to interpret the sensory information reaching area 17, the message must be sent on to the two secondary visual areas and areas 18 and 19. Area 18 is concerned exclusively with the recognition of objects, animate or inanimate, but is not concerned with the recognition of written or printed symbols of language. Area 19 is concerned with the recall of visual memory relating to objects but not to language symbols.

Two parallel routes carry visual information from the occipital lobe to the prefrontal lobe and the frontal eye fields. Fibers from these two routes distribute fibers to many other areas along each route before terminating in the prefrontal cortex and in the frontal eye fields. The first route is the superior route via the parietal and frontal lobes. The other route is the inferior route via the temporal and frontal lobes.

Summary

Since low vision is a condition in which visual acuity is reduced because of eye disease it is important to have a basic understanding of the anatomy and physiology of the eye and visual system. We urge readers who feel a need for more detail to refer to the Bibliography provided at the end of this chapter.

Bibliography

Moore KL. *Clinically Oriented Anatomy*. Baltimore, MD: Williams and Wilkins; 1980.

Moses RA. *Adler's Physiology of the Eye*. 7th ed. St. Louis, MO: CV Mosby Co; 1981.

Solomon H. *Binocular Vision: A Programmed Text*. London: William Heinemann Medical Books Ltd; 1978.

Three Component Model of Vision, Part One:
Visual Integrity

Mitchell Scheiman, OD, FCOVD, FAAO

The Three Component Model of Vision that will be described in Chapters Three through Five consists of three components:
1. Visual integrity (visual acuity, optics of the eye, and eye health)
2. Visual efficiency (accommodation, binocular vision, and eye movements)
3. Visual information processing (visual spatial, visual analysis, and visual motor integration skills)

Visual integrity, discussed in this chapter, involves the ability to see clearly at all distances and deals with the optical system and eye health.

Visual Acuity

Definition

Visual acuity is a measure of the resolving power of the eye. Because visual acuity testing is so popular, most people are familiar with the concept of 20/20 visual acuity. An individual with 20/20 acuity is considered to have normal ability to see small detail at the distance tested. The numerator refers to the testing distance at which the subject recognizes the stimulus, and the denominator refers to the distance at which the letter being viewed could be identified by a patient with normal visual acuity. For example, 20/100 suggests that a patient with normal visual acuity could identify the letter presented at a distance of 100 feet. The actual individual being tested could only see this letter at 20 feet, indicating that the visual acuity is reduced relative to the normal finding. In traditional vision screenings, visual acuity below the level of 20/30 to 20/40 is considered cause for referral. However, clinically, any deviation from 20/20 is considered a problem, and, in the course of the vision evaluation, the clinician must determine the basis for the loss of visual acuity.

Scheiman M
*Understanding and Managing Vision Deficits: A Guide for
Occupational Therapists, Third Edition* (pp 17-56)
© 2011 SLACK Incorporated

Figure 3-1. The standard Snellen Acuity Chart.

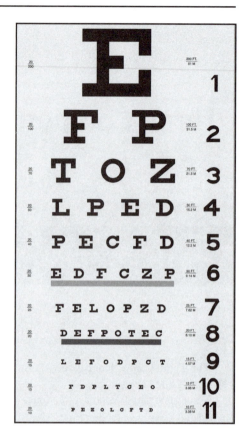

Classification of Visual Acuity Disorders

There is no classification of visual acuity disorders because these problems are actually always secondary to other conditions. Reduced visual acuity can occur secondary to a wide variety of conditions, including myopia, hyperopia, astigmatism, accommodative disorders, binocular vision disorders, amblyopia, eye disease, and psychogenic causes.

Clinical Assessment

Visual acuity testing is performed by every type of eye care professional and is repeated at every eye examination. In addition, visual acuity testing is often performed by family physicians, pediatricians, and school nurses. There are three methods of assessing visual acuity. The variable for these methods is the type of target used. The three methods are recognition acuity, resolution acuity, and detection acuity.

The recognition acuity format is a visual acuity task in which the patient is asked to "recognize" and identify a series of targets. Most people have experienced this type of visual acuity testing. The standard Snellen Acuity Chart (Figure 3-1) is an example of this format. In almost all clinical examinations, this is the general format used to assess visual acuity.

A second possible testing format would be to use resolution acuity. This is a task in which the patient is required to locate and "resolve" a difference between two targets. The most common example of this is called preferential looking. In this approach, the child is asked to resolve or differentiate a black-and-white striped stimulus from a homogeneous gray target.

Table 3-1		
Acuity Tests		
Test Type	*Name of Test*	*Appropriate for Age Group*
Traditional	Snellen Acuity Chart	6 years to adult
Limits verbal interaction	Tumbling E Test	5- to 6-year-old children
Limits verbal interaction	Broken Wheel Test	2½- to 6-year-old children, TBI and CVA patients
Limits verbal interaction	Lea Symbols Test	2½- to 6-year-old children, TBI and CVA patients
Limits verbal interaction	Allen Visual Acuity Chart	2½- to 6-year-old children
Limits verbal interaction	Teller Acuity Cards	18 to 36 months with operant conditioning
Eliminates need for verbal interaction	Teller Acuity Cards	1 to 18 months

CVA=cerebrovascular accident, TBI=traumatic brain injury.

The final general format is called a detection acuity task. In this approach, the patient is asked to "detect" and find a target. For example, the patient may have to find a small black dot on a white background. The smallest black dot that can be seen is considered the highest level of visual acuity for the patient. The detection acuity format is rarely used. It has potential value when assessment with a recognition acuity format is not possible.

There are many clinical tests available for visual acuity assessment. Most use the recognition format described previously. Visual acuity testing is generally a subjective evaluation in which the patient must identify visual stimuli presented at distance or at near. The test that is most widely used is the Snellen Acuity Chart (see Figure 3-1). This procedure is used for adults and children who can recognize and recall all the letters of the alphabet. Most children from first grade and above can be evaluated with the Snellen Acuity Chart. Children who have trouble with letter recognition or children who are nonverbal must be evaluated using other tests. Adults after cerebrovascular accident or traumatic brain injury are often difficult to evaluate with a standard Snellen Acuity Chart because of cognitive, perceptual, memory, and visual problems.

Three alternative approaches have been developed to enable clinicians to evaluate visual acuity in patients unable to respond to the Snellen Acuity Chart. These include the use of numbers, pictures, and charts that limit the number of letters; tests that minimize or eliminate verbal interaction; and tests that rely on the behavioral observation of the examiner. As Table 3-1 illustrates, clinical tests are now available that allow optometrists to assess the visual acuity of any patient regardless of age or cognitive ability. For example, infants can be evaluated as early as 1 month of age.

Figure 3-2 shows a test that uses pictures. The picture chart is called the Allen Visual Acuity Chart and is rather easy to administer. It has a serious flaw because it has not been shown to correlate well with the Snellen Acuity Chart, which is considered the standard measure.

Figures 3-3a through 3-3c illustrate other tests that limit the amount of verbal interaction during visual acuity testing. The Tumbling E Test (see Figure 3-3a) requires the child to point in the direction in which the "E" is pointing. The child simply points up, down, right, or left. Children who are 5 years old and younger often have difficulty with this test because of a poorly developed sense of direction.

The two tests that are most effective in the preschool population are the Broken Wheel Test and the Lea Symbols Test. These tests can be used when brain injury affects number and letter

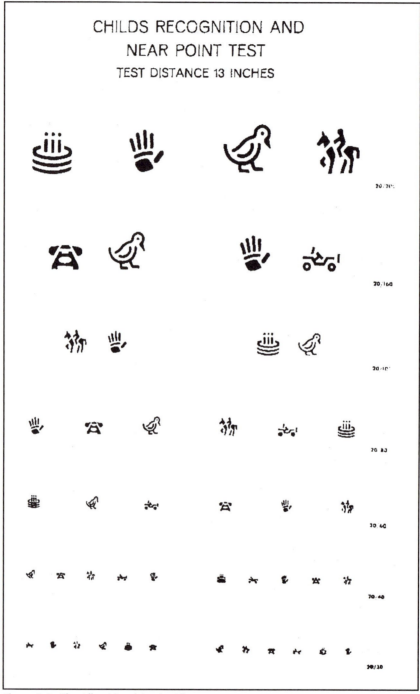

Figure 3-2. The Allen Visual Acuity Chart.

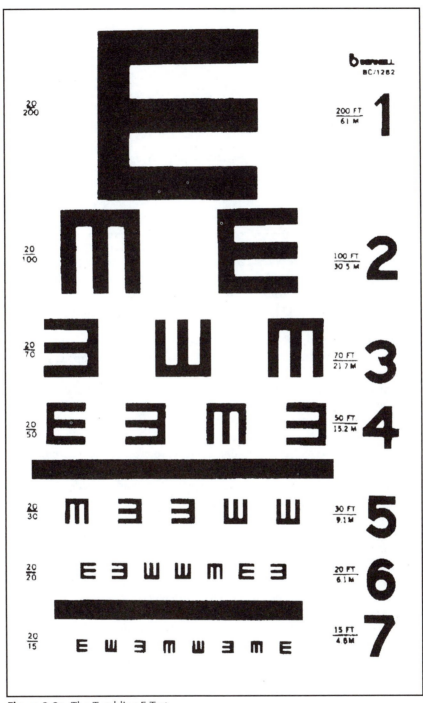

Figure 3-3a. The Tumbling E Test.

Figure 3-3b. The Broken Wheel Test.

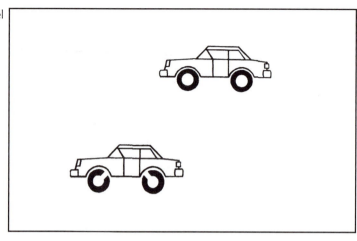

recognition. With the Broken Wheel Test (see Figure 3-3b), the examiner holds up two cards. One has a car with broken wheels while the other card has a picture of a car with intact wheels. If the child can see the small gap in the wheel, he or she is able to identify which card has the car with broken wheels. The child is taught to point to the car with broken wheels. The cars become smaller as does the gap in the wheel.

The Lea Symbols Test (see Figure 3-3c) is also extremely effective with children 2½ to 6 years of age. The examiner places the wooden puzzle with four pieces (apple, circle, square, and house) on the child's lap. The child is taught to point or hold up the block that matches the shape to which the examiner points. As soon as it is clear that the child understands the task, the examiner selects smaller and smaller targets until the child can no longer accurately match the shape. The Lea Symbols Test comes in several versions, allowing clinicians to select the version that is most appropriate for the patient's developmental level.

Figure 3-4 illustrates visual acuity testing in very young infants. The procedure is called forced-choice preferential looking, and the specific test displayed is the Teller Acuity Cards. This is an example of a resolution acuity task discussed above. The entire procedure is based on the fact that, when presented with two stimuli, infants will "prefer" to look at the stimulus with a pattern rather than a stimulus without a pattern. In order to evaluate acuity, the conditions must be ideal. The child must be comfortable, dry, well rested, and fed. The testing should be performed in a room without distractions, and it is preferable to use the setup illustrated in Figure 3-5. With the infant on the parent's lap and facing the examiner, the examiner holds up a card that has two stimuli. One has vertical lines, and the other matches the first stimulus in luminance but has no lines. If the infant can "see" the lines, he or she will be able to see a difference between the two stimuli and will, therefore, prefer to view the stimulus with lines. The examiner must observe the infant's behavior and will notice that the child tends to look at or prefer one stimulus over the other. The examiner continues to change the cards, choosing cards with narrower vertical lines until the child no longer appears to show a preference for one stimulus and spends an equal amount of time looking from one to the other. This test has been widely studied and is considered a reliable and valid assessment of visual acuity in the hands of an experienced clinician with the following exception[1]—researchers have reported that this test may overestimate the visual acuity in cases of strabismic amblyopia and macular disease.[2] In these cases, the results must be interpreted with caution.

Preferential looking acuity works well with young infants. However, around the age of 18 to 24 months, children no longer seem attracted enough to these stimuli to maintain attention during this task. Researchers and clinicians[3] have developed a modification called operant preferential looking to permit older infants and toddlers to be tested. This is illustrated in Figure 3-6. The key modification is the use of operant conditioning theory. The child is taught that if he or she points to

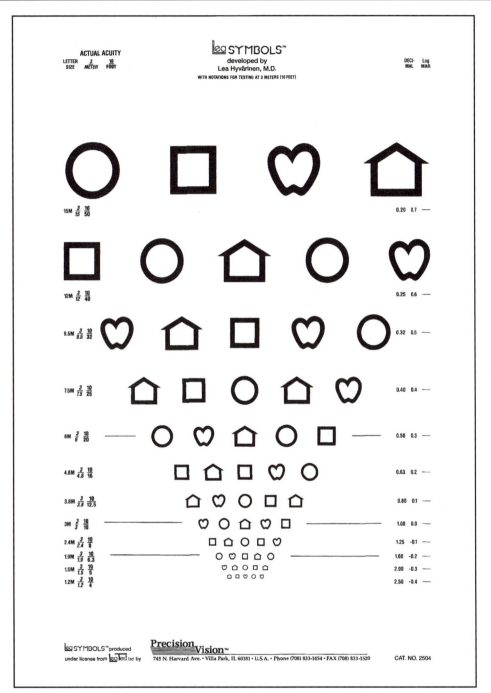

Figure 3-3c. The Lea Symbols Test. (Reprinted with permission from Vision Associates, www. visionkits.com.)

the stimulus with the stripes, he or she will receive a reward. Most clinicians use bits of cereal as a reward. Each time the child correctly identifies the stimulus with stripes, he or she receives the reinforcement. Studies have also demonstrated the effectiveness of this procedure. Forced-choice and operant preferential learning have also been used effectively with special populations such as mentally disabled adults.

Figure 3-4. The Teller Acuity Cards.

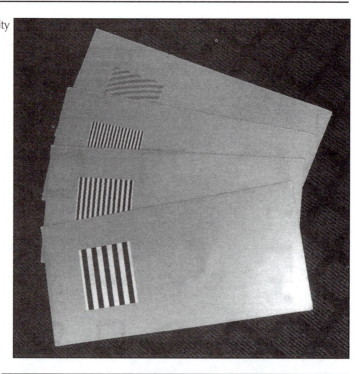

Figure 3-5. Preferential looking acuity procedure with the infant on the parent's lap and facing the examiner.

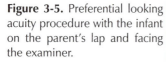

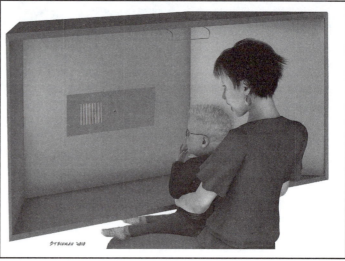

The important message is that optometrists now have the ability to evaluate visual acuity in virtually any patient regardless of age or cognitive ability.

Visual acuity can also be tested at near. Figure 3-7 illustrates a variety of near point visual acuity cards that are available. Essentially, they are simply reduced versions of the distance visual acuity charts.

Development of Visual Acuity

Researchers have used two different methods to study the development of visual acuity in infants and young children. One method is an electrophysiological approach using visually evoked potentials, and the other is the behavioral method called forced-choice preferential

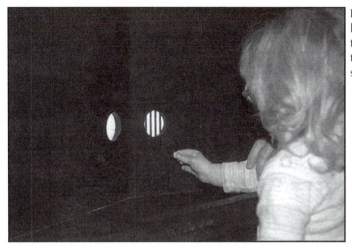

Figure 3-6. Operant preferential looking procedure. The child is taught that if he or she points to the stimulus with the stripes, he or she will receive a reward.

learning described previously. The electrophysiological approach simply requires the child to look at a video display of a flickering checkerboard pattern. The cortical response to this changing stimulus is recorded using electrodes placed on the scalp over the occipital pole.

There are significant differences between the results obtained from the two methods. Both approaches indicate that infants are born with very poor visual acuity and suggest that visual acuity is approximately 20/400 to 20/800 in newborns. The electrophysiological approach, however, suggests that the visual acuity reaches adult levels (20/20) by 6 months of age.[4,5] Studies using forced-choice preferential learning indicate that visual acuity is about 20/50 to 20/60 at 6 months, about 20/100 by 12 months, and slowly improves to 20/20 by 5 years of age.[6-8] Despite the differences in results, both research methods demonstrate that there is a very rapid period of development in visual acuity between birth and 6 months of age. The first 6 months of life are, therefore, very important in the development of visual acuity and many other aspects of the visual system.

When discussing the development of the visual system, it is important to mention the concept of plasticity and sensitivity. As described above, the infant is born with poor acuity. With normal stimulation during the first 5 years of life, however, acuity develops to adult levels. This time period has been referred to as the sensitive period of visual development, and it is the time frame during which the visual system is plastic and capable of developing normally. However, it is also the time period during which any disorder or interference will severely impact on the normal developmental process. The first 6 months of life is the period of most rapid development in acuity, accommodation, and binocular vision and is sometimes referred to as the critical period. This is the period of maximum sensitivity to interference.

The presence of uncorrected or undetected vision problems during the first 5 to 6 years of life will interfere with the development of visual acuity and binocular vision, and with other aspects of the visual system. This is the basis for the recent recommendation of the American Optometric Association (AOA). The AOA now recommends the first full eye examination by an optometrist at the age of 6 months, the second examination at age 3, and the next at 6 years of age.

Significance of Visual Acuity Disorders for Occupational Therapy

Reduced visual acuity does not occur as an isolated problem. Acuity that is less than expected for a given age level is always related to other vision problems or eye disease. Reduced visual acuity, therefore, can be thought of as a sign that another vision anomaly is present. The presence

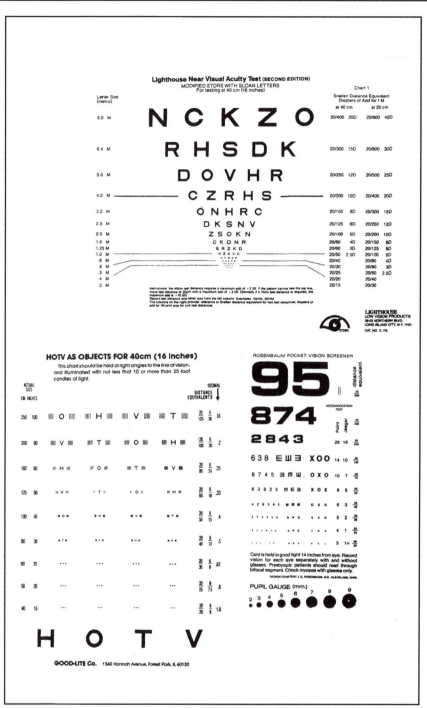

Figure 3-7. Variety of near point visual acuity cards.

of undetected poor visual acuity in both eyes in young children can have a devastating effect on development and on the child's ability to interact with his or her environment. It is important to understand that reduced visual acuity has this effect only if it is present in both eyes. If there is a loss of vision in only one eye, the child will use the eye with normal acuity, and generally there will

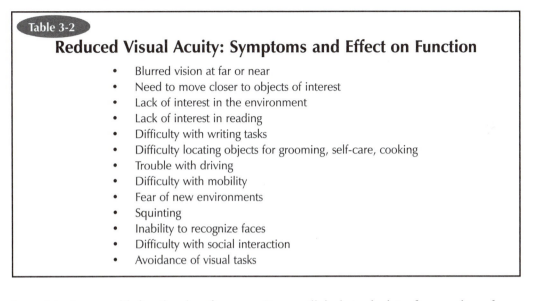

Table 3-2

Reduced Visual Acuity: Symptoms and Effect on Function

- Blurred vision at far or near
- Need to move closer to objects of interest
- Lack of interest in the environment
- Lack of interest in reading
- Difficulty with writing tasks
- Difficulty locating objects for grooming, self-care, cooking
- Trouble with driving
- Difficulty with mobility
- Fear of new environments
- Squinting
- Inability to recognize faces
- Difficulty with social interaction
- Avoidance of visual tasks

be no interference with functional performance. From a clinical standpoint, of course, loss of acuity in one eye, called amblyopia, is very significant and requires aggressive treatment. It does not affect the child's ability to interact with his or her environment, however, and would be unlikely to interfere with occupational therapy. It is also important to remember that the quality of the patient's vision is also critical for performance. It is possible for a patient to have reasonably good vision but still have significant and legitimate complaints about the quality of vision.

Reduced visual acuity will have a significant effect on rehabilitation of either a child or an adult. Reading, writing, and driving, for instance, are three tasks that are almost totally dependent on vision. Whether the occupational therapist is working with a developmentally delayed child or with a patient recovering from cerebrovascular accident or head trauma, reduced visual acuity will generally interfere with progress. It is critical for the therapist to be sensitive to this possibility and to make an appropriate referral for an evaluation and treatment of the reduced acuity.

Signs, Symptoms, and Significance of Visual Acuity Disorders for Occupational Therapy

The signs and symptoms of visual acuity are summarized in Table 3-2. The primary problems that therapists will observe are a need for the patient to move closer to objects of interest, lack of interest in the environment, difficulty with mobility, fear of new environments, squinting, and avoidance of visual tasks.

Contrast Sensitivity

Definition

An important topic that is related to visual acuity is contrast sensitivity. While visual acuity tests enable the therapist to estimate how well someone can see small high contrast objects, contrast sensitivity testing enables the therapist to estimate how well someone can see larger low contrast objects. Contrast sensitivity is related to visual acuity but provides information that is not as well captured by visual acuity measurement.[9] Contrast sensitivity is strongly associated with reading performance,[10] mobility,[11,12] driving,[13,14] face recognition,[14,15] and activities of daily living.[15,16] Contrast sensitivity testing tells us about the quality of the available vision when viewing larger objects. For instance, it is possible for a client to have reasonably good visual acuity but still complain of problems such as dim, foggy, or unclear vision or sensitivity to bright light. Visual acuity only allows us to evaluate one limited aspect of the person's ability to see. Contrast sensitivity is a measure of how faded or washed out an image can be before it becomes indistinguishable from a uniform field. A person with impaired contrast sensitivity might describe the problem by saying "it is like looking through a dirty windshield when I drive." People with reduced contrast sensitivity often are very particular about lighting. They usually are glare sensitive or can see best over only a very narrow range of light intensity.

Contrast sensitivity determines the lowest contrast level that can be detected by a client for a given size target. Contrast can vary from no contrast (0%) to highest contrast (100%). For example, high quality print has 85% to 95% contrast, while paper currency has only 55% to 60% contrast.

Examples of Low Contrast in Activities of Daily Living

- Communication: We need to use information from the faint shadows on people's faces to recognize facial expressions.

- Orientation and mobility: We need to see low contrast forms such as the curb, faint shadows, and the last step of carpeted stairs when walking. When driving, we need to function in low contrast conditions such as seeing in dusk, rain, fog, snow fall, and at night.

- Reading: When reading we may encounter poor quality copies, newsprint, and older books with poor contrast.

- Kitchen tasks: When cutting certain foods such as chicken, onion, or other light-colored objects on a white or light-colored cutting board we may encounter low contrast situations.

Classification of Contrast Sensitivity Disorders

There is no classification of contrast sensitivity disorders because these problems are always secondary to other conditions. Reduced contrast sensitivity can occur secondary to a wide variety of conditions, including amblyopia, and a wide variety of eye diseases.

Clinical Assessment

Contrast sensitivity testing can be performed at both distance and near using the instrumentation shown in Figures 3-8a through 3-8e. One test used for older children and adults is illustrated in Figure 3-8a. To use this device, the examiner asks the patient to observe the sample gratings at the bottom of the chart. The four possible responses (left, right, up, and blank) should be reviewed. With one eye occluded, the patient is instructed to begin with the top row and identify the orientation of as many of the circular patches as possible. This is repeated for all five rows of the chart. As Figure 3-8a illustrates, the contrast decreases as the patient views from left to right.

In recent years, however, letter contrast sensitivity testing has become the preferred method in clinical settings because it is easy to administer and clients are familiar with the use of letters to test vision.[17] The Pelli-Robson Contrast Sensitivity Chart has been a popular method of testing letter contrast sensitivity (see Figure 3-8b).[18] It is a large wall-mounted chart, arranged in eight rows of two triplets each. The three letters within each triplet have constant contrast, whereas the contrast across triplets, reading from left to right, and continuing on successive lines, decreases in contrast. The client reads the letters across and down the chart, as in standard letter acuity measurement. Instead of the letters decreasing in size, however, they decrease in contrast.

Although widely used by researchers it has not been widely used by clinicians for a variety of reasons.[17] First, it is inconvenient for testing in small clinical spaces, as it requires a large amount of wall space devoted to it. Second, it is difficult to arrange lighting that will illuminate such a large area uniformly. Third, a wall-mounted chart is difficult to keep clean and free of defects.[17]

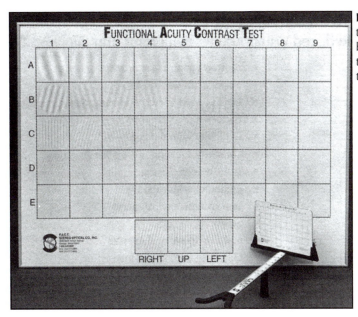

Figure 3-8a. Contrast sensitivity testing. The patient is instructed to begin with the top row and identify the orientation of as many of the circular patches as possible.

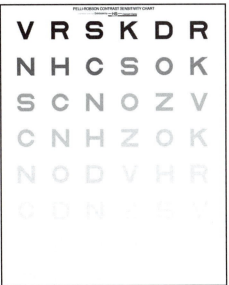

Figure 3-8b. The Pelli-Robson Contrast Sensitivity Chart. (Reprinted with permission from Scheiman M, Scheiman M, Whittaker SG. *Low Vision Rehabilitation: A Practical Guide for Occupational Therapists*. Thorofare, NJ: SLACK Incorporated; 2007.)

Recently, Arditi[17] reported on a new letter contrast sensitivity test called the Mars Letter Contrast Sensitivity Test (see Figure 3-8c). It is similar to the Pelli-Robson, but has greater accuracy due to its finer contrast decrements and scoring procedure, it is hand-held, with a recommended viewing distance of 50 cm, and is portable. These advantages may make this chart more desirable in a clinical setting.

Tests have also been developed in recent years to allow clinicians to evaluate contrast sensitivity in infants, young children, and developmentally or cognitively delayed patients.[19] Currently available tests include the Lea Symbols Contrast Sensitivity Chart (see Figure 3-8d) and the Hiding Heidi Contrast Sensitivity Chart (see Figure 3-8e). The Lea test uses the same Lea symbols described earlier for visual acuity testing. The child is asked to match the pictures at each contrast

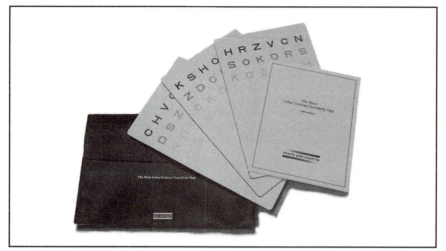

Figure 3-8c. The Mars Letter Contrast Sensitivity Test. (Reprinted with permission from Scheiman M, Scheiman M, Whittaker SG. *Low Vision Rehabilitation: A Practical Guide for Occupational Therapists*. Thorofare, NJ: SLACK Incorporated; 2007.)

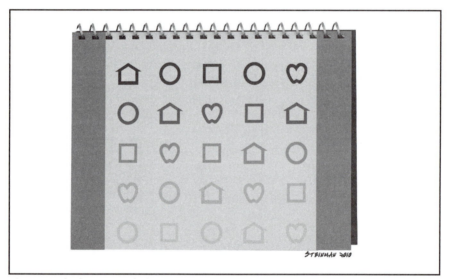

Figure 3-8d. The Lea Symbols Contrast Sensitivity Chart used to evaluate contrast sensitivity in infants, preverbal children, and developmentally and cognitively delayed patients.

level. This test is effective for children 3 years old or older. The Hiding Heidi Contrast Sensitivity Chart can be used with even younger children. It is a forced choice test. The child is shown two pictures, one with a homogeneous pattern and the other with a light contrast happy face. When a repeatable response is elicited to the light contrast figure, testing continues with reduced contrast figures.[19]

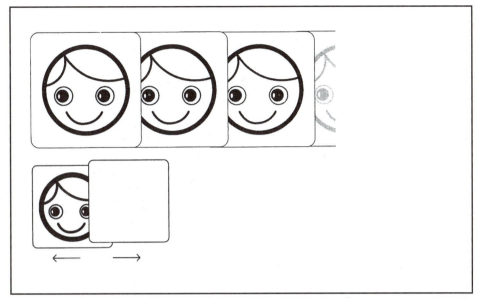

Figure 3-8e. The Hiding Heidi Contrast Sensitivity Chart used to evaluate contrast sensitivity in infants, preverbal children, and developmentally and cognitively delayed patients.

Significance of Contrast Sensitivity Disorders for Occupational Therapy

Contrast sensitivity problems can cause vision to seem hazy, dim, or cloudy and will interfere with activities of daily living such as shopping, driving, social interaction of any kind, and almost any activity in which identification of form and shape is important.

Refractive Disorders

Definition

Refraction is the term used to describe the evaluation of the optical system of the eye. We use the term *refractive error* to describe any disorder of refraction. When the optometrist performs the "refraction," he or she determines whether the individual is emmetropic (absence of refractive error), myopic (nearsighted), hyperopic (farsighted), or astigmatic. The refraction is the examination procedure used to determine if a patient will benefit from glasses and the exact prescription that is appropriate.

Etiology of Refractive Error

Within optometry, there is a debate about the etiology of refractive error. Traditional theory attributes refractive conditions such as myopia, hyperopia, or astigmatism to genetics and random biological variation. Children become nearsighted because they have parents who are nearsighted. Because refractive conditions are genetically determined, treatment involves correction of the refractive condition with appropriate lenses. Advocates of this theory dismiss any attempts to reduce or modify the problem using special lenses, prism, or vision therapy procedures.

Other models attribute the development of refractive problems and many other vision disorders to the extensive near work demands imposed by our society. The most popular model is Skeffington's near point stress model.[20] He suggests that refractive, binocular, and accommodative disorders develop because near work creates demands that are incompatible with our physiology. Proponents of this model have developed therapeutic regimens that stress prevention and remediation using special lens prescriptions, prism, and vision therapy.[21]

In spite of many years of research, this debate continues without a definitive answer. My philosophy at this time is that both theories are probably partially correct. I believe that there are certainly cases of refractive error that have a genetic basis. Usually, very high degrees of myopia, hyperopia, or astigmatism that have an early onset would fit into this category. Such cases are best treated in the traditional mode using corrective lenses without any attempt to eliminate or alter the refractive error. On the other hand, it is clear that there are also many cases in which the refractive condition may be secondary to environmental factors. Older children who develop myopia as they become heavily involved with reading or young adults who develop myopia in college or after entering the work force are examples of individuals who may have refractive disorders secondary to environmental demands. Studies have reported that there is a constellation of clinical findings that suggest when clinicians should attempt to prevent, control, or eliminate myopia using lenses, prism, or vision therapy.[22-25] This topic will be covered in more depth in Chapter Seven.

Classification of Refractive Conditions

EMMETROPIA

The word emmetropia is used to describe the condition in which there is an absence of refractive error. In emmetropia, the light rays entering the eyes focus right on the retina. Figure 3-9 illustrates how the light rays entering the eye are perfectly focused on the retina in emmetropia. In such a case, the patient is neither nearsighted nor farsighted and does not have astigmatism. Emmetropia is not necessarily considered normal, expected, or desirable. In fact, the average person is slightly hyperopic. A finding of emmetropia can be an indication that the patient's visual system is changing and is becoming myopic.

MYOPIA (NEARSIGHTEDNESS)

Myopia is a condition in which the light rays entering the eye focus in front of the retina. In myopia, the vision is blurred at distance but clear at near. Figure 3-10 illustrates the reason why a patient with myopia experiences blurred vision. The light rays entering the eye are focused in front of the retina because the optics of the eye are too strong relative to the length of the eye. The myopic eye has a longer axial length than the emmetropic or hyperopic eye. The human eye can make no internal adjustment to overcome the optical problem associated with myopia. An individual with myopia can squint, which actually does allow improved vision, but this is generally considered an unacceptable way to regain clarity because it can cause discomfort and is cosmetically unacceptable. Squinting helps compensate for the blur associated with myopia because it creates a pinhole effect. Any attempted focusing adjustment will simply make the blurred vision worse. Thus, a patient with myopia will have to move closer to the object he or she is trying to view. Table 3-3 lists the signs and symptoms associated with myopia.

Figure 3-9. Light rays entering the eye are perfectly focused on the retina in emmetropia. (Reprinted with permission from Scheiman M, Scheiman M, Whittaker SG. *Low Vision Rehabilitation: A Practical Guide for Occupational Therapists*. Thorofare, NJ: SLACK Incorporated; 2007.)

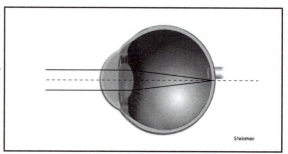

Table 3-3

Myopia: Symptoms and Effect on Function

- Blurred vision at far
- Need to move closer to objects of interest
- Lack of interest in the environment
- Squinting

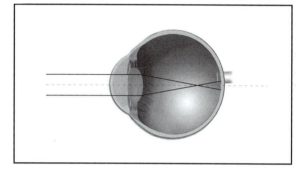

Figure 3-10. The light rays entering the eye are focused in front of the retina in myopia causing blurred vision. (Reprinted with permission from Scheiman M, Scheiman M, Whittaker SG. *Low Vision Rehabilitation: A Practical Guide for Occupational Therapists*. Thorofare, NJ: SLACK Incorporated; 2007.)

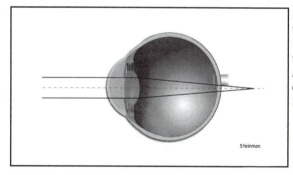

Figure 3-11a. The light rays entering the eye are focused behind the retina in hyperopia causing blurred vision. (Reprinted with permission from Scheiman M, Scheiman M, Whittaker SG. *Low Vision Rehabilitation: A Practical Guide for Occupational Therapists*. Thorofare, NJ: SLACK Incorporated; 2007.)

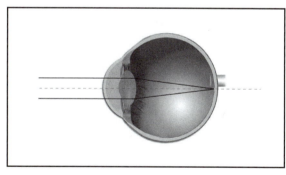

Figure 3-11b. To see clearly, a person with hyperopia must contract the ciliary muscle to change the shape of the lens in the eye and regain clarity. (Reprinted with permission from Scheiman M, Scheiman M, Whittaker SG. *Low Vision Rehabilitation: A Practical Guide for Occupational Therapists*. Thorofare, NJ: SLACK Incorporated; 2007.)

HYPEROPIA (FARSIGHTEDNESS)

Hyperopia is a condition in which light rays entering the eye focus behind the retina and the individual must accommodate to see clearly (Figure 3-11a). This need to accommodate requires the use of muscular effort. The amount of effort necessary is greater when the individual looks at near. Figure 3-11b illustrates that to see clearly, a person with hyperopia must contract the ciliary muscle to change the shape of the lens in the eye and regain clarity. Contraction of the ciliary muscle leads to a change in focus and is referred to as accommodation. The effort that is necessary to

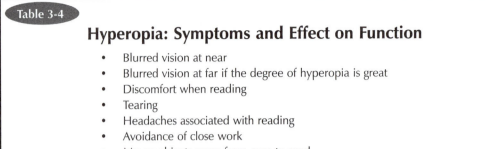

Table 3-4

Hyperopia: Symptoms and Effect on Function

- Blurred vision at near
- Blurred vision at far if the degree of hyperopia is great
- Discomfort when reading
- Tearing
- Headaches associated with reading
- Avoidance of close work
- Moves objects away from eyes to read

accommodate is directly related to the degree of hyperopia. A very high degree of hyperopia requires so much muscular effort that it cannot be overcome and results in blurred vision. If not corrected early, very high degrees of hyperopia can lead to amblyopia (loss of vision) and difficulty interacting with the environment. Moderate degrees of hyperopia can be overcome using accommodation. The constant need for accommodation, however, requires the use of muscular effort and leads to signs and symptoms, such as blurred vision, eyestrain, tearing, burning, inability to concentrate and attend, avoidance of visual tasks, and the need to move the object of interest closer or farther away. Small degrees of hyperopia are generally successfully overcome without symptoms. Remember that a low degree of hyperopia is considered normal, expected, and desirable. Table 3-4 lists the signs and symptoms associated with hyperopia.

ASTIGMATISM

Astigmatism is a condition in which vision is blurred and distorted at both distance and near. An astigmatic eye is not spherical. Rather, it has an oval shape, and this causes the light rays entering the eye to focus at two different points. Figure 3-12 illustrates the effect that astigmatism has on the light rays focusing on the retina. In order to see clearly, a person with astigmatism will attempt to accommodate. While accommodation may improve clarity, it is never completely successful for a person with astigmatism, and the effort that is necessary to accommodate may lead to discomfort. As discussed above for hyperopia, the degree of accommodation necessary is related to the degree and type of astigmatism. In some cases of astigmatism, accommodation has no beneficial effect on clarity. A very high degree of astigmatism generally cannot be overcome and results in blurred vision. If not corrected early, such problems can lead to amblyopia (loss of vision) and difficulty interacting with the environment. Moderate degrees of astigmatism can sometimes be overcome using accommodation. The constant need for accommodation, however, requires the use of muscular effort and leads to signs and symptoms, such as blurred vision, eyestrain, tearing, burning, inability to concentrate and attend, avoidance of visual tasks, and the need to move the object of interest closer or farther away. Small degrees of astigmatism are common and are generally successfully overcome without symptoms. Table 3-5 lists the signs and symptoms associated with astigmatism.

Figure 3-12. The affect of astigmatism on the light rays focusing on the retina. (Reprinted with permission from Scheiman M, Scheiman M, Whittaker SG. *Low Vision Rehabilitation: A Practical Guide for Occupational Therapists.* Thorofare, NJ: SLACK Incorporated; 2007.)

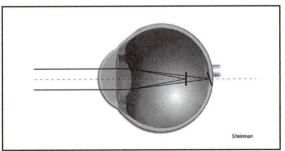

Steinman

Table 3-5	
Astigmatism: Symptoms and Effect on Function	

- Blurred vision at distance and near
- Discomfort when reading
- Tearing
- Headaches associated with reading
- Avoidance of close work
- Moves objects away from eyes to read

ANISOMETROPIA

Anisometropia is not another type of refractive error. Rather, the term refers to a condition in which there is a significant difference in the magnitude of the refractive error between the two eyes. Anisometropia can be present along with myopia, hyperopia, or astigmatism. The following are four common examples of anisometropia:

1. A patient has a mild degree of hyperopia in the right eye and a moderate or high degree of hyperopia in the left eye.

2. A patient has a mild degree of myopia in the right eye and a moderate or high degree of myopia in the left eye.

3. A patient has a mild degree of astigmatism in the right eye and a moderate or high degree of astigmatism in the left eye.

4. A patient has a mild to moderate degree of hyperopia in one eye and a mild to moderate degree of myopia in the other.

The significance of anisometropia is that the difference in refractive error between the two eyes interferes with binocular vision. The visual cortex receives images from each eye that differ in clarity and size, and this makes it difficult for the brain to fuse or merge the information from the two eyes. In such cases, the visual cortex generally will learn to suppress or ignore the information coming from the eye with the greater degree of refractive error. If the condition occurs during the sensitive period of visual development described earlier in the chapter, suppression will lead to loss of vision in the eye with the greater degree of refractive error. This loss of vision is referred to as amblyopia, which will be described in detail in Chapter Four.

Clinical Assessment

Like visual acuity, refraction is also a test that is performed by all eye care professionals. There are two general methods of evaluating the refractive status of the eye. These include objective and subjective methods. Subjective tests can only be successfully performed with cooperative, attentive patients with reasonable cognitive ability. These tests can generally be performed with any person with a developmental age of 7 years or older. Objective testing, however, can be successfully performed at any age and for virtually any patient.

Subjective Refraction Techniques

Most adults have had an eye examination at least once in their lives, and, if they have, they are likely to remember the subjective refraction portion of the examination. The instrumentation used is illustrated in Figure 3-13. This instrument, called the phoropter, contains numerous lenses and allows the optometrist to find the combination of lenses that will provide the best possible vision for any patient being examined. The procedure is very subjective, and the optometrist will ask questions such as, "Which is better, choice one or choice two?" or "Does this lens make the

Figure 3-13. The phoropter is an instrument used to find the combination of lenses that will provide the best possible vision for any patient being examined. (Reprinted with permission from Scheiman M, Scheiman M, Whittaker SG. *Low Vision Rehabilitation: A Practical Guide for Occupational Therapists*. Thorofare, NJ: SLACK Incorporated; 2007.)

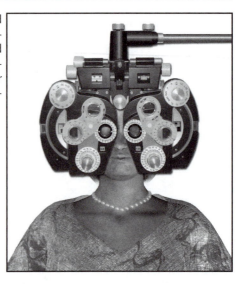

letters look clearer or just blacker and smaller?" This subjective approach works well for most of the population but is generally not used with children below the age of 6 or 7 or with patients who have attention problems, perceptual and cognitive disorders, or other special needs. It is clear, therefore, that many patients who are treated by occupational therapists will be unable to be evaluated using subjective refraction procedures. Fortunately, excellent objective techniques are available and produce accurate results in the hands of an experienced clinician.

Objective Refraction Techniques

The instrument illustrated in Figure 3-14 is called a retinoscope. This instrument permits the optometrist to accurately and objectively assess refractive status in virtually any patient. The optometrist directs the light from the retinoscope into the patient's eye and views the light that

Figure 3-14. The retinoscope can be used to accurately and objectively assess refractive status in virtually any patient. (Reprinted with permission from Scheiman M, Scheiman M, Whittaker SG. *Low Vision Rehabilitation: A Practical Guide for Occupational Therapists*. Thorofare, NJ: SLACK Incorporated; 2007.)

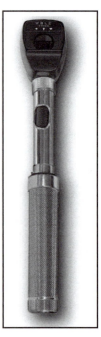

is reflected out of the eye. As the optometrist moves the retinoscope from side to side, he or she interprets the movement of the reflected light. Lenses are used to alter the movement of light and help the clinician determine the refraction and necessary eyeglass prescription. The procedure generally requires less than 1 minute per eye. It can be performed with or without eye drops. With a cooperative, intelligent patient with good attention, I always begin the refraction using retinoscopy. The subjective refraction is then performed to refine these results.

If a subjective refraction is not possible, clinical decisions can be made with confidence from the objective refraction alone. Thus, it is possible to determine if an individual has a refractive error such as myopia, hyperopia, or astigmatism even if he or she is unable to respond subjectively. A newborn child can be examined using this procedure, and an experienced clinician can confidently assess the refractive status of the eye.

Another objective refraction procedure can be performed using a computerized device called an automated refractor. The instrument is relatively expensive and provides the same type of information as the very inexpensive retinoscope. It also may require the patient to be attentive, to place his or her chin and forehead against the instrument, and to accurately fixate for a relatively long period of time. As a result, it has little value in the evaluation of patients unable to respond to subjective testing, even though this is an objective of the procedure. The typical patient seen by occupational therapists could not be tested with an automated refractor.

Refractive Error: Developmental Changes

The development of refractive error has been studied extensively. Before 1970, most of the research was performed with children starting from age 5 or so. In the past 20 years, however, new techniques have been developed that allow researchers and clinicians to evaluate vision in infants and preverbal children. This has led to a more complete understanding of the developmental changes that occur in the refractive status of the eye.

These studies have demonstrated that the most active period for changes in refractive error is the first 4 years of life. In particular, large fluctuations are common in astigmatism and anisometropia.[26] Studies have shown that large amounts of astigmatism are common in children below the age of 3 years.[26-29] In fact, Gwiazda et al[27] found that about 50% of infants between 9 and 32 weeks old have a significant degree of astigmatism. The magnitude of the astigmatism declines over the first few years of life so that the incidence of astigmatism is about 10% by 5 to 6 years of age.

All investigations show a bell-shaped curve distribution of refractive error with wide variability during infancy. This variability diminishes between the first and second years of life, with only small changes occurring thereafter.[30,31] Newborn infants tend to have a low to moderate degree of hyperopia with an incidence of about 35%. Most authors agree that hyperopia may increase during the first year of life, then there is a general reduction in the magnitude of hyperopia sometime after the age of 1 year.[19] Myopia is unusual in infants and preschool children, and at the age of 6 the incidence of myopia is only about 3.7%.[28] Children with very mild degrees of hyperopia or emmetropia at 5 or 6 years old develop mild to moderate myopia between ages 7 and 13. Others may develop mild myopia, or myopia may increase between ages 18 and 21.[32] Extreme ametropias are most often congenital and relatively stable.

Signs and Symptoms of Refractive Disorders and Significance of Refractive Disorders for Occupational Therapy

The significance of refractive disorders on progress in occupational therapy varies with the type of problem, the magnitude of the refractive error, and the age of the patient. In the adult population, most patients will have had several eye examinations, and as a general rule, any significant refractive error will already have been detected. In spite of this, it is important that the occupational therapist not assume that the glasses that were used before a stroke or head trauma are still appropriate. Studies have shown that changes in eyeglasses are sometimes necessary after cerebrovascular accident and traumatic brain injury, particularly for hyperopia and presbyopia, because of disorders of accommodation.[33,34] This issue is discussed in more detail in Chapters Nine and Ten.

For the pediatric population, the issue of refractive error and its effect on therapy is very significant. Studies have shown that children with these problems have a high incidence of refractive disorders. For example, the incidence of refractive disorders in children with mental retardation has been reported to be 50% to 80%; in children with cerebral palsy, 50% to 70%; and in children with Down syndrome, 43% to 65%.[35] In addition, a high percentage of children being seen by occupational therapists may never have had a comprehensive vision evaluation. Studies show that only about 31% of children between ages 6 and 16 are likely to have had an eye examination within the past year, while below the age of 6, only about 14% are likely to have had an eye examination.[36] Many parents still believe that between the pediatrician and school vision screenings, all of the vision care needs of their children are being met. This is an unfortunate misconception that may lead to late detection of significant vision disorders and negative effects on overall development. And certainly with children who have mentally and multi-handicapping conditions, the visual system should be functioning at the best possible level.

Researchers have studied the effect of correction of refractive error in mentally and multi-impaired people. These studies are very significant and demonstrate significant changes in ability to identify objects and people; improved eye-to-eye contact; improved performance in activities such as catching, kicking, and throwing a ball; improved posture while eating; and in fine motor control, such as reaching and grasping for objects, stacking blocks, stringing beads, and cutting paper.[37] Any occupational therapist would be thrilled to see such changes in his or her patient, and occupational therapy would certainly proceed more effectively.

HIGH DEGREES OF REFRACTIVE ERROR IN BOTH EYES

If a child has a high degree of refractive error in both eyes and it is not corrected with eyeglasses, amblyopia can develop, leading to difficulty seeing and problems with mobility. Any therapy task requiring good visual skills will be compromised. Amblyopia affects both far and near tasks.

MODERATE DEGREES OF REFRACTIVE ERROR IN BOTH EYES

Moderate degrees of refractive error present in both eyes and left uncorrected generally do not lead to a loss of vision. Rather, any task that requires good vision will be much more difficult for the patient because of the need to use excessive effort to overcome the refractive error. Symptoms related to this type of problem are generally directly related to the amount of detail in the task and the amount of sustained attention and concentration required of the patient to complete the task. The effects of moderate degrees of uncorrected refractive error may be more severe for adults than children because children have a greater ability to accommodate than adults.

SIGNIFICANT DEGREES OF REFRACTIVE ERROR IN ONLY ONE EYE

This condition is referred to as anisometropia and if undetected or untreated can lead to amblyopia in the eye. We call this condition anisometropic amblyopia. Although amblyopia is a serious vision problem with significant implications for the visual function in the affected eye, there are generally no effects on performance because the patient still has adequate vision in the dominant or good eye. Thus, with both eyes open, the patient is able to see clearly and has normal ocular motility function and accommodation. The only potential problems that might exist are a mild decrease in stereopsis (3-D vision) and other binocular vision skills. Although binocular vision is compromised in cases of anisometropic amblyopia, most people with this problem learn to ignore or suppress the information entering the amblyopic eye, and this prevents symptoms of double vision or eyestrain.

MYOPIA (NEARSIGHTEDNESS)

In the pediatric population, low (up to 1 diopter [D]) and moderate degrees (1 to 3 D) of myopia generally are insignificant in regard to their effect on therapy progress. Children with low to moderate myopia can often manage well by squinting and simply moving closer to the object of interest. Because these children tend to squint, they are generally easily identified as requiring help. High degrees (greater than 3 D) of myopia in young children, however, may interfere with motor development and lead to difficulty interacting with the environment. Children with undetected high myopia may be clumsy, fearful of activities involving movement through space, and slow to progress in therapy, and they may avoid all tasks that involve viewing distant objects. It is important to understand that even a child with a high degree of myopia may be able to see objects clearly if they are held very close to the eyes. Thus, holding objects very close to the face is a characteristic sign of uncorrected myopia. Because the negative effects of high myopia or other refractive error are so significant and easily treated, such problems certainly should be ruled out in all children with developmental, motor, or cognitive disorders.

In adults being treated after cerebrovascular accident or traumatic brain injury, the presence of refractive error must always be taken into consideration in treatment. In almost all cases, any significant myopia would have been previously detected and treated. Changes in refractive error occur after cerebrovascular accident or traumatic brain injury, and this has important implications for therapy. If an occupational therapist is working on activities of daily living such as cooking, shopping, writing checks, or driving, it is absolutely critical that the visual input be maximized. Visual information processing will certainly be compromised if the sensory input is affected. The occupational therapist should make sure that the patient is wearing his or her glasses correctly, and an eye examination should be performed to make sure that the prescription is up to date. Table 3-3 summarizes the signs and symptoms associated with myopia.

HYPEROPIA (FARSIGHTEDNESS)

In contrast to myopia, in which high degrees are of greater significance than low or moderate degrees of the disorder, with hyperopia, low (up to 1 D) and moderate degrees (1 to 3 D) of the condition can have a very deleterious effect on occupational therapy. Remember that an individual with hyperopia can accommodate to regain clear vision. Because the patient can regain clear vision with effort, he or she will be able to pass a typical vision screening that simply assesses visual acuity. Thus, an individual with low to moderate degrees of hyperopia will see clearly, but the effort that is necessary to accommodate can result in eyestrain, inability to attend and concentrate, headaches, and intermittent blurred vision. In some cases, the effort required to accommodate reflexively causes the eyes to turn inward (esophoria or esotropia), leading to intermittent or even constant double vision. The individual with low to moderate degrees of hyperopia, therefore, sees clearly but may feel uncomfortable and have difficulty sustaining attention. Because visual acuity is normal in such cases, the discomfort may not be attributed to a vision problem, and the individual may suffer for quite some time with an undiagnosed problem.

Occupational therapists often work with children with attention problems such as attention deficit hyperactivity disorder (ADHD). Because of their inability to concentrate and attend for reasonable periods of time, these children can be very difficult to successfully manage. In such cases, low to moderate degrees of hyperopia should certainly be ruled out as a possible contributing factor to the poor attention. Optometrists occasionally encounter patients who have been labeled as ADHD who have been functioning with moderate degrees of undetected hyperopia. When appropriate eyeglasses are prescribed, the attention problems dissipate.

Researchers have reported a significant relationship between hyperopia and visual perceptual skills.[38] These reports demonstrate a higher prevalence of visual perceptual disorders in children with moderate degrees of hyperopia than in children with myopia or emmetropia. Other studies have reported a higher prevalence of significant degrees of hyperopia in children with reading disorders.[39,40]

High degrees (greater than 3 D) of hyperopia cannot be overcome for extended periods of time and result in blurred vision. If not corrected early, such problems can lead to amblyopia (loss of vision) and difficulty interacting with the environment. Table 3-4 summarizes the signs and symptoms associated with hyperopia.

ASTIGMATISM

As with hyperopia, low (up to 1 D) and moderate degrees (1 to 3 D) of astigmatism can have a negative effect on occupational therapy. Patients with astigmatism may try to accommodate to regain clear vision. Unlike hyperopia, astigmatism can never completely be overcome by accommodating. The effort used to accommodate, however, can result in eyestrain, inability to attend and concentrate, headaches, and intermittent blurred vision. The individual with low to moderate degrees of astigmatism, therefore, will struggle with blurred vision and discomfort and may have difficulty sustaining attention. Because visual acuity is often borderline and may be just enough to pass a screening, the discomfort may not be attributed to a vision problem, and the individual may suffer for quite some time with an undiagnosed problem.

Low to moderate degrees of astigmatism should be ruled out as a possible contributing factor for any child with attention problems. High degrees (greater than 3 D) of astigmatism cannot be overcome and result in blurred vision. If not corrected early, such problems can lead to amblyopia (loss of vision) and difficulty interacting with the environment. Table 3-5 summarizes the signs and symptoms associated with astigmatism.

Eye Health Disorders

Classification

Eye health disorders are generally classified by the location of the disorder. The four main types of eye health problems are anterior segment, lenticular, posterior segment, and visual pathway disorders. Figure 3-15 is a cross-section of the human eye and illustrates the anterior and posterior portions of the eye. The anterior section includes all the structures from the front of the eye to the lens. The posterior segment includes all structures behind the lens to the optic nerve. Figure 3-16 is an illustration of the visual pathways from the optic nerve to the occipital cortex. Tables 3-6 through 3-9 summarize the most common eye disease conditions.

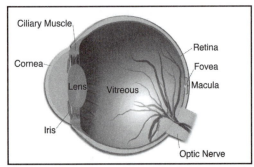

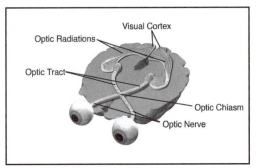

Figure 3-15. Cross-section of the human eye, illustrating the anterior and posterior portions of the eye. (Reprinted with permission from Scheiman M, Scheiman M, Whittaker SG. *Low Vision Rehabilitation: A Practical Guide for Occupational Therapists*. Thorofare, NJ: SLACK Incorporated; 2007.)

Figure 3-16. Illustration of the visual pathways from the optic nerve to the occipital cortex. (Reprinted with permission from Scheiman M, Scheiman M, Whittaker SG. *Low Vision Rehabilitation: A Practical Guide for Occupational Therapists*. Thorofare, NJ: SLACK Incorporated; 2007.)

Table 3-6

Anterior Segment Disease

Condition	Description	Anatomical Structure
Ptosis	Drooping eyelid.	Upper lid
Ectropion	Inferior eyelid does not make contact with the eyeball.	Lower lid
Entropion	Inferior eyelid turns inward and lashes rub against eye.	Lower lid
Basal cell carcinoma	Most common malignant tumor of the eyelid.	Eyelid
Chalazion or hordeolum	Common lid lump in which there is an infection of a gland in the eyelid. The external type is sometimes referred to as a sty.	Eyelid
Papilloma	Benign tumor of the eyelid.	Eyelid
Blepharitis	Inflammation of the eyelids. Common forms are bacterial, viral, or allergic blepharitis.	Eyelid
Conjunctivitis	Inflammation of the conjunctiva. Common forms are bacterial, viral, or allergic conjunctivitis.	Conjunctiva
Scleritis	Inflammation of the sclera.	Sclera
Keratitis	Inflammation of the cornea. Common forms are bacterial, viral, or allergic keratitis.	Cornea
Corneal abrasion	Injury to cornea. Usually caused by a foreign body or contact lenses overwear.	Cornea
Anterior uveitis	Inflammation of all or parts of the uvea including the iris and ciliary body.	Iris and ciliary body
Hyphema	Accumulation of blood in the anterior chamber.	Anterior chamber
Aniridia	Absence of the iris.	Iris

Clinical Assessment of Eye Health Disorders

To evaluate the integrity of the health of the eyes, clinicians use diagnostic drugs, along with a variety of instrumentation that provides variable illumination and magnification. Instrumentation can range from inexpensive hand-held instruments such as the ophthalmoscope to very expensive, computerized equipment such as the laser ophthalmoscope. Equipment is available to permit assessment of all external and internal structures of the eye. To evaluate the internal structures of the eyes, clinicians must use a series of drugs designed to dilate the pupil. Dilation of the pupil allows the clinician to view the retina and other internal structures through a wider opening.

Clinicians can also evaluate the visual system beyond the retina, even though it cannot be directly viewed. Disorders in the visual pathways lead to visual field deficits that can be detected

Table 3-7

Disease of the Lens

Condition	Description	Anatomical Structure
Cataract	An opacity occurring in the normally transparent lens, causing reduced visual acuity. It is generally related to the aging process but can also occur as a result of trauma.	Lens
Subluxation or dislocation of the lens	This can occur as a result of trauma or can be associated with a hereditary syndrome such as Marfan syndrome. The dislocation of the lens causes reduced visual acuity.	Lens

Table 3-8

Posterior Segment Disease

Condition	Description	Anatomical Structure
Optic nerve atrophy	Loss of nerve fibers in the optic nerve. This can be acquired due to a variety of diseases or congenital.	Optic nerve
Optic neuritis	Inflammation of the optic nerve head.	Optic nerve
Papilledema	Swelling or edema of the optic disc secondary to elevated intracranial pressure.	Optic nerve
Central retinal vein occlusion	A destructive retinal condition strongly associated with systemic disease or pressure on the optic nerve.	Retina
Central retinal artery occlusion	Sudden, painless loss of vision due to occlusion of central retinal artery. Can be secondary to emboli from atheromatous plaques from the internal carotid artery, cardiac lesions.	Retina
Diabetic retinopathy	Microaneurysms, retinal hemorrhages, and exudates due to disease of retinal vasculature secondary to diabetes.	Retina
Retinopathy of prematurity	Retinal disease due to oxygen used to treat prematurity, includes neovascularization, retinal dragging, scarring, retinal detachment.	Retina
Age-related macular degeneration	Number one cause of blindness in the United States in people over 60. Patient experiences loss of vision, usually bilateral.	Macula
Retinal detachment	The retina detaches from the choroid and leads to loss of vision if not repaired.	Retina

Table 3-9

Disease Affecting the Visual Pathways

Condition	Description	Anatomical Structure
Glaucoma	Visual field defects caused by damage to retinal nerve fiber bundles at the optic nerve head. The deficits are generally paracentral, arcuate scotomas, or nasal steps.	Optic nerve
Opacities of ocular media	Generalized depression of sensitivity due to corneal opacities, cataracts, or vitreous opacities.	Cornea, lens, vitreous
Optic nerve disease	Caused by monocular visual field defects. Common problems include papilledema, optic neuritis, compressive optic neuropathy, drusen.	Optic nerve
Optic chiasm disease	Characteristic bitemporal hemianopic defect commonly caused by a pituitary gland tumor.	Optic chiasm
Retrochiasmal visual pathway disease	Hemianopic field defects.	Optic tract, lateral geniculate body, optic radiations (temporal lobe, parietal lobe), visual cortex

using visual field testing equipment. Disease in the visual pathways can also affect fixation ability, eye movements, convergence, binocular vision, pupillary response, eyelid function, and visual information processing skills. All of the areas are assessed in a comprehensive vision/eye health evaluation, and this information can be used to determine the integrity of the visual pathways.

Development of Anatomical and Physiological Characteristics of the Eye

After birth, the size of the eye continues to grow, and the most rapid growth is during the first 2 years of life. Between 2 and 5 years, the growth rate is reduced, and a slow progression occurs up to about 13 years of age.[41] Most of the important characteristics of the adult visual system are established before birth and the first few years thereafter. During this time, the neurons of the retina and visual pathways differentiate and make their permanent synaptic connections.

The retina is not fully developed at birth. The entire retina, and in particular the fovea, continues to develop until age 4 or 5 years. This initial immaturity probably accounts for the reduced visual acuity at birth and early infancy.[42] The central 5 degrees of the retina is immature at birth, though peripheral regions appear well developed and mature. Over the first few years of life, especially the first 6 months, the central retina develops very rapidly. During this early stage in life, the visual system is very susceptible to interference.

The optic nerve and optic tract are also not fully developed at birth. Some nerve fibers are myelinated at birth, but myelination proceeds rapidly up to 2 years of age and less rapidly thereafter.[43] The evidence that is available from anatomical and physiological studies suggests that there is a plastic or sensitive period in human visual development of the visual cortex that lasts from birth to 7 to 10 years of age at least. Very little is known about the developmental details of the many extrastriate visual areas in the cerebral cortex or the complex neural circuitry responsible for eye movements and eye-body coordination.[44]

Common Eye Diseases

This section reviews the four most common eye diseases the occupational therapist is likely to encounter.

Age-Related Macular Degeneration

DESCRIPTION

Age-related macular degeneration (AMD) is a degenerative, acquired disorder of the central retina, the macula, which usually occurs in patients over age 55, results in progressive, sometimes significant, irreversible loss of central visual function from either fibrous scarring or atrophy of the macula. It is the leading cause of vision loss in the adult population.

The macula is located roughly in the center of the retina and is a small and highly sensitive part of the retina responsible for detailed central vision. The fovea is the very center of the macula. The normal macula has a characteristic appearance and is more heavily pigmented than the surrounding retina (Figure 3-17). The macula allows us to appreciate detail and perform tasks that require central vision such as reading, writing, recognizing faces, and driving. AMD is classified as either dry (nonexudative) or wet (exudative).

Dry (Nonexudative or Atrophic) Age-Related Macular Degeneration

Dry (nonexudative or atrophic) AMD accounts for 90% of all patients with AMD in the United States.[45] Most patients with dry AMD experience gradual, progressive loss of central visual function. This loss of vision is more noticeable during near tasks, especially in the early stages of the disease. In an estimated 12% to 21% of patients, dry AMD progresses to cause vision levels of 20/200 or worse.[46,47] Neovascularization is not present in dry AMD.

Wet (Exudative) Age-Related Macular Degeneration

Although wet AMD accounts for only 10% of patients with AMD, 90% of the AMD patients with significant vision loss have this form of the disease.[46,48] Wet AMD is characterized by the development of neovascularization in the choroid, leading to leakage of blood and subsequent elevation of the retinal pigment epithelium (Figure 3-18). Patients with wet AMD tend to notice a more profound and rapid decrease in central visual function. The leakage of blood from the new choroidal vessels causes distortion vision, central scotoma, and blurred vision.[49]

Figure 3-17. The normal macula has a characteristic appearance and is more heavily pigmented than the surrounding retina. (Reprinted with permission from Scheiman M, Scheiman M, Whittaker SG. *Low Vision Rehabilitation: A Practical Guide for Occupational Therapists.* Thorofare, NJ: SLACK Incorporated; 2007.)

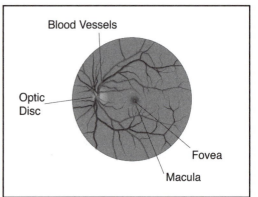

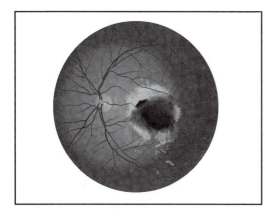

Figure 3-18. Wet macular degeneration with bleeding in the macular area. (Reprinted with permission from Scheiman M, Scheiman M, Whittaker SG. *Low Vision Rehabilitation: A Practical Guide for Occupational Therapists.* Thorofare, NJ: SLACK Incorporated; 2007.)

Risk Factors

Age is the most significant risk factor and clearly increases the risk of both developing AMD as well as of progressing to the late stages of the disorder.[50] Although age is a strong risk factor, AMD and vision loss do not inevitably occur with advancing age. People with an AMD-affected first-degree relative have a 50% lifetime risk of experiencing advanced AMD and vision loss, and tend to develop it earlier than those without a family history.[51] Smoking is associated with a four-fold increase in the risk of AMD and visual loss and, again, tends to promote earlier occurrence.[52] Studies have consistently implicated female gender as a risk factor. A relationship seems to exist between increased cumulative exposure to sunlight and ultraviolet radiation and wet AMD.[53] Weaker associations have been found with obesity, hypertension, macrovascular disease, raised cholesterol, and cataract surgery.

Dietary associations have also been found both with the signs of AMD and with progression to vision loss.[54-56] In a well-conducted, prospective study, dietary fat intake was systematically analyzed after correcting for other risk factors.[57] Vegetable fat intake had the strongest relationship with AMD progression, with a relative risk of 3.82 for the highest fat-intake quartile compared with the lowest quartile. Higher intakes of total fat and of saturated, monounsaturated, polyunsaturated, and trans-unsaturated fats all raised the relative risk of AMD progression about two-fold. Weekly fish intake and eating nuts two to three times a week were mildly protective. The implication is that a large shift away from vegetable oils, margarine, and fat-containing processed foods might reduce this epidemic of blindness in the elderly.

There is also evidence from a randomized controlled trial that high-dose dietary supplements of the antioxidants vitamin C, vitamin E, beta-carotene, and zinc can reduce the risk of progression from large or soft drusen to advanced AMD and visual loss by about 20% compared with controls over 6 years.[57] However, high-dose zinc can cause gastric irritation or anemia, and beta-carotene may possibly be associated with an increased risk of lung cancer among smokers. Uncontrolled studies suggest the antioxidants selenium, lutein, and zeaxanthin, which localize in the normal macula, may also help. There are as yet no studies to show whether dietary supplements are protective in patients in the early stages of dry AMD or in the 20% of patients who are at genetic risk. It is not yet known whether major dietary adjustment and/or introduction of dietary supplements for large numbers of elderly people will be justified in terms of preventing blindness.

Effect on Vision

Visual acuity varies with the extent of the degeneration and includes distortion, blurred vision (especially at near), and central scotoma. With dry AMD visual acuity can range from 20/20 to 20/400. Visual acuity with wet AMD is generally worse than 20/400. All patients with AMD have central visual field defects with normal peripheral vision. Patients with AMD almost never go

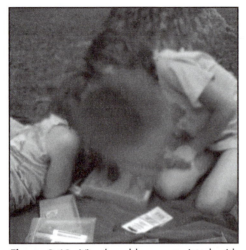

Figure 3-19. Visual problems associated with age-related macular degeneration and a macular scotoma. (Reprinted with permission from Scheiman M, Scheiman M, Whittaker SG. *Low Vision Rehabilitation: A Practical Guide for Occupational Therapists*. Thorofare, NJ: SLACK Incorporated; 2007.)

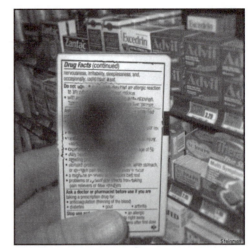

Figure 3-20. Visual problems associated with age-related macular degeneration and a macular scotoma. (Reprinted with permission from Scheiman M, Scheiman M, Whittaker SG. *Low Vision Rehabilitation: A Practical Guide for Occupational Therapists*. Thorofare, NJ: SLACK Incorporated; 2007.)

totally blind. However, if AMD occurs in both eyes, the visual acuity loss along with the central scotoma significantly impair a person's ability to engage in activities of daily living and quality of life. High-resolution tasks such as reading, writing, sewing, telling time, taking care of financial issues, driving, and distinguishing colors and facial expressions become problematic. The consequences of AMD lead to loss of independence, lowered self-esteem, decreased mobility, increased risk of injury due to falls, and depression. Figures 3-19 and 3-20 illustrate what a patient might see with AMD and a macular scotoma.

Some patients with AMD have a phenomenom called Charles Bonnet syndrome or visual hallucinations.[24] This is an occasional complaint of patients with bilateral AMD and may occur spontaneously with no known external cause.

TREATMENT

Treatment of AMD includes various medical procedures to slow the progression of the disease and low vision rehabilitation including optical and non-optical devices, environmental changes, education, support groups, and training in eccentric viewing, scanning, and reading.

Dry Age-Related Macular Degeneration

There is no medical treatment for dry AMD that can restore vision loss. Patients who have early retinal changes such as small drusen or mild pigmentation changes may experience no symptoms or may notice slowly progressive changes in visual function. These patients are generally seen by an eye doctor every 6 months. Patients are instructed to return for further examination within 24 hours of the onset of new symptoms because 10% of patients with dry AMD progress to wet AMD. Studies have shown that early treatment of wet AMD may limit the extent of damage and vision loss.

Wet Age-Related Macular Degeneration

The principal aim of treatment of wet AMD is to preserve visual acuity and reduce the risk of additional severe vision loss for as long as possible. Recently, a new treatment for wet AMD, injection of drugs called angiogenesis inhibitors, has been shown to be effective in randomized clinical trials. It is not a cure for wet AMD, but can prevent further loss of vision and may even improve vision to a small degree.

INJECTIONS WITH VASCULAR ENDOTHELIAL GROWTH FACTOR INHIBITOR

In December 2004, the Food and Drug Administration approved the latest treatment available for wet AMD using drugs known as vascular endothelial growth factor (VEGF) inhibitor. When these drugs (Lucentis [ranibizumab injection], Avastin [bevacizumab]) are injected into the vitreous humor of the eye, they have the capability of neutralizing a specific growth factor that promotes the growth of abnormal new blood vessels in eyes with AMD. The result is attack of both decrease of the vascular growth and leakage that are together responsible for the visual loss in wet AMD. These drugs have broad implications for treatment because it is effective in management of all types of new onset wet AMD. In fact, studies show that the use of these drugs can prevent severe visual loss (defined as loss of three lines of visual acuity on the Snellen eye chart) in as many as 70% of the treated patients during the period of follow-up.[58]

ANTIOXIDANTS

In a clinical trial researchers found that high levels of antioxidants and zinc significantly reduce the risk of advanced AMD and its associated vision loss.[57] In this study, patients at high risk of developing advanced stages of AMD lowered their risk by about 25% when treated with a high-dose combination of vitamin C, vitamin E, beta-carotene, and zinc. In the same high risk group the nutrients reduced the risk of vision loss caused by advanced AMD by about 19%. For those study participants who had either no AMD or early AMD, the nutrients did not provide an apparent benefit.[57] It is important to understand that these nutrients are not a cure for AMD, nor will they restore vision already lost from the disease. However, it may delay the onset of advanced AMD. It is also important to understand that there is no evidence that this AREDS formulation is effective for those diagnosed with early stage AMD. The study did not find that the formulation provided a benefit to those with early stage AMD.

LOW VISION REHABILITATION

Although, vision loss cannot be restored with medical treatment, low vision rehabilitation is an effective treatment that enables patients with dry AMD to function more effectively in activities of daily living and regain independence in spite of the visual deficit. The occupational therapist's role in low vision rehabilitation includes instruction in the use of optical and non-optical assistive devices; modification of lighting, contrast, and other environmental factors; treatment to learn adaptive eye movement patterns, scanning, and reading skills; education; and involvement in support groups.[59]

Diabetic Retinopathy

DESCRIPTION

Diabetic retinopathy is the most serious vision-threatening complication of chronic diabetes mellitus. Although there has been extensive research over several decades, knowledge about the etiology of diabetic retinopathy is still incomplete. The vascular complications of diabetes involve all organ systems including the eye. In the eye, these vascular changes lead to bleeding of small blood vessels and exudative material (inflammatory substance) flowing into the eye (Figure 3-21).

RISK FACTORS

Having diabetes puts an individual at risk of retinopathy. The risk of diabetic retinopathy increases the longer the person has the disease. The duration of the diabetes is also the major determinant of the severity of retinopathy and progression. Other risk factors for diabetic retinopathy include poorly controlled blood sugar levels, high blood pressure, high blood cholesterol, pregnancy, obesity, and kidney disease.

Figure 3-21. Vascular changes lead to bleeding of small blood vessels and exudative material (inflammatory substance) flowing into the eye in diabetic retinopathy. (Reprinted with permission from Scheiman M, Scheiman M, Whittaker SG. *Low Vision Rehabilitation: A Practical Guide for Occupational Therapists*. Thorofare, NJ: SLACK Incorporated; 2007.)

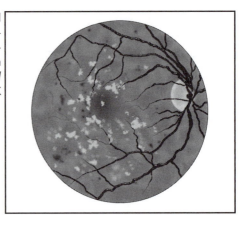

EFFECT ON VISION

Patients with diabetic retinopathy experience decreased, fluctuating, or distorted vision; focusing problems; loss of color vision; and floaters. They frequently have impaired contrast sensitivity as well because of cataracts, cloudy vitreous, and retinal edema and are very glare sensitive and particular about lighting. They may also have a central scotoma due to effects of the diabetic on the macular area (maculopathy), loss of peripheral vision, and difficulty in dim light. Treatments (described below) often leave a client with a small island of good vision. They may see individual numbers or letters but not words. The treatments also produce scotomas in the periphery, "Swiss cheese" vision. Figure 3-22 illustrates the visual problems of a patient with diabetic retinopathy.

TREATMENT

During the early stages of diabetic retinopathy, no treatment is needed, unless macular edema is present. The current approach in the early stage emphasizes the early recognition of retinopathy, vigorous control of blood glucose, and direct therapy with laser photocoagulation and vitreous surgery.

As the disease progresses the retinopathy is treated with laser surgery. This procedure is called laser photocoagulation treatment. Laser photocoagulation treatment helps to shrink the abnormal blood vessels.

Figure 3-22. Visual problems associated with diabetic retinopathy. (Reprinted with permission from Scheiman M, Scheiman M, Whittaker SG. *Low Vision Rehabilitation: A Practical Guide for Occupational Therapists*. Thorofare, NJ: SLACK Incorporated; 2007.)

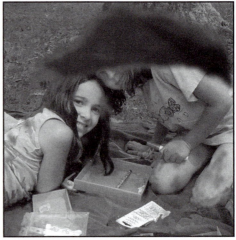

LOW VISION REHABILITATION

A hallmark of diabetic vision changes is impaired contrast sensitivity. Because of their fluctuating vision, these individuals usually respond well to electronic magnification, where contrast can be enhanced and magnification varied. Non-optical devices such as a glucose monitor and insulin-syringe aids are helpful to the patient.[59]

Glaucoma

DESCRIPTION

Glaucoma is a group of ocular diseases that cause an elevation of pressure in the eye (intra-ocular pressure) ultimately leading to progressive optic nerve damage and loss of peripheral visual function.

Figure 3-23 is an illustration of the front of the eye called the anterior chamber. The ciliary body is the structure that produces the fluid called aqueous fluid. This fluid is produced on a daily basis and flows to the front of the eye as illustrated in Figure 3-24. Because the eye is a closed structure, if new fluid is produced on a daily basis, an equal amount of fluid must drain out of the eye to maintain the proper intraocular pressure. Under normal conditions, the amount of aqueous fluid that is produced is equivalent to the amount that drains out on a daily basis, maintaining equilibrium and normal intraocular pressure. In glaucoma this equilibrium is disrupted. There are a number of reasons why a person may develop glaucoma, however, regardless of the cause, the ultimate problem is loss of this equilibrium causing a rise in intraocular pressure. When the intraocular pressure rises the nerve fibers exiting the eye through the optic nerve are compressed and damaged. The fibers that are generally affected in the beginning of the disease are those that carry information about our side vision (peripheral vision). Thus, in the initial stages of the disease,

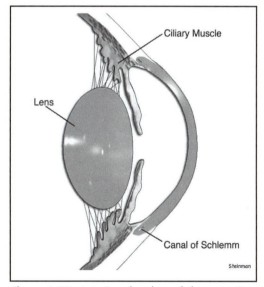

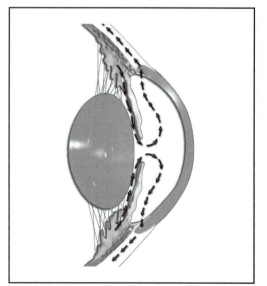

Figure 3-23. Anterior chamber of the eye. (Reprinted with permission from Scheiman M, Scheiman M, Whittaker SG. *Low Vision Rehabilitation: A Practical Guide for Occupational Therapists*. Thorofare, NJ: SLACK Incorporated; 2007.)

Figure 3-24. The ciliary body produces aqueous fluid that is produced on a daily basis and flows to the front of the eye. (Reprinted with permission from Scheiman M, Scheiman M, Whittaker SG. *Low Vision Rehabilitation: A Practical Guide for Occupational Therapists*. Thorofare, NJ: SLACK Incorporated; 2007.)

Figure 3-25. Peripheral visual field loss associated with glaucoma. (Reprinted with permission from Scheiman M, Scheiman M, Whittaker SG. *Low Vision Rehabilitation: A Practical Guide for Occupational Therapists*. Thorofare, NJ: SLACK Incorporated; 2007.)

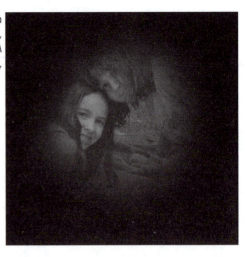

glaucoma leads to a gradual loss of peripheral vision. In most cases of glaucoma, the disease is painless because the rise in pressure is very gradual. As a result a person with glaucoma may be unaware of the problem until the loss of vision is advanced. Thus, routine eye examinations are important to rule out this disease and the best way to avoid the consequences of glaucoma.

RISK FACTORS

Age is a major risk factor for the development of glaucoma. The prevalence of glaucoma is 4 to 10 times higher in the older age groups than in persons in their 40s.[60,61] Race is another major risk factor for primary open angle glaucoma. African Americans develop the disease earlier, do not respond as well to treatment, are more likely to require surgery, and have a higher prevalence of blindness from glaucoma than Caucasians.[61] Finally, a family history of glaucoma is also a significant risk factor. Ocular factors include high intraocular pressure, thinness of the cornea, and abnormal optic nerve anatomy.

EFFECT ON VISION

Left uncorrected, glaucoma causes a reduction in visual field (Figure 3-25), which may progress to total blindness. Central vision is generally unaffected until the end stage of the disease.

TREATMENT

Treatment of glaucoma usually begins with medications (pills, ointments, or eyedrops) that help the eye either drain fluid more effectively or produce less fluid. Several forms of laser surgery can also help fluid drain from the eye.

Cataract

DESCRIPTION

A cataract is an opacification or clouding of the lens in the eye that affects vision. Cataracts are very common in older people and can occur in either or both eyes. Figure 3-26 is an illustration of a cataract.

RISK FACTORS

The main risk for developing cataracts is aging. By age 65 about half of all Americans have developed some degree of lens clouding, although it may not impair vision. Other significant factors are diabetes, a family history of cataracts, previous eye injury or inflammation, previous eye surgery, prolonged use of corticosteroids, excessive exposure to sunlight, and smoking.

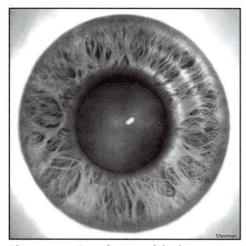

Figure 3-26. Opacification of the lens in cataract. (Reprinted with permission from Scheiman M, Scheiman M, Whittaker SG. *Low Vision Rehabilitation: A Practical Guide for Occupational Therapists*. Thorofare, NJ: SLACK Incorporated; 2007.)

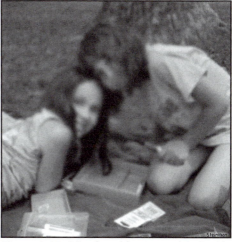

Figure 3-27. Visual problems associated with cataract. (Reprinted with permission from Scheiman M, Scheiman M, Whittaker SG. *Low Vision Rehabilitation: A Practical Guide for Occupational Therapists*. Thorofare, NJ: SLACK Incorporated; 2007.)

EFFECT ON VISION

A cataract usually develops slowly and causes no pain. As a result, most people are unaware of its development until it begins to interfere with everyday activities. Symptoms of a cataract include blurry vision, increasing difficulty with vision at night, sensitivity to light and glare, poor contrast sensitivity, halos around lights, the need for brighter light for reading and other activities, frequent changes in eyeglass or contact lens prescription, fading or yellowing of colors and double vision in a single eye. Figure 3-27 illustrates the effect of cataract on vision.

TREATMENT

The only effective treatment for a cataract is surgery to remove the clouded lens and replace it with a clear lens implant. The lens implant can correct refractive error as well. In some cases, one eye is corrected to focus at near and the other to focus at distance. Cataracts cannot be cured with medications, dietary supplements, exercise, or optical devices. However, in the early stages of cataract development the symptoms may be improved with new eyeglasses, brighter lighting, anti-glare sunglasses, or magnifying lenses. When these measures are no longer effective, surgery is necessary. Ophthalmologists treat cataract surgically when vision loss interferes with a person's activities such as working, driving, reading, or watching TV. Typically, if a person requires surgery on both eyes the surgery is performed on each eye at separate times, usually about 4 to 8 weeks apart.

Cataract removal is one of the most common, safest, and most effective types of surgery. Although cataract surgery is one of the most effective surgical procedures, there are potential risks including inflammation, infection, bleeding, swelling, retinal detachment, and glaucoma. Occasionally cataract surgery fails to improve vision because of conditions such as glaucoma or macular degeneration.

Visual Field Loss

The visual field is that portion of space where objects can be perceived while the individual is visually fixating on a single object in the straight ahead position. When looking straight ahead, the

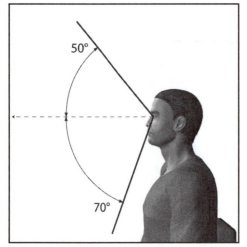

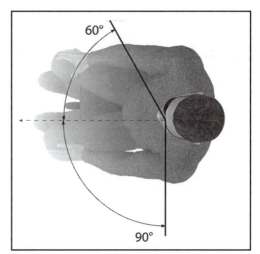

Figure 3-28. Vertical visual field is about 70 degrees in each eye. (Reprinted with permission from Scheiman M, Scheiman M, Whittaker SG. *Low Vision Rehabilitation: A Practical Guide for Occupational Therapists*. Thorofare, NJ: SLACK Incorporated; 2007.)

Figure 3-29. Horizontal visual field is about 150 degrees in each eye. (Reprinted with permission from Scheiman M, Scheiman M, Whittaker SG. *Low Vision Rehabilitation: A Practical Guide for Occupational Therapists*. Thorofare, NJ: SLACK Incorporated; 2007.)

normal visual field is 70 degrees vertically and 150 degrees horizontally with each eye individually (Figures 3-28 and 3-29). With both eyes open the vertically visual field remains the same while the horizontal visual field is now 180 degrees.

Visual field loss can occur after acquired brain injury that affects the visual pathway. This could be due to trauma, vascular causes, neoplasm, or it can occur secondary to surgical intervention for some other condition. Visual field disorders are among the most perplexing and difficult vision problems that therapists encounter. These problems affect mobility, reading, writing, activities of daily living, face recognition, and driving. The symptoms of visual field loss and its effect on performance are listed in Table 3-10.

As explained in Chapter Two, because of the anatomy of the visual pathway posterior to the optic chiasm (Figure 3-30), a common result is a complete or partial loss of sensitivity to one half of the visual field in each eye. This is referred to as a hemianopia meaning the patient is blind on one side of the visual field in both eyes. If the degree of loss of visual field is the same in both eyes it is referred to as a homonymous hemianopia. In some instances, a single quadrant is affected in which case it would be called a quadrantanopia.

Visual field loss is permanent and treatment is not designed to restore normal visual field. Rather treatment is designed to help the patient compensate for this permanent loss of vision.

Visual Inattention/Neglect

Visual inattention is a passive, diminished awareness of one side of field. It is generally not due to a localized lesion as in hemianopia. Often the cause unknown and visual inattention can be present along with a visual field defect, or it can be present alone. The presence of visual inattention has a significant effect on rehabilitation and activities of daily living. It may lead to deficits in localization of objects, scanning, fixation, orientation, eating, dressing, mobility, reading, and any other visually based activities of daily living.

Table 3-10

Visual Field Deficits: Symptoms and Effect on Function

- Walking: Inferior field loss causes difficulty with mobility, trouble seeing steps or curbs, shortened and uncertain stride when walking, poor balance, a tendency to trail behind others when walking, a tendency to walk next to wall and hold onto wall with hands, a tendency to be anchored to ground, and discomfort in the middle of a room. Patient does not turn head as much, frequently bumps into things, and is disoriented when moving whether in car or walking
- Trouble identifying visual landmarks
- Superior field deficit causes difficulty seeing signs, worse if in wheelchair
- Leaves food on half of plate
- Misidentification of details, misreading of long words
- Difficulty with reading, misreads words, reads inaccurately, reads slowly, has difficulty with page navigation, cannot stay on line
- Difficulty with writing, cannot stay on line, inaccurate
- Self-grooming: Cannot find necessary items
- Dressing: Cannot find necessary items
- Telephone: Cannot take accurate messages
- Driving: Cannot drive usually
- Shopping: Cannot drive; cannot find items
- Emotional problems: Anxiety, reduced self-confidence, increased passivity, social isolation

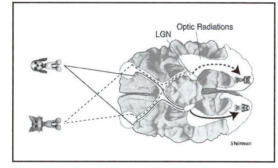

Figure 3-30. Anatomy of the visual pathway posterior to the optic chiasm. (Reprinted with permission from Scheiman M, Scheiman M, Whittaker SG. *Low Vision Rehabilitation: A Practical Guide for Occupational Therapists.* Thorofare, NJ: SLACK Incorporated; 2007.)

Cortical Visual Impairment

Cortical visual impairment is the leading cause of bilateral low vision in children. *Cortical visual impairment* replaces the term *cortical blindness* and is caused by a lesion in posterior visual pathways. This damage may be due to perinatal hypoxia-ischemia, infections (meningitis, encephalitis), or hydrocephalus. The diagnosis is based on physical findings, history, and neuroimaging. The majority of people with cortical visual impairment have some residual vision.

CHARACTERISTICS OF CORTICAL VISUAL IMPAIRMENT

Patients with cortical visual impairment may exhibit signs such as markedly short attention span, variable visual skills, frequent head turning when reaching for objects, close working distance, compulsive light gazing, photophobia (sensitivity to light), and eye pressing/poking.

PROGNOSIS IN CORTICAL VISUAL IMPAIRMENT

With early intervention some patients with cortical visual impairment may show improvement in visual skills.

Summary

Disorders of visual acuity, refraction, and eye disease are commonly diagnosed and treated by all eye doctors. Unfortunately, in many cases, an eye examination only includes an evaluation designed to detect these conditions. As the following two chapters will demonstrate, there are many more significant vision problems that must be considered.

References

1. Dobson V, MacDonald MA, Kohl P, et al. Visual acuity screening of infants and young children with the acuity card procedure. *J Am Optom Assoc.* 1986;57:284-289.
2. Mayer DL, Fulton AB, Rodier D. Grating and recognition acuities of pediatric patients. *Ophthalmology.* 1984;91:947.
3. Birch EE, Naegele J, Bauer JA, et al. Visual acuity of toddlers tested by operant preferential looking techniques. *Invest Ophthalmol Vis Sci.* 1980;20(Suppl):210.
4. Marg E, Freeman DN, Peltzman P, Goldstein PJ. Visual acuity development in human infants: evoked potential measurements. *Inv Ophthalmol.* 1976;15:150-153.
5. Sokol S. Measurement of infant visual acuity from pattern reversal evoked potentials. *Vision Res.* 1978;18:33-39.
6. Gwiazda J, Brill S, Mohindra I, Held R. Infant visual acuity and its meridional variation. *Vision Res.* 1978;18:1557-1564.
7. Dobson V, Teller DY. Visual acuity in human infants: a review and comparison of behavioral and electrophysiological studies. *Vision Res.* 1978;18:1469-1483.
8. Birch EE, Gwiazda J, Bauer JA, Naegele J, Held R. Visual acuity and its meridional variation in children aged 7-60 months. *Vision Res.* 1983;23:1019-1024.
9. Haegerstrom-Portnoy G, Schneck ME, Lott LA, Brabyn JA. The relation between visual acuity and other spatial vision measures. *Optom Vis Sci.* 2000;77:653-662.
10. Whittaker SG, Lovie-Kitchin J. Visual requirements for reading. *Optom Vis Sci.* 1993;70(1):54-65.
11. Marron JA, Bailey IL. Visual factors and orientation: mobility performance. *Am J Optom Physiol Opt.* 1982;59:413-426.
12. Kuyk T, Elliott JL. Visual correlates of mobility in real world settings in older adults with low vision. *Optom Vis Sci.* 1998;75:538-547.
13. Wood JM. Elderly drivers and simulated visual impairment. *Optom Vis Sci.* 1995;72:115-124.
14. Owsley C, Sloane ME. Contrast sensitivity, acuity, and the perception of "real-world" targets. *Br J Ophthalmol.* 1987;71:791-796.
15. West SK, Rubin GS, Broman AT, Munoz B, Bandeen-Roche K, Turano K. How does visual impairment affect performance on tasks of everyday life? The SEE Project. Salisbury Eye Evaluation. *Arch Ophthalmol.* 2002;120(6):774-780.
16. Rubin GS, Bandeen-Roche K, Prasada-Rao P, Fried. LP. Visual impairment and disability in older adults. *Optom Vis Sci.* 1994;71(12):750-760.
17. Arditi A. Improving the design of the letter contrast sensitivity test. *Invest Ophthalmol Vis Sci.* 2005;46:2225-2229.
18. Pelli DG, Robson JG, Wilkins AJ, The design of a new letter contrast chart for measuring contrast sensitivity. *Clin Vis Sci.* 1988;2:187-199.
19. Ciner EB, Appel S, Graboyes M, Zambone AM. Low vision special populations I: the multiply impaired patient. In: Appel S, Brilliant R, eds. *Essentials of Low Vision Practice.* Boston, MA: Butterworth-Heinemann; 1999.
20. Skeffington AM. *Introduction to Clinical Optometry.* Santa Ana, CA: Optometric Extension Program Foundation, Optometric Extension Program Postgraduate Courses. Vol 37, Oct. 1964-Sept 1965.
21. Birnbaum MH. *Optometric Management of Nearpoint Vision Disorders.* Boston, MA: Butterworth-Heinemann; 1993.
22. Goss DA. Effectiveness of bifocal control of childhood myopia progression as a function of near point phoria and binocular cross-cylinder. *J Opt Vision Dev.* 1995;26:12-17.
23. Gwiazda J, Hyman L, Hussein M, et al. A randomized clinical trial of progressive addition lenses versus single vision lenses on the progression of myopia in children. *Invest Ophthalmol Vis Sci.* 2003;44:1492-1500.
24. Gwiazda J, Hyman L, Norton T, et al and the COMET Group. Accommodation and related risk factors associated with myopia progression and their interaction with treatment in COMET children. *Invest Ophthalmol Vis Sci.* 2004;45:2143-2151.
25. Scheiman M and the COMET Group. PALs for children: can they slow myopia. *Rev Optom.* 2008;79:55-59.
26. Ciner EB. Management of refractive error in infants, toddlers, and preschool children. In: Scheiman M, ed. *Pediatric Optometry.* Philadelphia, PA: JB Lippincott; 1990.

27. Gwiazda J, Scheiman M, Mohindra I, Held R. Astigmatism in children: changes in axis and amount from birth to five years. *Invest Ophthalmol Vis Sci.* 1984;25:88-92.

28. Mohindra I, Held R, Gwiazda J, Brill S. Astigmatism in infants. *Science.* 1978;202:329-330.

29. Dobson V, Fulton AB, Sebris SL. Cycloplegic refraction of infants and young children. The axis of astigmatism. *Invest Ophthalmol Vis Sci.* 1984;25:83-87.

30. Mohindra I, Held R. Refraction in humans from birth to five years. *Doc Ophthalmol Proc Ser.* 1981;28:19-27.

31. Ingram RM, Barr A. Changes in refraction between the ages of one and three-and-a-half. *Br J Ophthalmol.* 1979;63:339-342.

32. Baldwin WR. Refractive status of infants and children. In: Rosenbloom AA, Morgan MW, eds. *Principles and Practice of Pediatric Optometry.* Philadelphia, PA: JB Lippincott; 1990:104-112.

33. Gianutsos R, Ramsey G, Perlin RR. Rehabilitative optometric services for survivors of acquired brain injury. *Arch Phys Med Rehabil.* 1988;69:573-578.

34. Zost MG. Diagnosis and management of visual dysfunction in cerebral injury. In: Maino D, ed. *Diagnosis and Management of Special Populations.* St. Louis, MO: CV Mosby; 1995.

35. Scheiman M. Assessment and management of the exceptional child. In: Rosenbloom AA, Morgan MW, eds. *Pediatric Optometry.* Philadelphia, PA: JB Lippincott; 1990:388-419.

36. Poe GS. Eye care visits and use of eyeglasses or contact lenses: United States 1979 and 1980. In: *Vital Health Statistics.* Hyattsville, MD: Department of Health and Human Services; 1984. Publication PHS 84-1573. Series 10, No. 45.

37. Bader D, Woodruff ME. The effects of corrective lenses on various behaviors of mentally retarded persons. *Am J Optom Physiol Opt.* 1980;57:447-459.

38. Rosner J, Rosner J. Comparison of visual characteristics in children with and without learning difficulties. *Am J Optom Physiol Opt.* 1987;64:531-533.

39. Young FA. Reading, measures of intelligence and refractive errors. *American Journal of Optometry and Archives of the American Academy of Optometry.* 1963;49:257-264.

40. Eames TH. The influence of hypermetropia and myopia on reading achievement. *Am J Ophthalmol.* 1955;39:375-377.

41. Larson JS. The sagittal growth of the eye. IV. Ultrasonic measurement of the axial length of the eye from birth to puberty. *Acta Ophthalmol.* 1971;49:872-878.

42. Boothe RG, Dobson V, Teller DY. Postnatal development of vision in human and nonhuman primates. *Ann Rev Neurosci.* 1985;8:495-503.

43. Maggon EH, Robb RM. Development of myelin in human optic nerve and tract. *Arch Ophthalmol.* 1981;99:655-661.

44. Beauchamp R. Normal development of the neural pathways. In: Rosenbloom AA, Morgan MW, eds. *Pediatric Optometry.* Philadelphia, PA: JB Lippincott; 1990:46-65.

45. Klein R, Klein BEK, Linton K. Prevalence of age-related maculopathy. The Beaver Dam Study. *Ophthalmology.* 1992;99:933-943.

46. Hyman LG, Lilienfeld AM, Ferris FL 3rd, Fine SL. Senile macular degeneration: a case control study. *Am J Epidemiol.* 1983;118:213-227.

47. Murphy RP. Age-related macular degeneration. *Ophthalmology.* 1986;93:969-971.

48. Ferris FLI, Fine SL, Hyman LA. Age-related macular degeneration and blindness due to neovascular maculopathy. *Arch Ophthalmol.* 1984;102:1640-1642.

49. Fine AM, Elman MJ, Ebert JE, Prestia PA, Starr JS, Fine SL. Earliest symptoms caused by neovascular membranes in the macula. *Arch Ophthalmol.* 1986;104:513-514.

50. Hirvela H, Luukinen H, Laara E, et al. Risk factors of age-related maculopathy in a population 70 years of age or older. *Ophthalmology.* 1996;103(6):871-877.

51. Klaver CC, Wolfs RC, Assink JJ, van Duijn CM, Hofman A, de Jong PT. Genetic risk of age-related maculopathy. *Arch Ophthalmol.* 1998;116:1646-1651.

52. Klein R, Klein BE, Franke T. The relationship of cardiovascular disease and its risk factors to age-related maculopathy. The Beaver Dam Eye Study. *Ophthalmology.* 1993;100(3):406-414.

53. Newsome D. Medical treatment of macular diseases. *Ophthalmol Clin North Am.* 1993;6:307-314.

54. Cho E, Hung S, Willett WC, et al. Prospective study of dietary fat and the risk of age-related macular degeneration. *Am J Clin Nutr.* 2001;73(2):209-218.

55. Seddon JM, Cote J, Rosner B. Progression of age-related macular degeneration: association with dietary fat, transunsaturated fat, nuts, and fish intake. *Arch Ophthalmol.* 2003;121(12):1728-1737.

56. Seddon JM, Rosner B, Sperduto RD, et al. Dietary fat and risk for advanced age-related macular degeneration. *Arch Ophthalmol.* 2001;119(8): 1191-1199.

57. Age-Related Eye Disease Study Research Group. A randomized, placebo-controlled, clinical trial of high-dose supplementation with vitamins C and E, beta carotene, and zinc for age-related macular degeneration and vision loss: AREDS report no. 8. *Arch Ophthalmol.* 2001;119(10):1417-1436.

58. Azab M, Benchaboune M, Blinder KJ, et al. Verteporfin therapy of subfoveal choroidal neovascularization in age-related macular degeneration: meta-analysis of 2-year safety results in three randomized clinical trials: treatment of age-related macular degeneration with photodynamic therapy and verteporfin in photodynamic therapy study report no. 4. *Retina*. 2004;24(1):1-12.

59. Scheiman M, Scheiman M, Whittaker SG. *Low Vision Rehabilitation: A Practical Guide for Occupational Therapists*. Thorofare, NJ: SLACK Incorporated; 2007.

60. Hollows FC, Graham PA. Intraocular pressure, glaucoma, and glaucoma suspects in a defined population. *Br J Ophthalmol*. 1966;50:570-586.

61. Tielsch JM, Sommer A, Katz J, Royall RM, Quigley HA, Javitt J. Racial variations in the prevalence of primary open-angle glaucoma. The Baltimore Eye Survey. *JAMA*. 1991;266:369-374.

Chapter Four

Three Component Model of Vision, Part Two:
Visual Efficiency Skills

Mitchell Scheiman, OD, FCOVD, FAAO

Visual Efficiency Skills

Definition and Classification of Visual Efficiency Disorders

Visual efficiency refers to the effectiveness of the visual system to clearly, efficiently, and comfortably allow an individual to gather visual information at school, work, or play. The various component skills that are important in this process are called visual efficiency skills and include the subcategories of accommodation, binocular vision, and ocular motility. Table 4-1 illustrates a classification system of visual efficiency disorders.

Accommodation Disorders

Definition and Description

Assuming that any refractive error has been corrected with eyeglasses, the normal human visual system is physiologically focused for objects at distances of 20 feet and greater. If an object is brought closer than 20 feet, a focusing adjustment must be made or the object will appear blurred. This focusing adjustment is referred to as accommodation. Accommodation is the ability to change the focus of the eye so that objects at different distances can be seen clearly. The accommodative system of the human eye generally works so well that most people are totally unaware that they even have a focusing system until about the age of 40 to 45 when there is a natural decline in accommodative ability that begins to cause blurred vision when reading.

Accommodation occurs by stimulating the smooth muscle of the ciliary body in the eye to contract, thereby enabling the lens to change its shape. Figure 4-1a is a cross-section of the human eye showing the lens and the ciliary muscle in its relaxed state. The light rays entering the eye are focused behind the retina, which would cause blurred vision. In Figure 4-1b, the ciliary muscle has contracted and allows the light rays to focus on the retina.

Scheiman M
Understanding and Managing Vision Deficits: A Guide for
Occupational Therapists, Third Edition (pp 57-78)
© 2011 SLACK Incorporated

Table 4-1

Classification of Visual Efficiency Disorders

Accommodative Disorders

- Accommodative insufficiency
- Accommodative excess
- Accommodative infacility
- Presbyopia

Binocular Vision Disorders

STRABISMIC BINOCULAR VISION DISORDERS

- Esotropia
- Exotropia
- Hypertropia
- Noncomitant strabismus

NONSTRABISMIC BINOCULAR VISION DISORDERS

- Esophoria
- Exophoria
- Hyperphoria

Amblyopia

- Strabismic amblyopia
- Anisometropic amblyopia
- Isometropic amblyopia
- Stimulus deprivation amblyopia
- Hysterical amblyopia

Ocular Motility Disorders

- Saccadic dysfunction
- Pursuit dysfunction
- Disorders of fixation (nystagmus)

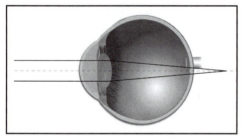

Figure 4-1a. A cross-section of the human eye showing the lens and the ciliary muscle in its relaxed state with the light rays focused behind the retina. (Reprinted with permission from Scheiman M, Scheiman M, Whittaker SG. *Low Vision Rehabilitation: A Practical Guide for Occupational Therapists*. Thorofare, NJ: SLACK Incorporated; 2007.)

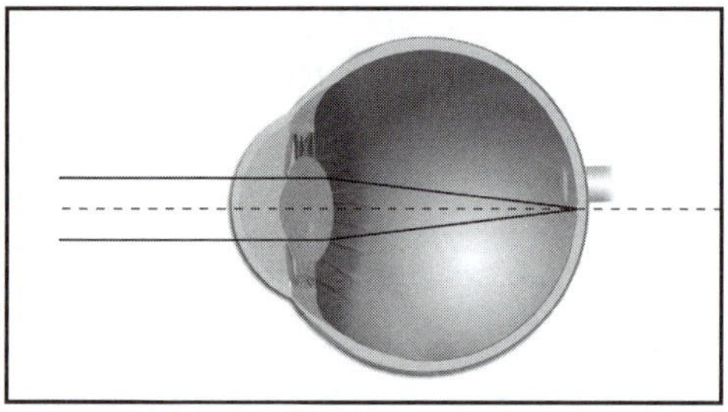

Figure 4-1b. The ciliary muscle has contracted and allows the light rays to focus on the retina. (Reprinted with permission from Scheiman M, Scheiman M, Whittaker SG. *Low Vision Rehabilitation: A Practical Guide for Occupational Therapists*. Thorofare, NJ: SLACK Incorporated; 2007.)

A blurred image on the fovea of the eye is the stimulus for accommodation and initiates a signal that is received at area 17 of the occipital cortex and continues to area 19. This acts as a stimulus for motor signals that will cause contraction of the ciliary muscle. The projection from area 19 to the midbrain complex is not well established. The actual innervation of the ciliary muscle is carried in the autonomic fibers of the third cranial nerve. These are axons of neurons originating in the Edinger-Westphal nuclei of the oculomotor complex. During accommodation, not only does the lens focus, but the pupil constricts as well. Both of these actions are mediated by parasympathetic components of the third cranial nerve.

The accommodative ability of an individual is inversely related to age. We use the term *accommodative amplitude* to refer to the total amount of accommodation available for a particular patient. Young children have very large amplitudes of accommodation, and this declines with age. This relationship between age and accommodative amplitude is so consistent across the population that it is possible for an optometrist to predict a patient's age within several years simply by measuring the amplitude of accommodation. The accommodative amplitude declines gradually with age, and by 40 to 45 years of age, the decline is significant enough to interfere with the ability to see small print held at reading distance. This is why most people begin wearing reading glasses or bifocals once they reach about 40 to 45 years of age. This is referred to as presbyopia and is described later in the chapter.

Clinically, we are not only interested in the amount of accommodation available, but also in the facility and sustaining ability of the accommodative response. This is called accommodative facility. Facility testing is designed to assess a number of key factors. The first is referred to as the latency of the accommodative response and refers to the amount of time it takes for the accommodative system to begin to respond once a stimulus is presented. The second factor is the velocity of the response or how fast the system can fully accommodate to the demand presented. The final factor assessed during accommodative facility testing is the ability to change accommodation over time or sustaining ability. The reason for the interest in accommodative facility is that studies have shown that there is a significant relationship between patient symptoms and problems with accommodative facility.

Accommodative disorders are commonly encountered in the general population. A recent study found that approximately 6% of children between 6 and 18 years old had clinically significant accommodative problems.[1] Accommodative problems are more common in physically, mentally, and developmentally delayed children, learning disabled children and adults, and children who have had cerebrovascular accident or traumatic brain injury. The presence and nature of accommodative problems in these populations are discussed in detail in Chapters Eight, Nine, and Eleven.

Classification of Accommodative Disorders

There are four primary types of accommodative disorders (see Table 4-1).[1] Accommodative insufficiency is a condition in which the amount of accommodation available (amplitude of accommodation) is less than expected for the individual's age. The result is that when a child attempts to accommodate when reading, for example, he or she experiences intermittent blurred vision. In an attempt to regain clear vision, the child exerts extra effort to stimulate additional accommodation. This effort may lead to the signs and symptoms listed in Table 4-2.

Presbyopia is a condition in which near visual acuity is decreased because of an age-related decline in accommodative ability. There is a universal decline in the amplitude of accommodation with age. For instance, at 10 years of age, the normal amplitude of accommodation is about 20 D. This declines to 10 D at age 20, 7 D by age 30, and 4 to 5 D by age 40. As accommodative ability declines with age, it eventually becomes difficult to read and perform other close work. This is the reason why most adults need to use reading glasses or bifocals at around 40 to 45 years of age. All adults after the age of 45 or so have the condition called presbyopia and require reading glasses or some modification of their eyeglasses to account for this condition. Both presbyopia and accommodative insufficiency are problems in which the amplitude of accommodation is reduced, but presbyopia is an age-related disorder with an onset around 40 to 45 years of age, whereas accommodative insufficiency generally affects children and young adults. The signs and symptoms of presbyopia are identical to those of accommodative insufficiency.

Another common accommodative disorder is called accommodative excess. This is a condition in which the amplitude of accommodation is normal, but the ciliary muscle has a tendency to spasm. Typically, the problem is intermittent and variable. The individual may report that after

Table 4-2

Accommodative Disorders: Symptoms and Effects on Performance

Accommodative Infacility

These symptoms are generally related to the use of the eyes for reading or other near tasks:
- Blurred vision particularly when looking from near to far or far to near
- Headaches
- Eyestrain
- Reading problems
- Fatigue and sleepiness
- Loss of comprehension over time
- A pulling sensation around the eyes
- Movement of the print
- Avoidance of reading and other close work
- Difficulty with activities of daily living that require sustained close work

Accommodative Insufficiency and Presbyopia

These symptoms are generally related to the use of the eyes for reading or other near tasks:
- Blurred vision
- Headaches
- Eyestrain
- Reading problems
- Fatigue and sleepiness
- Loss of comprehension over time
- A pulling sensation around the eyes
- Movement of the print
- Avoidance of reading and other close work
- Difficulty with activities of daily living that require sustained close work

Accommodative Excess

These symptoms are generally related to the use of the eyes for reading or other near tasks:
- Blurred vision, worse after reading or other close work
- Headaches
- Eyestrain
- Difficulty focusing from far to near
- Sensitivity to light
- Difficulty with activities of daily living that require sustained close work

reading for a period of time, he or she experiences blurred vision when looking at a distant object. He or she may also experience some of the other symptoms listed in Table 4-2.

The fourth accommodative problem is called accommodative infacility. This is a condition in which the amplitude of accommodation is normal, but the speed of the response is reduced. The most common complaint associated with accommodative facility is blurred vision when looking from near to far or far to near.

Clinical Assessment

While accommodative testing is routinely performed by most eye care professionals, there is a great deal of variability in the extent of testing performed from one doctor to another. The test performed by most eye doctors is measurement of the amplitude of accommodation. This is a very simple and quick test to perform and is described in Chapter Six as one of the standard screening tests for occupational therapists. Evaluation of accommodative amplitude can generally be performed from about 2 to 3 years of age. The unit of measure used for accommodative amplitude is the diopter (D). A natural decline in the amplitude of accommodation occurs with age.

Too many eye doctors limit their evaluation of accommodation to this one measure. However, of the four accommodative disorders described previously, only accommodative insufficiency and presbyopia can be detected using accommodative amplitude testing alone. The other two conditions cannot be diagnosed unless additional testing is performed. Two additional tests are very important to enable the doctor to adequately evaluate accommodation.

To evaluate accommodative speed and sustaining ability, optometrists perform a test called accommodative facility testing. The test probes the individual's ability to change accommodation rapidly and for a sustained period of time. It is considered a key test, is very sensitive to mild to moderate accommodative problems, and is the only method of detecting the condition called accommodative infacility.

Another important method of evaluating accommodation is called near point retinoscopy. Using an instrument called the retinoscope, the clinician is able to objectively evaluate the accommodative system. This test allows us to determine how accurately the patient accommodates and is an important test for detecting the condition called accommodative excess.

Development of Accommodation

Accommodation is very poorly developed at birth. Newborns are unable to accommodate, and their focus appears to be set at about 30 cm from their eyes. Like visual acuity, however, there is a very rapid development, and by 6 months of age, accommodation appears to reach adult levels.[2]

As described above, an interesting fact about accommodation is the natural and expected decline that occurs with age. At about the age of 40 to 45 years, accommodation has declined to the point that reading becomes difficult and uncomfortable. This condition is called presbyopia. By the age of about 65 years, accommodation is virtually absent, and we become dependent on eyeglasses to help us focus.

Significance of Accommodative Disorders for Occupational Therapy

Table 4-2 lists the symptoms of accommodative problems. Accommodative disorders will interfere whenever an occupational therapist asks a patient to engage in an activity that requires visual concentration on small objects or print at a close distance.

Binocular Vision Disorders

Definition and Description

The human visual system works so well and reliably that most people take it for granted that when we look at the world with two eyes, we receive one single impression of the external world. When a problem is encountered, however, it becomes apparent that the system that allows single vision to occur is very elaborate, requiring a delicate balance of neural and muscular processes. Binocular vision is the ability of the visual system to fuse or combine the information from the right and left eyes into one image. Visual information that enters the right and left eyes remains monocular as it passes from the optic nerve through the chiasm, the optic tract, the lateral geniculate body, and the optic radiation. At the level of the visual cortex (area 17), the information finally reaches cortical cells capable of binocular processing.

For binocular vision to occur, the information arriving from each eye must be identical and approximately equal in clarity and size. To satisfy these requirements, the two eyes must be aligned so that they point at the same object at all times, and the optics or refractive error of the two eyes must be approximately equal. Problems with either alignment or refractive equality will cause binocular vision disorders. The hallmark symptom of a binocular vision disorder is double vision (diplopia).

When the two eyes actually lose alignment, it is referred to as strabismus. When strabismus occurs and the eyes either drift in, out, up, or down, each eye views a different part of the environment and sends different information to the visual cortex. The result is the perception of diplopia. Because diplopia is intolerable, the visual system attempts to eliminate the problem through one of two mechanisms: by trying to overcome the problem and restore normal alignment using muscular effort or by adapting to the misalignment of the eyes. In some cases, the tendency for the eye to turn can be overcome with muscular effort. In such cases, patients often successfully eliminate double vision and experience binocular vision, but may be uncomfortable. They report eyestrain, headaches, the inability to sustain attention for long periods of time, intermittent blurred vision, and occasional diplopia. The other option is to allow the eye to turn but to eliminate diplopia by either ignoring the information coming from the eye that turns (suppression) or by altering the neurophysiology of the eye (anomalous correspondence). Until the age of about 6 years, the human visual system has been shown to have an extraordinary plasticity and ability to adapt to strabismus. Age affects adaptation; generally, younger children adapt more quickly than older children and adults. It is also more likely to occur if the eye turn is a constant, rather than an intermittent, problem.

The human visual system has two modes of adaptation. The first is called suppression and, in such cases, the information entering the eye that turns is ignored at the cortical level. Suppression eliminates diplopia, but as a result of this adaptation, normal visual development does not occur, leading to a loss of vision called amblyopia. The second mode of adaptation demonstrates the high level of plasticity of the human visual system during the sensitive period and is called anomalous correspondence. Under normal conditions, similar anatomical points on each retina correspond neurophysiologically with the retina of the fellow eye (Figure 4-2). When these two "corresponding" retinal points are stimulated, the brain experiences single vision. The visual system is born with this normal correspondence between similar points on the retinas of the two eyes. As long as visual experience is normal, this correspondence remains stable throughout life. However, if strabismus occurs during the first 5 to 6 years of life, resulting in diplopia, the visual system must make a choice to overcome the eye turn with muscular effort or to allow the eye turn to exist and to try to adapt to it. The second possible adaptation is for the normal correspondence to be altered. In such cases, the neurophysiology of the visual system makes an adjustment to the new alignment of the eyes, and the corresponding points of the two retinas are altered to allow single vision to occur in spite of the strabismus. This is called anomalous correspondence and only occurs if the eye turn develops early, is small to moderate in size, is stable and constant, and is present for a long period of time.

If the individual overcomes the eye turn by adapting either with suppression or anomalous correspondence, the strabismus becomes more difficult to eliminate with treatment, and additional problems such as loss of vision in the eye that turns (amblyopia) and several other significant secondary conditions may occur.

If a strabismus develops after the age of 6 years or so, the option of adaptation is no longer viable. The age of 6 is an approximation, and there is certainly individual variation in the end of the period of visual plasticity. The important concept, however, is that the visual system is incapable of adapting to a strabismus that develops in older children or adults. Thus, late-onset strabismus will generally result in either constant or intermittent double vision. This is the reason why adults experiencing strabismus after traumatic head injury will have double vision.

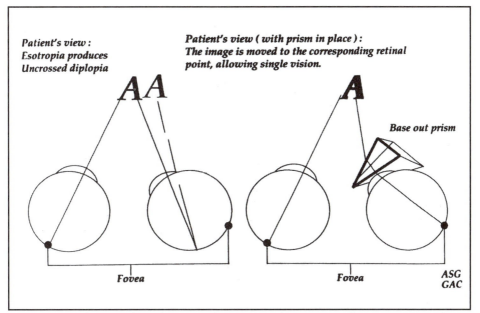

Figure 4-2. Under normal conditions, similar anatomical points on each retina correspond neurophysiologically with the retina of the fellow eye. In this figure, the corresponding points illustrated are the foveas of the two eyes.

Prevalence of Binocular Vision Disorders

Other than refractive error, the most common vision problems encountered in clinical practice are binocular vision disorders. In a study of a clinical pediatric population, Scheiman et al[3] found that about 25% of children from 6 months to 18 years old had significant binocular vision disorders. Similar prevalence data have been found in adult populations.[4] Binocular vision problems are more common in physically, mentally, and developmentally delayed children; learning disabled children; and adults who have had a cerebrovascular accident or traumatic brain injury.[5-9] These studies have shown that convergence insufficiency (a binocular vision problem) is the most common vision disorder after acquired brain injury on both the civilian population[5,6] and soldiers returning from the wars in Iraq and Afghanistan.[7-9]

Classification of Binocular Vision Disorders

There are two main types of binocular vision disorders: strabismic and nonstrabismic binocular disorders (Tables 4-3 and 4-4).

STRABISMUS

Strabismus is a condition in which the eyes are misaligned. It occurs in about 3% to 5% of the general population and is often very obvious cosmetically. Other terms used to describe strabismus include *heterotropia*, *tropia*, *squint*, *cross-eyed*, and *wall-eyed*. Strabismus can also be categorized based on four characteristics:

1. Direction: Whether the eyes turn in, out, or up.
2. Frequency: The percentage of time the eye is misaligned.
3. Laterality: Whether one eye always turns or if the two eyes alternate.
4. Comitancy: Whether the magnitude of the eye turn is the same in all positions of gaze.

Table 4-3

Classification of Strabismic Binocular Vision Disorders

Direction

- Esotropia: Eyes turn in
- Exotropia: Eyes turn out
- Hypertropia: One eye turns up

Each of these conditions are also classified based on the following characteristics.

Frequency

- Intermittent esotropia or constant esotropia
- Intermittent exotropia or constant exotropia
- Intermittent hypertropia or constant hypertropia

Laterality

- Right esotropia, left esotropia, or alternating esotropia
- Right exotropia, left exotropia, or alternating exotropia
- Right hypertropia, left hypertropia, or alternating hypertropia

Comitancy

- Comitant or noncomitant esotropia
- Comitant or noncomitant exotropia
- Comitant or noncomitant hypertropia

Table 4-4

Classification of Nonstrabismic Binocular Vision Disorders

Direction

- Esophoria: Eyes have a tendency to turn in
- Exophoria: Eyes have a tendency to turn out
- Hyperphoria: One eye has a tendency to turn up
- Nonstrabismic binocular vision disorders can also be classified based on the relationship between the magnitude of the phoria at distance and the magnitude of the phoria at near.

Distance to Near Relationship

- Magnitude equal at distance and near: Basic esophoria
  Basic exophoria
- Magnitude greater at distance: Divergence excess (exophoria)
  Divergence insufficiency (esophoria)
- Magnitude greater at near: Convergence insufficiency (exophoria)
  Convergence excess (esophoria)

Direction

The three most common types of strabismus are esotropia (eyes turn in), exotropia (eyes turn out), and hypertropia (one eye turns up). Combinations of these are possible and often occur. For example, the right eye could turn up and out or down and in. The direction of the strabismus has some significance in terms of prognosis for treatment using different treatment modalities. For example, the prognosis for the treatment of exotropia using vision therapy is good to excellent, while with esotropia it is only fair.

Frequency

Strabismus can be classified according to the percentage of time it is present. Strabismus present 100% of the time is called constant strabismus, while strabismus present less than 100% of the time is referred to as intermittent strabismus. This characteristic has very significant clinical implications. If the strabismus is intermittent, it means that binocular vision is still present at least some of the time. Rehabilitation using vision therapy is considerably easier and more effective if binocular vision has been present even part of the time. The prognosis, therefore, is excellent for elimination of an intermittent strabismus using vision therapy. If the strabismus is constant and has been present for a long period of time, normal binocular vision will be absent, and adaptations such as suppression and anomalous correspondence, described above, may have developed. These adaptations make it considerably more difficult to restore normal binocular vision and reduce the prognosis for vision therapy.

Laterality

Another important characteristic is called laterality and refers to whether the same eye always turns or whether the two eyes alternately turn. A strabismus in which the right or left turns all of the time is called a unilateral strabismus. If the right eye and left eye turn alternately, it is called an alternating strabismus. The laterality of the strabismus also has significant clinical implications. A unilateral, constant strabismus will generally cause the development of amblyopia or loss of vision in the eye that turns. If the strabismus is alternating, amblyopia does not develop, and the visual acuity remains normal in each eye because each eye continues to receive normal stimulation.

Comitancy

Figure 4-3 illustrates the nine positions of gaze that are generally tested in a clinical evaluation. A strabismus is referred to as comitant if the size of the strabismus remains relatively constant in all nine positions of gaze. It is important to understand that comitancy testing takes place at a constant

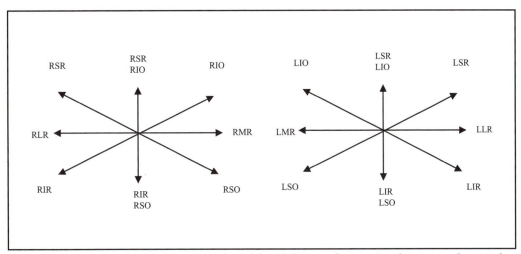

Figure 4-3. Positions of gaze that are evaluated by clinicians when testing the extraocular muscles. (RSR=right superior rectus, RLR=right lateral rectus, RIR=right inferior rectus, RSO=right superior oblique, RMR=right medial rectus, RIO=right inferior oblique, LSR=left superior rectus, LLR=left lateral rectus, LIR=left inferior rectus, LSO=left superior oblique, LMR=left medial rectus, LIO=left inferior oblique.)

working distance from the patient. For example, a clinician measures the size of the strabismus in the nine positions of gaze at 40 cm or at 6 m. The size of the strabismus is not compared from one distance to another, only from one position of gaze to another at the same distance. Thus, if the strabismus is 20 prism D (prism D is the unit of measurement for strabismus) at 6 m and 60 prism D at 40 cm, this is not an indication of noncomitancy. However, if the strabismus is 20 prism D in right gaze and 60 prism D in left gaze, with both measurements taken at 40 cm from the patient, the strabismus is noncomitant. The three most common causes of adult-onset noncomitant strabismus are trauma, vascular problems, and neoplasm. In children, the three most common causes are congenital, trauma, and acute viral infection.[10] Occupational therapists frequently encounter noncomitant strabismus in patients with traumatic brain injury and stroke.

NONSTRABISMIC BINOCULAR VISION DISORDERS

Remember that strabismus is a condition in which the eyes are actually misaligned at least 1% of the time. If the eyes have a tendency to turn in, out, or up but this tendency is controlled at all times, the deviation is categorized as a nonstrabismic binocular vision disorder. Other frequently used terms to describe this condition are *heterophoria* and *phoria*. The tendency for the eyes to misalign in cases of heterophoria can vary from very slight to very large. In fact, in the average person, a slight tendency for the eyes to drift outward is expected. We become concerned about heterophoria when the tendency becomes moderate to large and, in addition, the patient's ability to compensate is inadequate. For example, if the individual's eyes have a tendency to drift out, we are clinically interested in his or her ability to converge or pull the eyes in. If the ability to converge is not sufficient to comfortably control the tendency for the eyes to drift outward, symptoms occur.

The most common method of categorizing heterophoria is by direction of the deviation. The three most common types of heterophoria according to this classification are exophoria (the eyes have a tendency to turn out), esophoria (the eyes have a tendency to turn in), and hyperphoria (one eye has a tendency to turn up).

Another popular way of classifying nonstrabismic binocular vision disorders is by comparing the size of the problem at 6 m to the size of the disorder at 40 cm. This system only applies to esophoria or exophoria, not hyperphoria. The phoria may be equal at distance and at near, or the problem may be greater at near than at distance or greater at distance than at near. This leads to six different possibilities listed in Table 4-4. The two most common types of heterophoria according to this classification system are convergence insufficiency and convergence excess.

Convergence insufficiency is probably the most common nonstrabismic binocular vision disorder that occupational therapists will encounter. It is a condition in which the eyes have a tendency to drift outward when being used for near work such as reading, while at a far distance the eyes work well together. This is one of the leading causes of eyestrain and discomfort. In the general population, convergence insufficiency is present in about 5% of the population, while in the populations managed by occupational therapists the prevalence is considerably greater. Convergence insufficiency is one of the most common vision problems that occurs after cerebrovascular accident or traumatic brain injury in both civilian[5,6,11-15] and military populations.[7-9]

Convergence excess also affects close vision, but in this case the eyes have a tendency to turn inward rather than outward. Again, if the patient can control this tendency all of the time, the problem is called a phoria. Convergence excess has been found to be slightly more prevalent than convergence insufficiency in a clinical population.

Clinical Assessment of Binocular Disorders

The clinical assessment of binocular vision is divided into two major areas: the motor fusion evaluation and the sensory fusion evaluation. In reference to the visual system, the term *fusion* is used to refer to the process of uniting the information received from the two eyes into one single image. The neural and muscular mechanism that brings the eyes into alignment on the object of

Table 4-5

Tests Used to Evaluate Motor and Sensory Fusion

Motor Fusion Testing

- Cover test
- Near point of convergence
- Comitancy testing
- Fusional vergence amplitude testing
- Fusional vergence facility testing

Sensory Fusion Testing

- Stereopsis testing
- Suppression testing (Worth 4 Dot)
- Anomalous correspondence testing (Bagolini Striated Lenses, After Image Test)

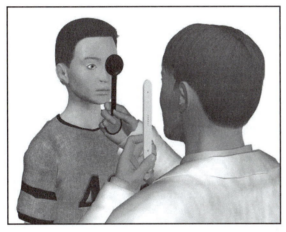

Figure 4-4. The cover test using a plastic cover paddle and a fixation target.

interest is called motor fusion, while the activity within the cerebral cortex that allows a single perception to be achieved is called sensory fusion.[16]

MOTOR FUSION EVALUATION

Several tests are used to evaluate the neural and muscular mechanism that brings the eyes into alignment on the object of interest. While the equipment used for this part of the evaluation is simple and inexpensive, advanced clinical skills and significant clinical experience are required to interpret the patient's responses. At least the five tests listed in Table 4-5 must be performed to properly assess motor fusion. Many clinicians consider the cover test to be the most important test in this group. This test is illustrated in Figure 4-4 and involves the use of a plastic cover paddle and a fixation target. Using this simple equipment, the clinician is able to determine many key binocular vision characteristics, including the magnitude, direction, frequency, laterality, and comitancy of the deviation. The cover test is an objective test and can, therefore, be effectively used with patients of any age including infants and patients who are nonverbal, mentally disabled, and autistic.

A test that many occupational therapists may already be aware of is the measurement of the near point of convergence. This procedure is illustrated in Figure 4-5 and only requires the use of a small penlight target. This test probes the ability of the individual to converge the eyes and to maintain their alignment as an object is brought closer and closer to the eyes. This is one of the key tests used to reach the diagnosis of convergence insufficiency. The normal response is to be able to

Figure 4-5. Measurement of the near point of convergence using a small penlight target.

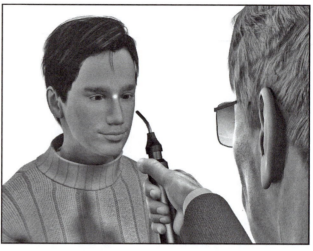

converge to about 2 to 4 inches from the eyes. This test is part of the vision screening described in detail in Chapter Six.

Comitancy is evaluated by asking the patient to follow a light as it is moved in the nine diagnostic positions of gaze illustrated in Figure 4-3. The clinician observes the relationship of the eyes as in the various positions of gaze. Ruling out a noncomitant strabismus is a critical part of the examination because such a condition may suggest a serious underlying etiology for the binocular vision disorder.

The final two critical tests are used to assess the ability of the patient to compensate for the strabismus or heterophoria that is present. This characteristic is called fusional vergence, and the testing is referred to as fusional vergence testing. As a general rule, if the problem is an esodeviation (the eyes tend to turn in), clinicians are most interested in the ability of the patient to diverge or move the eyes outward, whereas if the problem is an exodeviation, clinicians are most interested in the ability of the patient to converge or move the eyes inward. Again, very simple equipment is required as illustrated in Figure 4-6. Two measurements are important: the fusional vergence amplitude and fusional vergence facility. This is comparable to the assessment of accommodation in which we are also interested in both amplitude and facility.

While some binocular vision testing is routinely performed by most eye care professionals, there is a great deal of variability in the extent of testing performed from one doctor to another. If an occupational therapist is looking to develop a referral relationship with an optometrist, it is critical to determine the type and extent of the evaluation he or she performs. An incomplete evaluation will often result in a lack of identification of important binocular vision problems. Table 4-5 can be used by occupational therapists to evaluate the type of testing performed by the optometrist.

Sensory Fusion Evaluation

The evaluation of the activity within the cerebral cortex that allows a single perception to be achieved is called sensory fusion. The tests listed in Table 4-5 are often performed to assess this function. While the evaluation of motor fusion requires advanced clinical training to properly interpret patient responses, the same is not true of all aspects of the evaluation of sensory fusion. In addition, good sensory fusion is one indication of adequate motor fusion. These two points have great significance for professionals who want to perform a visual screening. Because sensory fusion is dependent on motor fusion and because some of this type of testing is rather easy to interpret, it becomes an ideal screening test for the evaluation of binocular vision. It is

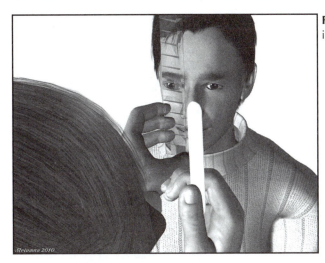

Figure 4-6. Fusional vergence testing using a prism bar.

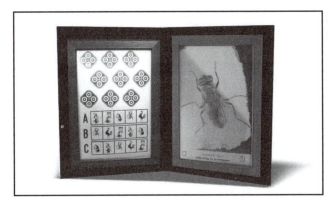

Figure 4-7a. Stereopsis testing equipment (Stereofly Test).

important to understand, however, that it is possible to have normal sensory fusion and still have a significant binocular vision disorder. For example, sensory fusion testing may be very close to normal in cases of significant heterophoria.

A very popular probe of sensory fusion is stereopsis testing. Several different tests are illustrated in Figures 4-7a and 4-7b. These tests are inexpensive, simple to administer, and easy to interpret, making them excellent screening tests. Stereopsis testing will be described in detail in Chapter Six.

Other tests are used to probe for suppression (Worth 4 Dot) and anomalous correspondence (Bagolini Striated Lenses, After Image Test).

Development of Binocular Vision

Although the neurophysiology for binocular vision is present at birth, it is not fully developed and requires normal stimulation for proper development to occur. For the first month of life, alignment of the eyes may be variable with occasional strabismus occurring. By 1 month, however, alignment should be normal. Strabismus occurring after the age of 1 month is considered to be a problem. Stereopsis (3-D vision) is the ability to appreciate depth based on binocular input. It is one of the most important clinical indications of normal binocular vision. Stereopsis can be measured in very young infants, and researchers have found that it is absent at birth but reaches adult levels by about 16 to 20 weeks of age.[17]

Figure 4-7b. Stereopsis testing equipment (Randot Stereo Test). (Reprinted with permission from Scheiman M, Scheiman M, Whittaker SG. *Low Vision Rehabilitation: A Practical Guide for Occupational Therapists*. Thorofare, NJ: SLACK Incorporated; 2007.)

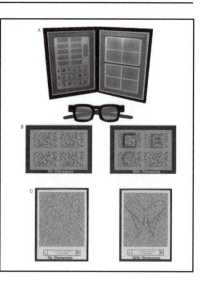

Significance of Binocular Vision Disorders for Occupational Therapy

Table 4-6 provides a summary of the significance of binocular vision disorders for occupational therapy. If we consider strabismus to be the most extreme or severe binocular vision problem and heterophoria to be the least severe, an interesting phenomenon becomes apparent. The most significant symptoms related to binocular vision problems are associated with the least severe binocular vision problems. Strabismus is the most severe binocular vision problem, yet it has the fewest and least significant symptoms associated with it in all populations except for the traumatic brain injury/cerebrovascular accident population. Heterophoria, which is the least severe binocular vision problem, at least from a standpoint of neurophysiology and cosmetic appearance, may be associated with the most severe symptoms. This is because children develop adaptations to long-standing, early-onset strabismus that eliminate all bothersome symptoms. Adults who have experienced traumatic brain injury or cerebrovascular accident and have developed strabismus as a result cannot make these adaptations and are, therefore, frequently bothered by symptoms associated with strabismus and heterophoria.

A common misconception that I often hear as an optometrist is concern on the part of a referring occupational therapist that the presence of a very obvious strabismus must be affecting a child's performance and ability to learn. A strabismus may be very apparent to the observer who sees a very obvious crossed eye, for example. The adaptations that occur after the onset of strabismus, however, eliminate any symptoms and any impact on performance or learning. This does not mean that the child should not be referred if a strabismus is present. A referral is certainly appropriate in such cases. However, the concern is related to the negative effects of the strabismus on the development of the visual system and not to performance or learning. In many cases, children with strabismus may also have a number of other vision anomalies that do have a negative effect on performance and function, such as ocular motility and accommodative and visual perceptual problems.

Nonstrabismic binocular vision problems, which are the less severe form of binocular vision disorder, are related to the most significant symptoms. Because patients can overcome a phoria using neuromuscular effort, the eyes never appear misaligned in such cases. Thus, the child's visual cosmetic appearance is normal. The neuromuscular effort required to overcome the phoria, however, causes a host of symptoms that can have a very severe impact on function and performance.

> **Table 4-6**
>
> ## Binocular Vision Disorders: Symptoms and Effect on Performance
>
> *Strabismic*
> - Cosmetic problem, the eyes look crossed or "wall-eyed"
> - If intermittent, may cause double vision that can interfere with eye-hand and mobility tasks
> - If intermittent, may cause eyestrain
> - Loss of vision if left untreated and the strabismus is unilateral
>
> *Nonstrabismic*
> These symptoms are generally related to the use of the eyes for reading or other near tasks:
> - Blurred vision
> - Headaches
> - Eyestrain
> - Reading problems
> - Fatigue and sleepiness
> - Loss of comprehension over time
> - A pulling sensation around the eyes
> - Movement of the print
> - Avoidance of reading and other close work
> - Difficulty with activities of daily living that require stereopsis (driving, near tasks involving reaching for objects, pouring liquids)

Amblyopia

Definition and Description

Amblyopia is a condition in which the visual acuity is less than 20/20, and this loss of visual acuity cannot be attributed to refractive error or observable eye disease. This means that even after prescribing the best possible eyeglasses, the patient has reduced vision in one or both eyes. Amblyopia is not an optical problem, rather it is a neurophysiological problem in which the visual pathway from the eye to the visual cortex does not develop normally or deteriorates due to some type of interference during the sensitive period.

Most people are familiar with amblyopia, which is commonly called "lazy eye" by the public. The term *lazy eye* is a misnomer and does not really describe the condition well. The eye is not lazy; it simply has not received proper stimulation for one of several reasons described next. The classic treatment is use of an eye patch to force the child to use the weaker eye.

Classification of Amblyopia

The classifications of amblyopia are listed in Table 4-1. The most common type of amblyopia is caused by refractive error problems. There are two types of refractive error problems that can cause amblyopia. The most common of these is called anisometropic amblyopia. This problem, which is described in Chapter Three, is a condition in which the prescription in one eye is considerably stronger than the prescription in the fellow eye. The inequality in vision and size of the images in the two eyes creates difficulty for the visual cortex in its attempt to fuse the two images. Because the two images are incompatible, the brain cannot fuse them and tends to ignore the input from the eye with the more significant refractive error. If this occurs before 5 to 6 years of age or so, visual development does not proceed normally. The result is reduced visual acuity, which we call amblyopia.

Another refractive disorder that can lead to the development of amblyopia is called isometropic amblyopia. This is a condition in which there is a very high refractive error in both eyes. For example, both eyes may have a very high degree of astigmatism, hyperopia, or myopia. If left uncorrected during the first 5 to 6 years of life, amblyopia can occur.

Another common form of amblyopia is caused by strabismus. If one eye always turns in, out, or up and the problem begins during the first 5 to 6 years of life, amblyopia will occur. When one eye turns at all times during the sensitive period of development, the child will initially experience double vision because of the misalignment of the eyes. Because double vision is intolerable, the child's visual system will make one or more adaptations to eliminate this double vision. These adaptations are generally successful in eliminating the double vision. However, they lead to deterioration or lack of development of visual acuity.

Two other forms of amblyopia are considerably less common. The first is called stimulus deprivation amblyopia and occurs when a very young infant has a problem, such as a congenital cataract or some type of corneal scar, that interferes with the ability of visual information to enter one eye. The second unusual form is called hysterical amblyopia. This type of amblyopia is caused by emotional factors, and there are no actual physical or physiological changes. Generally, patients with this type of amblyopia present with poor vision, and the eye doctor is unable to find a cause during the examination. Often in such cases, the child is under a great deal of emotional stress because of personal or family problems.

Clinical Assessment

Amblyopia is detected during the course of any traditional eye examination using visual acuity testing. The cause of the amblyopia must then be determined using tests designed to evaluate refraction, binocular vision, and eye health.

Significance of Amblyopia for Occupational Therapy

Unless the amblyopia is present in both eyes, the condition has little significance for occupational therapists. If the visual acuity is reduced in one eye, the other eye still sees well, and the patient generally does not experience any functional deficits.

Ocular Motility Disorders

Definition and Description

We use the term *ocular motility disorders* to refer to eye movement problems in any one or more of the following areas: fixation, saccades, and pursuits (see Table 4-1). Other terms used to describe ocular motility disorders are *eye movement disorders*, *tracking problems*, and *visual scanning problems*. Visual scanning is particularly popular in the rehabilitation and occupational therapy literature. Warren[18] stresses the importance of identifying visual scanning deficits in adults after acquired brain injury. She defines visual scanning as one of the primary means by which the central nervous system obtains visual information from the environment and describes scanning as a function that involves both eye movements and fixation. The optometric literature, on the other hand, stresses the three component model of eye movements, and authors generally refer to disorders of fixation, saccades, and pursuits.[1]

Eye movement disorders are an important diagnostic and management concern because of the effect such problems may have on the functional capability of an individual. Much of the emphasis of both researchers and clinicians has been on the relationship between eye movements and reading. During reading, the three important components of eye movements are saccades, fixations, and regressions. Saccades take up approximately 10% of the reading time. The average saccade is about eight to nine character spaces.[19] The duration of the saccade is a function of the distance covered. For instance, a 2 degree saccade takes about 25 to 30 msec, and a 5 degree saccade takes about 35 to 40 msec.[19] Between saccades, the eye is relatively still in a fixational pause. For normal readers, the average duration of the fixation is 200 to 250 msec. The third important characteristic of reading eye movements is the regression. A regression is a right to left movement and occurs 10% to 20% of the time in skilled readers. Regressions occur when the reader overshoots the target, misinterprets the text, or has difficulty understanding the text.

Because eye movement deficiencies intuitively seem to be so closely linked with reading, numerous studies have investigated this relationship. Two basic viewpoints have evolved about the relationship between eye movements and reading. The first suggests that eye movement disorders can cause below-average reading ability.[20-29] Investigators using a variety of methods to assess eye movements have found that poor readers tend to make more fixations and regressions than normal readers. The second position is that the random and unskilled eye movement skills observed with poor readers are secondary to deficient language skills that cause reading disorders. Thus, the reading difficulty itself leads to erratic and inconsistent eye movements.[30-34] A third perspective is probably most likely to be correct and is essentially a combination of the first two viewpoints. This alternative suggests that, in some cases, problems with fixation and saccadic abilities may be a primary interference in a patient's ability to read quickly, comfortably, and with adequate comprehension.[35] In other cases, the eye movement deficiencies observed during reading may simply be a reflection of poor reading ability.

Another important background issue is that during reading, eye movements are integrated with higher cognitive processes including attention, memory, and the utilization of the perceived visual information.[36-38] Some optometrists believe that there is a relationship between poor ocular motor skills and attention problems.[39-41] When such a relationship exists, treatment of eye movement disorders may lead to improvement in attention and concentration.

Eye movement problems have also been reported to be one of the more common and problematic vision problems secondary to acquired brain injury.[18,42-45] Problems with saccades after head trauma can interfere with occupational therapy. Warren[18] suggests that visual scanning deficits contribute to the failure of some adults to regain independence in many daily activities including self-care, reading, arithmetic, and driving. Strano[46] also describes the importance of saccades for driving and suggests that abnormal saccades greatly affect quick and accurate fixation on a target in the periphery and ability to return to the traffic ahead.

There have been several studies of the prevalence of eye movement disorders in children with learning and reading disabilities. In a sample of 50 children with learning disabilities between the ages of 6 and 13 years old, Sherman[47] found that 96% had problems with ocular motor inefficiency (saccadic and pursuit problems). Hoffman[48] reported on a larger sample of 107 children with learning problems. The children's ages ranged from 5 to 14 years old. His results revealed that 95% of the sample had ocular motor problems. It is interesting to note that both Sherman and Hoffman found that ocular motor dysfunction was the most prevalent vision disorder in their samples of learning disabled children.

In my experience, and in the studies described above, eye movement disorders are rarely present in isolation. Rather, they are generally found associated with accommodative, binocular, and visual information processing dysfunctions. As a result, treatment of eye movement deficiencies should not occur in isolation, instead such treatment should take place within the context of an overall treatment approach designed to deal with other problems as well.

Classification of Ocular Motility Disorders

Ocular motility disorders can be divided into three distinct areas: fixation stability, saccadic function, and pursuit function. Ocular motility disorders can reflect serious underlying central nervous system disease or functional/developmental problems. It is always important to consider the possibility that abnormalities in fixation stability, saccades, and pursuits may require additional consultation.

Assessment of fixation is an important part of the routine examination. An individual with inadequate fixation ability may look away from the task more often than other children. This "off-task" behavior may give the impression that the person is inattentive or impulsive. Asking the patient to fixate on a target during the initial evaluation is sufficient to evaluate fixation status. All patients, except the very young, anxious, hyperactive, or inattentive, should be able to sustain precise fixation with no observable movement of the eyes for 10 seconds.[49,50] A variety of disorders of fixation can occur and may represent organic or functional anomalies. A very significant disorder of fixation commonly seen by occupational therapists is nystagmus.

Nystagmus is a condition in which there are involuntary, rhythmic oscillations of one or both eyes. It may be a sensory problem due to very poor visual acuity or a disorder of ocular motor control. Nystagmus can be thought of as a disorder of the mechanisms that keep fixation stable. The pursuit, optokinetic, and vestibular systems act to maintain a steady image on the retina. Any lesion that creates an imbalance in these neurological systems can cause nystagmus by making the eyes drift off target. Nystagmus affects about one in every 5000 to 10,000 people. It is much more prevalent in patients who have certain ocular and/or systemic health conditions. For example, a large percentage of people with cerebral palsy have nystagmus, and approximately 10% to 15% of visually impaired school-age children have nystagmus. Nystagmus will be discussed in detail in Chapter Eleven.

Saccadic dysfunction is a condition in which the accuracy and speed of saccadic eye movements are reduced relative to expected findings for the individual's age. Saccades are eye movements that enable us to rapidly redirect our line of sight so that the point of interest stimulates the fovea. Saccades are the fastest eye movement with velocities as high as 700 degrees per second.[51] The ideal saccade is a single eye movement that rapidly reaches and abruptly stops at the target of interest. Saccades may be inaccurate, however, in two ways. The most common inaccuracy is a slight undershoot. In most cases, the saccade is slightly short of the target, and the eye "glides" to alignment but, in more extreme cases, a second, smaller saccade is made to reach the target. A less common inaccuracy is an overshoot of the target.

Saccadic fixation problems can lead to the signs and symptoms listed in Table 4-7. Problems with fixation and saccadic abilities may be a primary factor interfering with a child's ability to read quickly, comfortably, and with adequate comprehension. As described above, there may be a relationship between poor saccadic ability and attention problems. Saccadic problems have also been reported to be one of the more common and problematic vision problems secondary to acquired brain injury.

Pursuit dysfunction is a condition in which the individual is unable to accurately follow a moving object. Pursuit eye movements enable continuous clear vision of moving objects. This visual following reflex ideally produces eye movements that ensure continuous foveal fixation of objects moving in space. Pursuit movements are affected by age, attention, and motivation. Because pursuit eye movements are only involved when a target is moving, they are more difficult to relate to reading and school performance than saccades. However, pursuits may play a more significant role in other activities of daily living, such as driving and sports, and any other activities in which the individual is moving or the object of regard is moving.

Clinical Assessment

Examination of eye movements involves three distinct steps: Assessment of stability of fixation, saccadic function, and pursuit function. To evaluate fixation stability, we simply ask the patient to fixate on a target during the initial evaluation. All patients, except the very young,

---

Table 4-7

Ocular Motility Disorders: Symptoms and Effect on Performance

- Excessive head movement
- Frequent loss of place
- Skips lines
- Poor attention span
- Copying is slow and coloring and drawing results are poor
- Difficulty with activities of daily living that require frequent change in fixation and accurate eye movements (driving, reading, writing)

---

anxious, hyperactive, or inattentive, should be able to sustain precise fixation with no observable movement of the eyes for 10 seconds.

The purpose of saccadic testing is to assess the quality and accuracy of saccadic function. A variety of assessment procedures have been developed to evaluate saccades. Tests may involve direct observation by the clinician, timed or standardized tests involving a visual-verbal format, and objective eye movement recording using electro-oculographic instruments. There are problems associated with all of these methods, however. Electro-oculographic procedures are expensive, time consuming, and difficult to use with young elementary school children and patients with cognitive or attention problems. Subjective techniques involving observation of the patient's eye movements have been developed along with rating scales. These rating scales are highly subjective, and inexperienced clinicians may have difficulty learning to effectively use them. A study by Maples and Ficklin[52] did show that the rating scale used in their study was reliable and repeatable. An important advantage of subjective rating scales is that they can be used with some of the more challenging populations managed by occupational therapists. This method of evaluating eye movement can be used with nonverbal, intellectually challenged, autistic, and low functioning adults after acquired brain injury.

Direct observation tests require the subject to look from one object to another while the clinician observes the patient's saccades. Several rating scales have been developed to create better uniformity in observation. One of these rating scales is described in detail in Chapter Six.

Another alternative is the use of tests using a visual-verbal format. These tests are inexpensive, easily administered, and provide a quantitative evaluation of eye movements in a simulated reading environment.[53] They assess ocular motor function on the basis of the speed in which a series of numbers can be seen, recognized, and verbalized with accuracy. The most popular test of this type is the Developmental Eye Movement (DEM) test. This test requires the subject to be functioning at a 6-year-old level at least.

The second method described above is the use of timed and standardized tests. The most widely used test today is the DEM test. The patient is asked to call off a series of numbers as quickly as possible without using a finger or pointer as a guide. The response times and number of errors are then compared to tables of expecteds. This test is also described in detail in Chapter Six.

The third approach to the assessment of saccades is objective eye movement recording. Currently, the clinical device available for this purpose is the Visagraph ([Figure 4-8] Stockholm, Sweden). This system consists of a computer unit and goggles. Objective eye movement recording has several advantages over direct observation and timed or standardized tests. The Visagraph system provides a permanent recording of the evaluation, is an objective procedure, and does not depend on the skill of the examiner. The information gained from objective recording is also more sophisticated. It provides information about number of fixations, regressions, duration of fixations, reading rate, relative efficiency, and grade equivalence. All of this information can be compared to established norms for elementary school children through adulthood. The disadvantage of the

Figure 4-8. The Visagraph used for objective eye movement recording.

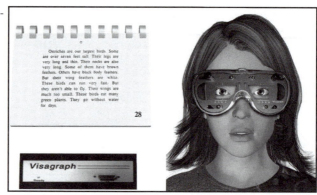

Visagraph is the expense of the instrument. It is also difficult to use with patients who are inattentive or hyperactive or who have poor fixation. Most clinicians use a combination of direct observation using rating scales like those described in Chapter Six along with the DEM test.

The purpose of pursuit testing is to assess the quality and accuracy of pursuit function. There are not as many testing alternatives for pursuits as there are for saccades. Direct observation of the patient following a moving target is the most commonly used clinical technique. Several rating scales have been developed for direct observation of pursuit movements. We suggest using the one described in Chapter Six.

Development of Ocular Motility

Unlike visual acuity, accommodative, and binocular vision skills that reach adult levels of development very early in infancy, clinical assessment indicates that eye movement development is considerably slower, continuing through the early elementary school years.[54,55] Because of the long developmental process for eye movement control, slow development can leave a child with inadequate skills to meet the demands of the classroom.

Significance of Ocular Motility Disorders for Occupational Therapy

Table 4-7 provides a summary of the symptoms of ocular motility disorders and their effect on performance. Problems with fixation and saccadic abilities may be a primary factor interfering with a patient's ability to read quickly, comfortably, and with adequate comprehension. There may be a relationship between poor saccadic ability and attention problems. Eye movement disorders may even interfere with the ability of the patient to perform well during vision information processing testing. Pursuit problems may play a significant role in activities of daily living such as driving and sports and any other activities in which the individual is moving or the object of regard is moving.

Summary

Visual efficiency problems are highly prevalent in the populations served by occupational therapists. The possible effects on a patient's performance are very significant, and if left uncorrected, visual efficiency problems will interfere with progress in occupational therapy. In spite of the significance of visual efficiency problems, they are often undetected even after a professional eye examination. If these problems are suspected, it is incumbent upon occupational therapists to make a referral to an eye care professional who will perform the type of testing battery that can detect these disorders.

References

1. Scheiman M, Wick B. *Clinical Management of Binocular Vision*. 3rd ed. Philadelphia, PA: JB Lippincott; 2008.
2. Brookman KE. Ocular accommodation in human infants. *Am J Optom Physiol Opt*. 1980;60:91-95.
3. Scheiman M, Gallaway M, Ciner EB, et al. Prevalence of vision disorders in a pediatric population. *J Am Optom Assoc*. 1996;67:193-202.
4. Hokoda SC. General binocular dysfunctions in an urban optometry clinic. *J Am Optom Assoc*. 1985;56:560-562.
5. Suchoff IB, Kapoor N, Waxman R, Ference W. The occurrence of ocular and visual dysfunctions in an acquired brain-injured patient sample. *J Am Optom Assoc*. 1999;70:301-308.
6. Ciuffreda KJ, Kapoor N, Rutner D, et al. Occurrence of oculomotor dysfunctions in acquired brain injury: a retrospective analysis. *Optometry*. 2007;78:155-161.
7. Goodrich GL, Kirby J, Cockerham G, Ingalla SP, Lew HL. Visual function in patients of a polytrauma rehabilitation center: a descriptive study. *J Rehab Res Dev*. 2007;44:929-936.
8. Brahm KD, Wilgenburg HM, Kirby J, Ingalla S, Chang CY, Goodrich GK. Visual impairment and dysfunction in combat-injured servicemembers with traumatic brain injury. *Optom Vis Sci*. 2009;86:817-825.
9. Stelmack JA, Frith T, Van Koevering D, Stelmack TR. Visual function in patients followed at a Veterans Affairs polytrauma network site: an electronic medical record review. *Optometry*. 2009;80:419-424.
10. Caloroso E, Rouse MW. *Clinical Management of Strabismus*. Santa Ana, CA: Optometric Extension Program Foundation; 1993.
11. Krohel GB, Kristan RW, Simon JW, Barrows NA. Post-traumatic convergence insufficiency. *Ann Ophthalmol*. 1986;18:101-104.
12. Pratt-Johnson JA, Tillson G. Acquired central disruption of fusional amplitude. *Ophthalmology*. 1979;86:2140-2142.
13. Padula WV, Shapiro JB, Jasin P. Head injury causing post trauma vision syndrome. *N Engl J Optom*. 1988;Dec/Winter:16-21.
14. Harrison RJ. Loss of fusional vergence with partial loss of accommodative convergence and accommodation following head injury. *Bin Vis*. 1987;2:93-100.
15. Cohen M, Groswasser Z, Barchadski R, Appel A. Convergence insufficiency in brain injured patients. *Brain Inj*. 1989;3:187-191.
16. Solomons H. *Binocular Vision. A Programmed Text*. London: Heinemann; 1978.
17. Birch EE, Gwiazda J, Held R. Stereoacuity development for crossed and uncrossed disparities in human infants. *Vision Res*. 1982;22:507-510.
18. Warren M. Identification of visual scanning deficits in adults after cerebrovascular accident. *Am J Occup Ther*. 1990;44:391-399.
19. Rayner K. Eye movements in reading and information processing. *Psych Bull*. 1978;85:618-660.
20. Zangwill OL, Blakemore C. Dyslexia. Reversal of eye movements during reading. *Neuropsychologica*. 1972;10:371-373.
21. Rubino CA, Minden H. An analysis of eye movements in children with a reading disability. *Cortex*. 1973;9:217-220.
22. Griffin DC. Saccades as related to reading disorders. *J Learn Disab*. 1974;7:50-58.
23. Goldrich SG, Sedgwick H. An objective comparison of oculomotor functioning in reading disabled and normal children. *Am J Optom Physiol Opt*. 1982;59:82P.
24. Raymond JE, Ogden NA, Fagan JE, et al. Fixational stability in dyslexic children. *Am J Optom Physiol Opt*. 1982;65:174-179.
25. Jones A, Stark L. Abnormal patterns of normal eye movements in specific dyslexia. In: Rayner K, ed. *Eye Movements in Reading. Perceptual and Language Processes*. New York, NY: Academic Press; 1983:481-498.
26. Pavlidis GT. Eye movement differences between dyslexics, normal, and retarded readers while sequentially fixating digits. *Am J Optom Physiol Opt*. 1985;62:820-832.
27. Pavlidis GT. Eye movements in dyslexia. Diagnostic significance. *J Learn Disabil*. 1985;18:42.
28. Flax N. Problems in relating visual function to reading disorder. *American Journal of Optometry and Archives of American Academy of Optometry*. 1970;47:366-372.
29. Ludlam WM, Twarowski C, Ludlam DP. Optometric visual training for reading disability: a case report. *Am J Optom Arch Am Acad Optom*. 1973;50:58-66.
30. Heath EJ, Cook P, O'Dell N. Eye exercises and reading efficiency. *Acad Therapy*. 1976;11:435-445.
31. Pierce JR. Is there a relationship between vision therapy and academic achievement? *Rev Optom*. 1977;114:48-63.
32. Getz D. Learning enhancement through vision therapy. *Acad Therapy*. 1980;15(4):457-466.
33. Adler-Grinberg D, Stark L. Eye movements, scanpaths, and dyslexia. *Am J Optom Physiol Opt*. 1978;55:557-570.
34. Brown B, Haegerstrom-Portney G, Adams A, et al. Predictive eye movements do not discriminate between dyslexic and control children. *Neuropsychologica*. 1983;21:121-128.

35. Olson RK, Kliegl R, Davidson BJ. Dyslexic and normal readers eye movements. *J Exp Psych (Hum Percept)*. 1983;5:816-825.

36. Stanley G, Smith GA, Howell EA. Eye movements and sequential tracking in dyslexic and control children. *Br J Psych*. 1983;74:181-187.

37. Black JL, Collins DWK, DeRoach JN, Zubrick SR. Dyslexia: a detailed study of sequential eye movements for normal and poor reading children. *Percept Mot Skills*. 1983;59:423-434.

38. Grisham D, Simons H. Perspectives on reading disabilities. In: Rosenbloom AA, Morgan MW, eds. *Principles and Practice of Pediatric Optometry*. Philadelphia, PA: JB Lippincott; 1990:518-559.

39. Garzia RP, Richman JE, Nicholson SB, Gaines CS. A new visual-verbal saccade test: the Developmental Eye Movement test (DEM). *J Am Optom Assoc*. 1990;61:124-135.

40. Richman JE. Use of a sustained visual attention task to determine children at risk for learning problems. *J Am Optom Assoc*. 1986;57:20-27.

41. Simon MJ. Use of a vigilance task to determine school readiness in preschool children. *Percept Mot Skills*. 1982;54:1020-1022.

42. Warren M. A hierarchical model for evaluation and treatment of visual perceptual dysfunction in adult acquired brain injury. *Am J Occup Ther*. 1993;47:42-54.

43. Schlageter K, Gray B, Hall K, et al. Incidence and treatment of visual dysfunction in traumatic brain injury. *Brain Inj*. 1993;7:439-448.

44. Bouska MJ, Gallaway M. Primary visual deficits in adults with brain damage: management in occupational therapy. *Occup Ther Pract*. 1991;3:1-11.

45. Baker RS, Epstein AD. Ocular motor abnormalities from head trauma. *Surv Ophthalmol*. 1991;35:245-267.

46. Strano CM. Effects of visual deficits on ability to drive in traumatically brain injured population. *J Head Trauma Rehabil*. 1989;4:35-43.

47. Sherman A. Relating vision disorders to learning disability. *J Am Optom Assoc*. 1973;4:140-141.

48. Hoffman LG. Incidence of vision difficulties in children with learning disabilities. *J Am Optom Assoc*. 1980;51:447-451.

49. Higgins JD. Oculomotor system. In: Barresi BJ, ed. *Ocular Assessment*. Boston, MA: Butterworth; 1984:208.

50. Grisham D, Simons H. Perspectives on reading disabilities. In: Rosenbloom AA, Morgan MW, eds. *Pediatric Optometry*. Philadelphia, PA: JB Lippincott; 1990:518-559.

51. Leigh RJ, Zee DS. *The Neurology of Eye Movement*. Philadelphia, PA: FA Davis Co; 1983.

52. Maples WC, Ficklin TW. Interrater and test-retest reliability of pursuits and saccades. *J Am Optom Assoc*. 1988;59:549-552.

53. Richman JE, Walker AJ, Garzia RP. The impact of automatic digit naming ability on a clinical test of eye movement functioning. *J Am Optom Assoc*. 1983;54:617-622.

54. Borish IM. *Clinical Refraction*. 3rd ed. Chicago, IL: Professional Press; 1970.

55. Rouse R. Clinical examination in children. In: Rosenbloom AA, Morgan MW, eds. *Pediatric Optometry*. Philadelphia, PA: JB Lippincott; 1990.

Chapter Five

Three Component Model of Vision, Part Three:
Visual Information Processing Skills

Mitchell Scheiman, OD, FCOVD, FAAO

Visual Information Processing Skills

Visual information processing, or visual perception, is an area in which both occupational therapy and optometry are actively involved. The goal of this chapter, therefore, is not to teach occupational therapists how to evaluate visual information processing skills. Most occupational therapists already evaluate and treat such problems. Rather, this chapter is designed to help the occupational therapist better understand the way optometrists think about and evaluate visual information processing skills. I believe that most occupational therapists will recognize some differences as well as similarities between the approach presented in this chapter and their own clinical practice. As we learn more about these differences and similarities, we will be able to work together more effectively for the benefit of our patients.

Definition and General Concepts

A vision problem could still be present even if an individual has good visual acuity; no refractive error or eye health disorder; and normal accommodation, binocular vision, and ocular motility. Vision is more than just seeing clearly and comfortably. An individual must also be able to analyze, interpret, and make use of the incoming visual information in order to interact with the environment. We refer to this final aspect of our three-part model as visual information processing. Visual information processing refers to a group of visual cognitive skills used for extracting and organizing visual information from the environment and integrating this information with other sensory modalities and higher cognitive functions.[1] Other terms such as *visual perception*, *visual perceptual-motor*, and *visual processing* have been used to describe similar skills.

Visual processing involves the ability to extract and select information from the environment. So much information reaches the visual system that a selection process must occur. The person must select the incoming information that is most relevant to the task he or she is performing. This selection is dependent on prior experience and development.[2] Once information is extracted or selected from the environment, meaning has to be attached to the visual stimuli. This process involves a complex interaction between visual processing and cognitive factors that are influenced by past experiences, motivation, and development.[1] In the model presented in this chapter, perception and cognition are considered overlapping concepts that influence each other in the processing of visual information and are not seen as distinct entities. Essentially, perception provides visual cognitive information that is used in higher-order cognitive functions. As a result, the term *visual information processing* is used to describe the visual processing skills evaluated by optometrists.[1]

The model presented in this book is based on an approach recommended by Scheiman and Rouse.[3] This model divides visual information processing into three components: visual spatial, visual analysis, and visual motor. Each of these components relates to specific skills an individual could perform.

Visual Spatial Skills: Definition and Description

These skills allow the individual to develop normal internal and external spatial concepts and are used to interact with and organize the environment. They allow the individual to make judgments about location of objects in visual space in reference to other objects and to the individual's own body. Visual spatial skills develop from an awareness within the individual's body of concepts such as left and right, up and down, and front and back. Visual spatial skills are important for the development of good motor coordination, balance, and directional senses when reading and writing. Component skills include bilateral integration, laterality, and directionality.

Bilateral Integration

Bilateral integration is the ability to be aware of and use both sides of the body separately and simultaneously.

Laterality

Laterality is the ability to be internally aware of and identify right and left on one's self.

Directionality

Directionality is the ability of the individual to interpret right and left directions in three separate components of external space.

Visual Analysis Skills: Definition and Description

These skills contribute to the individual's ability to analyze and discriminate visually presented information, to determine the whole without seeing all of the parts, to identify more important features and ignore extraneous details, and to use visual imagery to recall past visual information. Visual analysis skills include the ability of the child to be aware of the distinctive features of visual forms, including shape, size, color, and orientation. Early in life, a child uses visual analysis skills to recognize familiar faces, toys, or objects in the house. As the child approaches preschool age, he or she begins using visual analysis skills to analyze and comprehend more abstract shapes, such as the visual symbols we use to represent sounds and quantities. These analysis skills represent one of the basic foundational skills that enable a child to learn to recognize letters, numbers, and eventually whole words. These skills are also important for the development of math concepts.

Clinically, we subclassify visual spatial dysfunction into four categories: visual discrimination, visual figure ground, visual closure, and visual memory and visualization.

Visual Discrimination

This is the ability of the child to be aware of the distinctive features of forms, including shape, orientation, size, and color.

Visual Figure Ground

This is the ability of the child to attend to a specific feature or form while maintaining an awareness of the relationship of this form to the background information.

Visual Closure

This is the ability of the child to be aware of clues in the visual stimulus that allow him or her to determine the final percept without the necessity of having all the details present. In reading, for example, visual closure allows us to perceive an entire word accurately when we may only have seen part of the word.

Visual Memory and Visualization

This is the ability of the child to recognize and recall visually presented information. Spelling requires recall of visual information, as does word recognition in reading when we try to match the word on the page with an image that is stored in the brain. Visualization, or the ability to mentally manipulate a visual image, is important in reading comprehension and math.

VISUAL MOTOR SKILLS: DEFINITION AND DESCRIPTION

These skills are related to the individual's ability to integrate visual information processing skills with fine motor movement. Another term for visual motor integration is eye-hand coordination. A very concrete example of a task requiring eye-hand coordination is catching a ball. A child must make a number of visual judgments about the ball including speed and direction and then translate the visual judgments into appropriate motor responses of his or her hand and body. If the visual motor integration is accurate, the child will catch the ball.

Handwriting is a more abstract and higher-level example of visual motor integration. As a child begins to write a letter, no external stimulus guides his or her hand. Rather, he or she must use his or her "mind's eye" to guide his or her hand in the desired direction and pattern. As the written product emerges, the child must continuously use visual analysis skills to judge whether the shape or size of the letter is appropriate. He or she must also use fine motor skills to manipulate the pencil. If he or she can accurately integrate (or combine) his or her visual analysis skills and fine motor skills, the desired letter will be successfully completed. Thus, visual motor skills are a necessary prerequisite for learning good handwriting and keyboard skills as well as throwing and catching a ball.

The two subskills in this category are visual motor integration and fine motor coordination.

Visual Motor Integration Skills

These skills are related to the individual's ability to integrate visual information processing skills with fine motor movement.

Fine Motor Coordination Skills

These skills are related to the ability to manipulate small objects or a pencil or pen.

Clinical Assessment of Visual Information Processing Skills

The assessment battery includes tests to evaluate the three diagnostic categories described above and is based on the testing approach recommended by Scheiman and Rouse.[3] Although this is a popular approach used by many optometrists, it is important to understand that visual information processing or visual perceptual motor anomalies can be assessed and subclassified in many ways. If the reader is interested in full details about these tests, references and addresses are provided in Appendix A.

The testing approach described below makes extensive use of standardized objective tests. Standardized objective testing has several important characteristics:

• Subjective judgments by the clinician are minimized, although not excluded.

• Testing is performed in a uniform way, and theoretically every trained observer would achieve the same result.

• Scoring follows specific rules, and performance is compared to normative data.

Using standardized testing, we can more confidently know what we are measuring, and we are better able to communicate our results to other professionals. For the less experienced clinician or

Table 5-1

Visual Information Processing Problems: Symptoms and Effect on Performance

Visual Spatial Dysfunction

- Poor athletic performance
- Difficulty with rhythmic activities
- Lack of coordination and balance
- Clumsy, falls and bumps into things often
- Tendency to work with one side of the body while the other side does not participate
- Difficulty learning left and right
- Reverses letters and numbers when writing or copying
- Writes from right to left

Visual Analysis Dysfunction

- Has trouble learning the alphabet, recognizing words, and learning basic math concepts of size, magnitude, and position
- Confuses likenesses and minor differences
- Mistakes words with similar beginnings
- Cannot recognize the same word repeated on a page
- Cannot recognize letters or simple forms
- Cannot distinguish the main idea from insignificant details
- Overgeneralizes when classifying objects
- Has trouble writing and remembering letters and numbers

Visual Motor Dysfunction

- Difficulty copying from the board
- Sloppy drawing or writing skills
- Poor spacing and inability to stay on lines
- Erases excessively
- Can respond orally but not produce answers in writing
- Difficulty completing written assignments in allotted period of time
- Seems to know the material but does poorly on tests
- Difficulty writing numbers in columns for math problems

for students learning to evaluate visual information processing for the first time, these characteristics are highly desirable. While experienced clinicians can sometimes make meaningful decisions about visual information processing simply by watching the patient in an unstructured task, less experienced clinicians are unable to do so.

There is evidence that even an experienced clinician's subjective and intuitive judgments may not always be reliable or valid.[4] Solan and Groffman[4] state, "There will always be some persons whose quality of judgment enables them to make more accurate estimates than others. Unfortunately, there are also persons who tend to utilize intuitive judgments based on inadequate data and whose conclusions are not accurate." The use of standardized objective testing eliminates this problem.

The case history helps direct the evaluation of the child with learning problems. Children with visual information processing disorders present with a characteristic case history. Specific signs and symptoms also suggest problems in certain aspects of visual information processing. Table 5-1 lists the various diagnostic categories along with their characteristic signs and symptoms. If a patient presents with a chief complaint of difficulty with handwriting and copying skills, for example, the most likely clinical hypothesis would be a visual motor integration problem as indicated in Table 5-1. A problem with reversals and learning left and right would suggest a clinical hypothesis of a visual spatial problem. Although knowledge of the symptoms and signs of the various diagnostic categories may allow the clinician to predict the results of the evaluation, we still recommend evaluation of all three areas discussed below.

VISUAL SPATIAL SKILLS

Component skills in this category include bilateral integration, laterality, and directionality. Tests are used to probe each one of these areas.

Evaluation of Bilateral Integration

Standing Angels in the Snow (for 3 to 8 year olds). This test probes the child's ability to be aware of and use both sides of the body separately and simultaneously. The examiner sits and the child stands directly in front of the examiner. The examiner's legs should be separated so that the child is standing midway between them (Figure 5-1). The examiner asks the child to make a very specific series of arm and leg movements. The movements range from very simple to complex. It is important for the examiner to not only observe if the correct movements are made, but also to watch for motor overflow, inappropriate movement, and other indications of performance breakdowns.

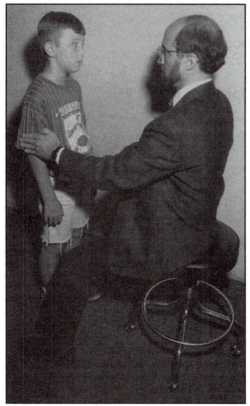

Figure 5-1. For the Standing Angels in the Snow test, the examiner sits and the child stands directly in front of the examiner.

Table 5-2

Piaget Test of Left-Right Concepts: Questions Asked

Section A

Subject's body parts: Ask the child the following questions and record the responses:
- Show me your right hand.
- Show me your left leg.
- Touch your left ear.
- Show me your left hand.
- Show me your right leg.
- Point to your right eye.

Section B

Examiner's body parts: Sit opposite the child.
- Show me my left hand.
- Point to my right ear.
- Show me my left leg.
- Show me my right hand.
- Point to my left ear.
- Show me my right leg.

Section C

Place a coin on the table to the left of a pencil in relation to the child.
- Is the pencil to the right or to the left of the coin?
- Is the coin to the right or to the left of the pencil?

Now have the child walk around to the opposite side of the table.
- Is the pencil to the right or to the left of the coin?
- Is the coin to the right or to the left of the pencil?

Section D

Sit opposite the child with a coin in your right hand and a watch or bracelet on your left arm.
- Do you see this coin? Do I have it in my right hand or my left hand?
- Is this bracelet on my right arm or my left arm?

Section E

Place three objects in front of the child: A pencil to the left, a key in the middle, and a penny to the right.
- Is the pencil to the left or to the right of the key?
- Is the pencil to the left or to the right of the penny?
- Is the key to the left or to the right of the penny?
- Is the key to the left or to the right of the pencil?
- Is the penny to the left or to the right of the pencil?
- Is the penny to the left or to the right of the key?

Evaluation of Laterality

Piaget Test of Left-Right Concepts (for 5 to 11 year olds). This test evaluates the child's ability to differentiate right from left on his or her own body (laterality), on another person, and on the location of objects in space (directionality). The examiner and child sit in chairs facing each other, and the examiner asks the child a series of questions designed to probe his or her knowledge of right and left. The questions asked are listed in Table 5-2.

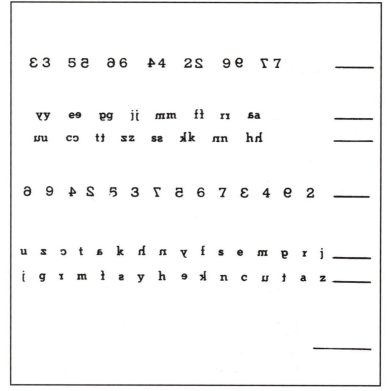

Figure 5-2. For the Gardner Reversal Frequency Test: Recognition Subtest, the child is asked to mark off those letters and numbers that are written backward or reversed.

Evaluation of Directionality

The Gardner Reversal Frequency Test: Recognition Subtest (for 5 to 15 year olds). This test consists of three subtests that assess different aspects of directionality. We include two of the three tests in our test battery. This test evaluates the existence, nature, and frequency of occurrence of receptive letter and number reversals (reversals that the patient can recognize). In this test, the patient is asked to mark off those letters and numbers that are written backward or reversed (Figure 5-2). Once seated properly, the patient is asked to carefully work through the six lines of the test worksheet and cross out the numbers or letters that appear backward. The test is untimed, and the patient is allowed to erase. Nevertheless, it is important for the examiner to observe and take into consideration the amount of time it takes and the ease with which the patient completes this task. For example, if one 7-year-old patient completes the test in 2 minutes with five errors and a second patient completes the test in 8 minutes with five errors, certainly the qualitative difference in performance must be noted.

Gardner Reversal Frequency Test: Execution Subtest (for 5 to 15 year olds). This test evaluates the existence, nature, and frequency of occurrence of expressive letter and number reversals (reversals that the patient actually makes during a writing task). In this test, the patient is asked to write letters and numbers as they are dictated. As with the recognition subtest, it is important to seat the patient so that he or she cannot observe books and other written material that may provide information about letter and number orientation. Give the patient a pencil with an eraser, place the test sheet in front of him or her, and ask him or her to print the numbers and letters you dictate. These numbers and letters are dictated one by one, and there is no time limit to this test. The letters must be reproduced as lowercase letters.

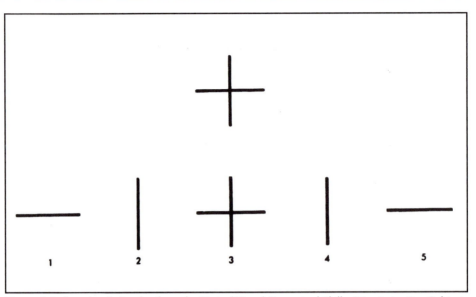

Figure 5-3. Sample of stimulus from the Test of Visual Perceptual Skills: Discrimination Subtest. (Reprinted with permission from Psychological and Educational Publications Inc.)

As with the recognition subtest, it is important to remember that although the test is untimed, the amount of time and ease with which the patient performs this task may suggest qualitative differences in performance that are important in diagnosis and treatment.

VISUAL ANALYSIS SKILLS

Clinically, we subclassify visual analysis dysfunction into four categories: visual discrimination, visual closure, visual figure ground, and visual memory.

Evaluation of Visual Discrimination
Test of Visual Perceptual Skills: Discrimination, Form Constancy, and Spatial Relationships (for 4-year-old to adult level). These three subtests evaluate the ability of the patient to be aware of the distinctive features of forms including shape, orientation, and size. The three subtests are identical in their construction, administration, and scoring. Each test is made up of 16 different plates with stimuli that become more complex. Figures 5-3 through 5-5 are illustrations of one of the early stimuli used in each of these tests. The patient must choose the matching figure from among five choices.

Evaluation of Visual Closure
Test of Visual Perceptual Skills: Visual Closure (for 4-year-old to adult level). This subtest evaluates the ability of the patient to be aware of clues in the visual stimulus that allow him or her to determine the final percept without the necessity of having all the details present. The test is made up of 16 different plates with stimuli that become more complex. Figure 5-6 is an illustration of one of the early stimuli used in this test. The patient is asked to look at the picture on top and to find the one that would look like the top form if the lines were connected or completed.

Evaluation of Visual Figure Ground
Test of Visual Perceptual Skills: Figure Ground (for 4-year-old to adult level). This subtest evaluates the ability of the patient to attend to a specific feature or form while maintaining an awareness of the relationship of this form to the background information. The test is made up of 16 different plates with stimuli that become more complex. Figure 5-7 is an illustration of one of

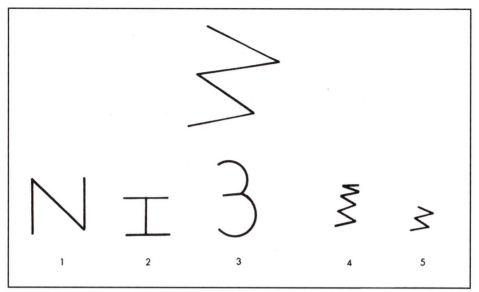

Figure 5-4. Sample of stimulus from the Test of Visual Perceptual Skills: Form Constancy Subtest. (Reprinted with permission from Psychological and Educational Publications Inc.)

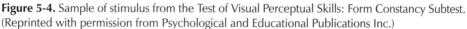
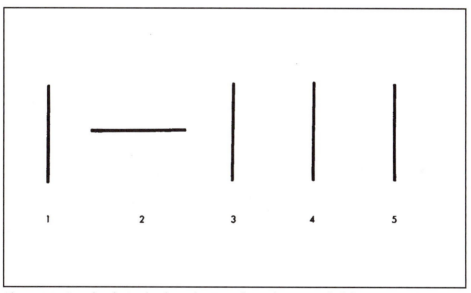

Figure 5-5. Sample of stimulus from the Test of Visual Perceptual Skills: Spatial Relationships Subtest. (Reprinted with permission from Psychological and Educational Publications Inc.)

the early stimuli used in this test. The patient is asked to look at the picture on top and to find the exact form from among the forms below.

Evaluation of Visual Memory

Test of Visual Perceptual Skills: Visual Memory (for 4-year-old to adult level). This subtest evaluates the ability of the patient to recognize and recall visually presented information. The test is made up of 16 different plates with stimuli that become more complex. Figure 5-8a is an illustration of one of the early stimuli used in this test. The patient is asked to look at an isolated picture for 5 seconds. After the stimulus is removed, he or she is asked to select the one that looks the same from among five choices (Figure 5-8b).

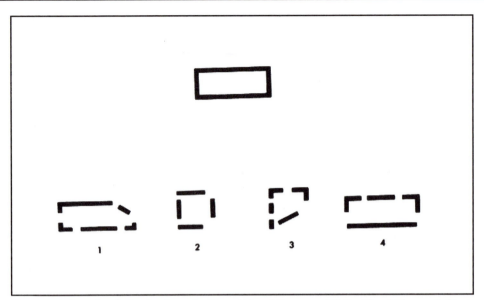

Figure 5-6. Sample of stimulus from the Test of Visual Perceptual Skills: Visual Closure Subtest. (Reprinted with permission from Psychological and Educational Publications Inc.)

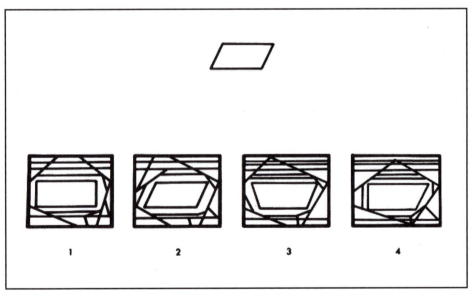

Figure 5-7. Sample of stimulus from the Test of Visual Perceptual Skills: Figure Ground Subtest. (Reprinted with permission from Psychological and Educational Publications Inc.)

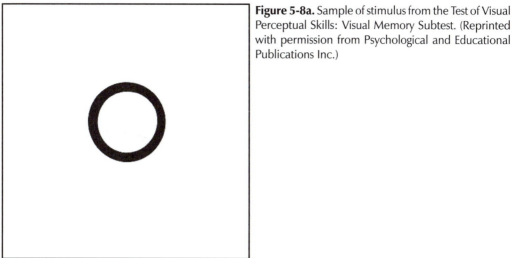

Figure 5-8a. Sample of stimulus from the Test of Visual Perceptual Skills: Visual Memory Subtest. (Reprinted with permission from Psychological and Educational Publications Inc.)

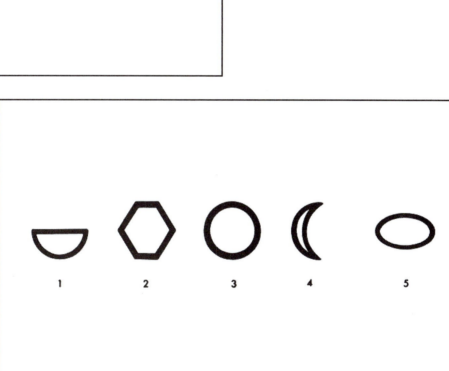

Figure 5-8b. Sample of stimulus from the Test of Visual Perceptual Skills: Visual Memory Subtest. (Reprinted with permission from Psychological and Educational Publications Inc.)

Test of Visual Perceptual Skills: Visual Sequential Memory (for 4 to 13 year olds). This subtest evaluates the ability of the patient to recognize and recall visually presented information when sequence is important, such as in spelling. The test is made up of 16 different plates with stimuli that become more complex. Figure 5-9a is an illustration of one of the early stimuli used in this test. The patient is asked to look at a series of pictures for 5 seconds. After the stimulus is removed, he or she is asked to select the one that has the same sequence from among four choices (Figure 5-9b).

Figure 5-9a. Sample of stimulus from the Test of Visual Perceptual Skills: Visual Sequential Memory Subtest. (Reprinted with permission from Psychological and Educational Publications Inc.)

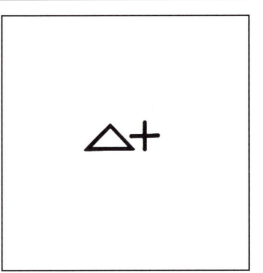

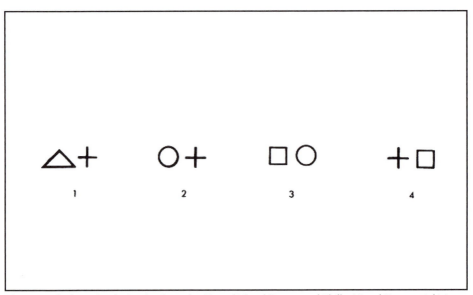

Figure 5-9b. Sample of stimulus from the Test of Visual Perceptual Skills: Visual Sequential Memory Subtest. (Reprinted with permission from Psychological and Educational Publications Inc.)

VISUAL MOTOR INTEGRATION SKILLS

The two subskills in this category are visual motor integration and fine motor coordination.

Evaluation of Visual Motor Integration

Developmental Test of Visual Motor Integration (Beery) (for 4 to 18 year olds). This test evaluates the patient's ability to integrate visual information processing and fine motor skills by assessing his or her ability to accurately copy a visual stimulus. The patient is presented with pictures of increasing complexity and is asked to reproduce the pictures as accurately as possible. Figure 5-10 is a sample of some of the forms used in this test. To score the test, clinicians must use the very detailed scoring criteria included in the scoring manual.

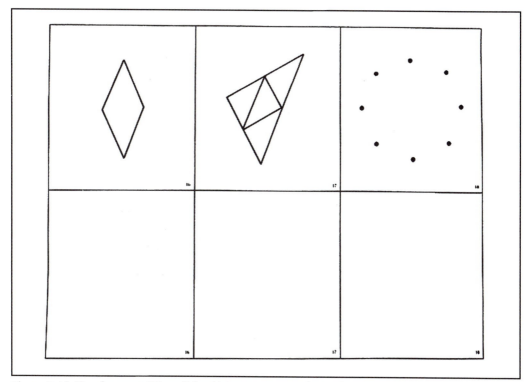

Figure 5-10. Developmental Test of Visual Motor Integration by Keith E. Beery and Norman A. Buktenica. © 1989 Modern Curriculum Press. (Reprinted with permission from Simon and Schuster Elementary.)

Wold Sentence Copy Test (for school-aged children). This test evaluates the patient's fine motor and visual motor integration skills. The Wold Sentence Copy Test is a timed test used to determine a patient's speed and accuracy in copying a sentence from the top to the bottom of a page (Figure 5-11). The test is comparable to a common school task of copying from a book to a notebook and provides the clinician with a sample of the patient's handwriting skill.

To administer this test, the test is placed in front of the patient, and the patient is told to copy the sentence on the blank lines on the bottom of the test sheet. The patient is instructed to go as fast as he or she can, but to be as neat as possible.

Evaluation of Fine Motor Skills

Grooved Pegboard Test (for kindergarten to fifth-grade children). This test evaluates the patient's fine motor skills. Other skills that are indirectly evaluated are visual attention, concentration, and directionality. The test requires the patient to place pegs in a pegboard as quickly as possible (Figure 5-12). Prior to administration of the test, hand dominance is established by asking questions about how the patient brushes his or her teeth, hammers a nail, cuts with a scissors, writes with a pencil, and throws a ball. The examiner tries to establish which hand is used for these activities. The dominant hand is the one that is used for the majority of the tasks.

Once the dominant hand is determined, the patient is told to place the pegs in the holes by matching the groove of the peg to the groove of the hole. Let the patient try the first row to demonstrate that he or she understands the task. Once he or she understands the task, ask the patient to place all of the pegs in the holes as quickly as possible.

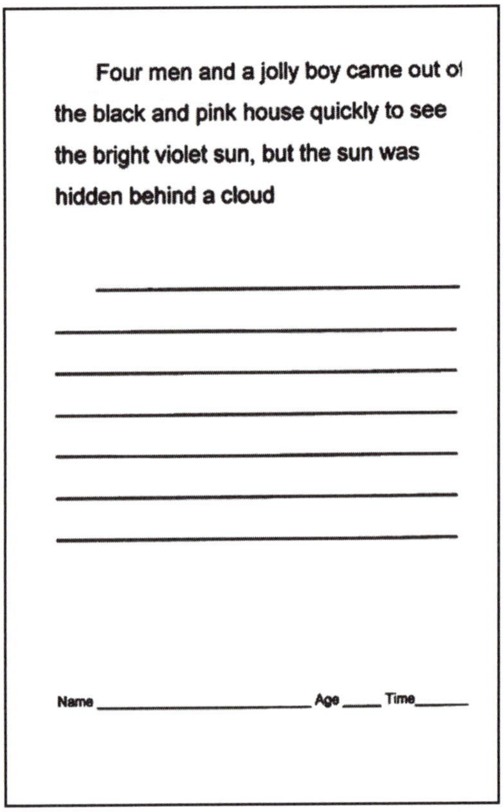

Figure 5-11. The Wold Sentence Copy Test is a timed test used to determine a child's speed and accuracy in copying a sentence.

Four men and a jolly boy came out of the black and pink house quickly to see the bright violet sun, but the sun was hidden behind a cloud

_____

_____
_____
_____
_____
_____
_____

Name _____ Age _____ Time_____

Figure 5-12. Grooved Pegboard Test used to evaluate a child's fine motor skills.

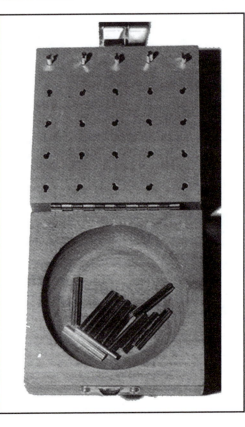

Development of Visual Information Processing Skills

The rate of development of visual processing skills is not uniform during infancy, preschool, and school-aged years. In the early years, the rate of development is more rapid than that seen in the later years. The difference between a 4-year-old child and a 5-year-old child is much greater than the difference between a 12-year-old child and a 13-year-old child.[1] This is important when comparing performance among different age groups, because a 1-year delay at 5 years of age is much more significant than a 1-year delay at 13 years of age.

VISUAL SPATIAL SKILLS

These skills allow the individual to develop normal internal and external spatial concepts and are used to interact with and organize the environment. Preschool children who are 3 to 4 years of age can correctly identify front and back and up and down on themselves and on objects.[5] The correct identification of right and left on self is usually seen at 6 to 7 years of age,[5,6] and identification of right and left directions on objects in space develops between 7 and 12 years of age.[5,6]

Reversal of letters and numbers is a common finding in children just entering school. These errors should decline in frequency, and most reversals should cease by the middle of the second grade.[7]

VISUAL ANALYSIS SKILLS

The development of form perception and discrimination in infants and young children has been extensively studied. Research indicates that face recognition, size, and shape consistency are present by 6 months.[8-10] Even though infants possess many of the basic form perception skills, they are unable to use them efficiently. During the preschool- and school-aged years, the ability to make feature comparisons and to search and explore patterns in a complete and systematic way becomes the crucial components of form perception development.[1] The ability to efficiently use these form perception skills probably does not reach adult levels until early adolescence.[1]

VISUAL MOTOR INTEGRATION SKILLS

These skills are related to the individual's ability to integrate visual information processing skills with fine motor movement. These skills begin in early infancy. White and Held[11] found that infants begin swiping with a closed fist at objects at about 2 to 3 months of age. By 5 months, the infant is able to integrate the eye and the hand. During the preschool years, the use of visual motor skills to reproduce visual form begins to develop. The first attempts at drawing usually occur around 1½ to 2 years of age. At 3 years of age, a child can draw a circle; at 4½ years of age, a square; at 5 to 5½ years of age, a triangle; and at 8 years of age, a diamond.[12]

Significance of Visual Information Processing Skills for Occupational Therapy

Table 5-1 provides a summary of the significance of visual information processing skills for occupational therapy. The effect of these problems on occupational therapy will obviously be directly related to the demand the activity places on visual information processing skills. Visual information processing problems will have greatest effect when the patient must make decisions about directional orientation, if the task involves symbol and word recognition, matching of shapes, visual memory, visualization, and copying of visual stimuli.

Summary

Of the three components in our model of vision, visual information processing disorders are the most likely to be neglected by eye care professionals. In my experience, these problems are rarely found in isolation. It is more common for there to be a combination of visual efficiency and visual information processing disorders. It is important for occupational therapists to realize that normal visual information processing or visual perceptual function depends on normal visual acuity and visual efficiency. This hierarchical relationship has been discussed in both the optometric[3] and occupational therapy literature.[13,14] Warren[13] and Bouska et al[14] have both developed models that emphasize this point. They discuss the importance of detecting and treating ocular motor, accommodative, and binocular vision disorders before the management of visual processing disorders. This is why it is so critical that occupational therapists have a comprehensive understanding of all aspects of all three components of the model of vision presented in this book.

References

1. Borsting E. Overview of visual and visual processing development. In: Scheiman M, Rouse MW, eds. *Optometric Management of Learning Related Vision Problems*. 2nd ed. St. Louis, MO: CV Mosby; 2006:35-68.
2. Blankenship E. A first primer in visual perception. *J Learn Disabil*. 1971;10:39-42.
3. Scheiman M, Rouse MW. *Optometric Management of Learning Related Vision Problems*. 2nd ed. St. Louis, MO: CV Mosby; 2006.
4. Solan HA, Groffman S. Understanding and treating developmental and perceptual motor disabilities. In: Solan HA, ed. *The Treatment and Management of Children With Learning Disabilities*. Springfield, IL: Charles C. Thomas; 1982.
5. Ilg FL, Ames LB. *School Readiness*. New York, NY: Harper & Row; 1972:159-189.
6. Laurendeau M, Pinard A. *The Development of the Concept of Space in the Child*. New York, NY: International Universities Press; 1970:278-309.
7. Gardner RA. *The Objective Diagnosis of Minimal Brain Dysfunction*. Cresskill, NJ: Creative Therapeutics; 1979.
8. Fantz RL, Fagen JF, Miranda SB. Early visual selectivity. In: Cohen LB, Salapatek P, eds. *Infant Perception: From Sensation to Cognition*. New York, NY: Academic Press; 1975.
9. Fagen JF. Infant's recognition of invariant features of faces. *Child Dev*. 1976;47:627-638.
10. Goldstein EB. *Sensation and Perception*. Belmont, CA: Wadsworth Publishing; 1989:333-337.
11. White BL, Held R. Observations on the development of visually directed reaching. In: Hellmuth J, ed. *Exceptional Infant*. Seattle, WA: Special Child Publications; 1967.
12. Beery KE. *The Developmental Test of Visual Motor Integration*. Cleveland, OH: Modern Curriculum Press; 1982.
13. Warren M. Identification of visual scanning deficits in adults after cerebrovascular accident. *Am J Occup Ther*. 1990;44:391-399.
14. Bouska MJ, Kauffman NA, Marcus SE. Disorders of the visual perceptual system. In: Umphred DA, Jewell MJ, eds. *Neurological Rehabilitation*. St. Louis, MO: CV Mosby; 1985:552-585.

Chapter Six

Screening for Visual Acuity, Visual Efficiency, and Visual Information Processing Problems

Mitchell Scheiman, OD, FCOVD, FAAO

In the first five chapters, I have tried to establish the importance of vision and the various ways in which vision can possibly interfere with occupational therapy progress. It is critical that an occupational therapist be aware of the characteristics of the visual system of any patient he or she is treating. Ideally, this information should be readily available before treatment begins. In most cases, however, no information or very limited information will be available. In a school system, the child may have been screened in the past by the school nurse. School screenings generally consist of only a test to screen for visual acuity problems, myopia, and high degrees of hyperopia and astigmatism. Early day care centers will often have medical records available that may include a screening performed by the pediatrician. This will most often consist of only an evaluation of eye health. In a hospital setting, an ophthalmological consultation may occur before the occupational therapist treats a patient. Even if this has been done, it is very likely that the only aspects of the visual system that will have been tested will be visual acuity, refractive error, and eye health. Very little attention is paid to binocular vision, accommodation, eye movements, and visual fields in acute care or rehabilitation hospitals.[1-4] Gianutsos,[2] a well-respected researcher and clinician in the area of rehabilitation of acquired brain injury, states:

> *Generally, after brain injury, the visual system is not comprehensively evaluated, sometimes because there is a lack of articulated complaints due to impaired subjective experience or reduced cognition. Visual system evaluations are frequently neglected. Often referrals, if they are made at all, are made to ophthalmologists, reflecting the medical orientation of the delivery system. Ophthalmologists, however, are primarily concerned with the physiologic health of the eye. Important as this is for the survivor of brain trauma, further issues of concern for visual information processing pertain to the function of the full visual system.*

Table 6-1

Questions to Ask the Eye Doctor Before Referring a Patient

- Do you have experience working with learning disabled children?
- Do you have experience working with developmentally delayed, multiply handicapped, autistic, and physically impaired children?
- Do you have experience working with patients with acquired brain injury?
- Do you test accommodative amplitude and facility?
- Do you evaluate fusional vergence amplitude and facility?
- Do you evaluate visual information processing skills?
- Do you offer vision therapy as a service in your practice?

Thus, information about vision will be limited and, when available, may be incomplete. It is advantageous for an occupational therapist to be able to gather information about the three different aspects of vision covered in our model. This can be accomplished using a series of simple screening tests. While such a screening is not a substitute for a comprehensive examination by an optometrist, it can be helpful in establishing the need for such an examination. It also helps the therapist to plan his or her therapy program, taking vision into consideration. Because the prevalence of vision disorders is so high in the types of patients seen by occupational therapists, all patients should have a full vision examination before therapy begins. Remember that the absence of symptoms should not be the criterion for deciding whether or not to refer a patient for a vision evaluation. It is well established that patients who have experienced changes in their functional skills have difficulty accepting or acknowledging new and unwanted vision deficits or may actually be totally unaware of these changes. For example, partial visual field loss is rarely experienced for what it is by the patient. This failure to experience partial visual field loss has been termed the *completion effect*.[2]

When a referral for a comprehensive vision examination is made, it is critical that the doctor to whom the referral is made practices with a full appreciation of the complexity of vision. I suggest that therapists call eye doctors in their area and determine if the model of vision is comparable to that described in this book. Table 6-1 is a series of questions the therapist can ask the doctor before making a referral. If the eye doctor does not answer yes to each of these questions, I suggest looking elsewhere. Using this system, you will invariably find that the eye doctor to whom you refer patients will be an optometrist with some advanced education in vision therapy. A good resource is the College of Optometrists in Vision Development (COVD) directory of fellow and associate members. The address and phone number for the COVD are provided in Appendix A. COVD members are more likely than others to practice in a manner consistent with the philosophy described in this book.

Preliminary Issues

Age and Developmental Level of the Patient

A comprehensive vision evaluation can be successfully performed by an experienced optometrist regardless of the age, verbal skills, or cognitive level of the patient. To be successful, however, the examiner must have a great deal of experience with objective testing and specialized equipment. The screening battery described in this chapter will only be useful with patients functioning at about a 3-year-old level and above. The patient will have to interact with the therapist either verbally or nonverbally and will have to be able to attend for short periods of time. If the patient is unresponsive or inattentive, a vision screening may not be possible. That does not mean, however, that vision testing cannot be performed by an experienced optometrist. In virtually all cases, testing can be successfully accomplished. If you are unable to successfully perform a vision screening, it is wise to refer for a comprehensive vision evaluation.

Lighting

The room lighting is very important in all visual testing. The lighting does not have to be excessively bright, but the room should be well illuminated. It is important to eliminate glare and reflections off the stimuli that are being used.

Positioning

The posture of the patient during the screening is very important, and the therapist should ensure that patients with poor head, neck, or trunk control have appropriate support. For the visual screening, the patient should be positioned so that the head is vertically erect, if possible.

Glasses

If the patient wears glasses, the glasses should be used for the screening. When glasses are worn full-time by the patient, they should be used for all screening tasks. If the glasses are used only for a specific distance, such as near or far, they should be used for tests administered at the same distance. When a patient is wearing bifocal glasses, make sure that he or she looks through the top portion for all distance testing and the bottom portion for all near testing.

Symptom Questionnaire

An important part of the screening is completion of the symptom questionnaire. Two sample questionnaires are included in this chapter. The first (Table 6-2) is useful for preschool- and school-aged children, and the second (Table 6-3) is designed for adults after acquired brain injury. In some cases, the patient can complete these questionnaires. In most situations, the therapist will have to complete the questionnaire by talking with the patient, parent, and/or spouse; by observing the patient; and by reviewing the questions with others. Occasionally, a screening may not be possible due to age, attention, or cognitive problems. In such cases, the therapist can base his or her decision about referral for a comprehensive vision evaluation on the results of the symptom questionnaire.

Visual Acuity

Visual acuity is an important screening test. Reduced visual acuity may suggest the presence of significant degrees of myopia, astigmatism, or hyperopia and can help detect amblyopia. Near visual acuity testing is an indirect method of assessing accommodation. Visual acuity testing is particularly important in patients with acquired brain injury.

Distance Visual Acuity for Preverbal Children, Nonverbal Adults

Standard visual acuity testing with a letter or number eye chart cannot be used with this population. Instead, it is important to have a technique that does not require any verbal response from the patient. A number of tests have been developed that simply require a matching response. The test that I have found most useful for this population is the Lea Symbols Test. As illustrated in Figures 6-1a and 6-1b, the test consists of four easily recognizable symbols: a square, circle, house, and apple.

Table 6-2

Symptom Questionnaire: Children

Patient's full name: _____

Birthdate __/__/__   Date __/__/__   Age: _____

Please place a check mark next to any problem that seems to occur often for this child.

Signs of Eye Teaming Problems

Covers or closes one eye when reading	
Rubs eyes	
Child complains of eyestrain	
Child complains of headaches	
Child complains of double vision	
Child complains of words moving on the page	
Inattentive	
Poor reading comprehension	
Loses place	

Signs of Focusing Problems

Child complains of blurred vision	
Child complains of blurred vision when looking from desk to board	
Child complains of eyestrain	
Child complains of headaches	
Rubs eyes	
Inattentive	
Poor reading comprehension	
Is tired at the end of the day	
Holds things very close	

Signs of Tracking Problems

Loses place often	
Must use finger or guide to keep place	
Skips lines and words often	
Poor reading comprehension	
Short attention span	

Signs of Visual Processing Disorders

Trouble learning left from right	
Reverses letters and numbers	
Mistakes words with similar beginnings	
Cannot recognize the same word repeated on a page	
Trouble learning basic math concepts of size, magnitude	
Poor reading comprehension	
Poor recall of visually presented material	
Trouble with spelling and sight vocabulary	
Sloppy writing skills	
Trouble copying from board to book	
Erases excessively	
Can respond orally but not in writing	
Seems to know material but does poorly on written tests	

EQUIPMENT NEEDED

- #A2506 Single Symbol Book
Vision Associates
295 NW Commons Loop, Suite 115-312
Lake City, FL 32055
Phone: 407-352-1200
Fax: 386-752-7839
www.visionkits.com

Table 6-3

Symptom Questionnaire: Acquired Brain Injury

Patient's name _____   Date_____

General

- Do you wear glasses? Bifocals? Trifocals?
- Do your glasses work as well now as before the trauma, stroke?
- Do you have blurry vision? Is the difficulty at far or near?

Binocular Vision

- Do you ever see double? See overlapping or shadow images?
- Do you ever have to close one eye?
- Do you experience eyestrain, headaches when using your eyes?
- Do you have difficulty concentrating on tasks?

Accommodation

- Do you have trouble focusing from one distance to another?
- Do your eyes burn or water?
- Do you have difficulty concentrating on tasks?

Ocular Motility

- Do you find yourself losing your place or skipping words or lines when reading?
- Do you have difficulty following moving objects?
- Do letters jump around on the page while you are reading?

Visual Fields

- Do you bump into chairs, objects?
- Do you have any difficulty seeing at night?
- Do you need to hold onto walls, objects, or people when walking?
- Do you ever find that when you reach for an object that you knock it over or your hand misses?
- Are portions of a page or any objects missing?
- Do people or things suddenly appear from one side that you didn't see approaching?

Setup and Testing Strategy

Typically when an optometrist assesses visual acuity, each eye is tested individually. In a routine optometric examination it is important to know if there is a difference between the two eyes. However, the purpose of visual acuity screening for an occupational therapist is different. The goal is to determine if there is a visual acuity problem with both eyes open that might be affecting the patient's ability to engage in various activities of daily living. It is not important to know if one eye is worse than the other. This will have minimal impact on activities of daily living. What is of primary importance is the visual acuity with both eyes together. Thus, for all of the following visual acuity tests the recommendation is to test with both eyes open.

When testing children or adults with cognitive and perceptual problems, it is wise to test at near before distance. It is easier to hold the patient's attention and teach the procedure at near than at far. It is helpful to create a play- or game-like situation with children. Before testing begins, it is also important to determine the best method of communication with the patient. Some patients will be able to verbally name the object, while others may have to find or point to the matching block. Once the patient has demonstrated an understanding of the procedure, you can begin the

Figure 6-1a. Lea Symbols Book used to test preverbal children and nonverbal adults.

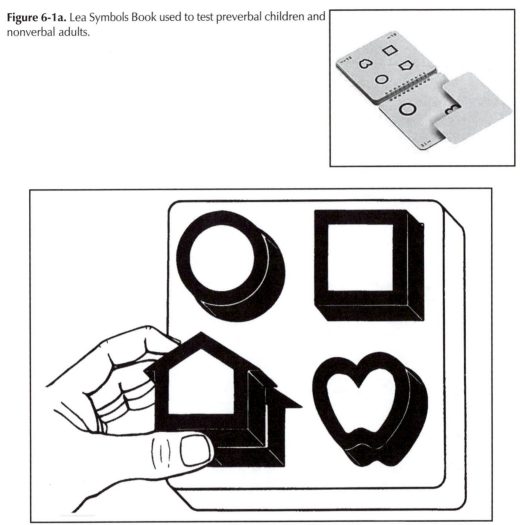

Figure 6-1b. Three-dimensional Lea Symbols Blocks used by a patient to match symbols on the test chart. (Reprinted with permission from Vision Associates, www.visionkits.com.)

actual testing. Positioning is important, and the occupational therapist should try to find the best positioning that permits the patient to attend and concentrate on the task.

PROCEDURE

1. With a patient, create a pleasant play situation.
2. Establish the best method of communication.
3. Before beginning the actual testing procedure, make sure that the patient understands the task and can either verbally identify all four test objects when held at a close distance or can successfully match all four symbols on a consistent basis.
4. Test with both eyes open.
5. Place the 3-D blocks on the patient's lap.
6. Hold the test chart at 10 feet, and point to a target. Ask the patient to verbally identify the symbol or find the block that matches the symbol.
7. If the patient seems confused by all the symbols on one page, isolate one line at a time.

8. Acuity is recorded as the last line on which at least three of the five symbols are identified correctly.

9. If the patient is inattentive when the chart is held at 10 feet, perform the testing at a closer working distance (move to 80, 60, or 40 inches, if necessary).

10. Make sure you record the distance at which you tested distance visual acuity.

EXPECTED FINDINGS AND POSSIBLE RESPONSES

We expect to find 20/20 visual acuity. A referral is necessary if vision is 20/40 or worse.

Distance Visual Acuity for Verbal/Literate Children and Adults

EQUIPMENT NEEDED

• Chronister Portable Acuity Test (CPAC Test)
  Gulden Ophthalmics
  225 Cadwalader Ave
  Elkins Park, PA 19027
  Phone: 800-659-2250
  www.guldenophthalmics.com

SETUP AND TESTING STRATEGY

Test with both eyes open.

PROCEDURE

1. Hold the CPAC at 20 feet (Figure 6-2), and ask the patient to verbally identify the letter on the 20/40 line.

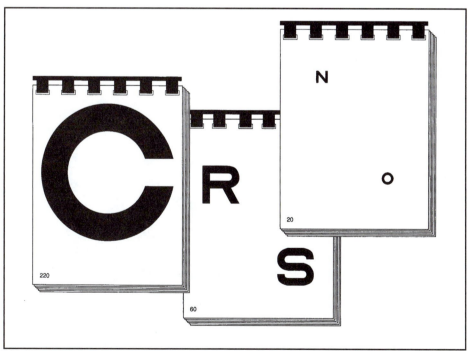

Figure 6-2. The Chronister Portable Acuity Test used to test distance visual acuity in verbal and literate children and adults. (Reprinted with permission of Gulden Ophthalmics.)

2. If the patient has trouble with letters, attempt to test visual acuity using the Lea Symbols Test.

3. Continue until the patient misses more than 50% of the letters at any size.

4. Record acuity as the last line in which the patient can successfully identify more than 50% of the letters.

EXPECTED FINDINGS AND POSSIBLE RESPONSES
We expect to find 20/20 visual. A referral is necessary if vision is 20/40 or worse.

Binocular Vision

To screen for binocular vision problems, it is important to test for both eye alignment and sensory fusion. The screening tests described below will enable the occupational therapist to detect a large phoria, poor convergence, and suppression.

Alignment of the Eyes

EQUIPMENT NEEDED
• Binocular Vision Screening Software (BVA) OT Version
Home Therapy System
Phone: 800-346-4925
www.homevisiontherapy.com

• Computer (either PC or Mac)

SETUP AND TESTING STRATEGY
Positioning is important, and the occupational therapist should try to find the positioning that best permits the patient to attend and concentrate on the task. For binocular vision testing, the patient's head should be vertically erect.

The software is loaded onto the computer that will be used for the vision screening (Figure 6-3). Once it is loaded you select "NEW TEST," enter the patient's name and begin the screening. The initial screen will allow you to select various testing procedures. The recommended tests for this screening are:

• Worth 4 Dot

• Phoria

• Fusional vergence

Figure 6-3. BVA binocular vision screening software.

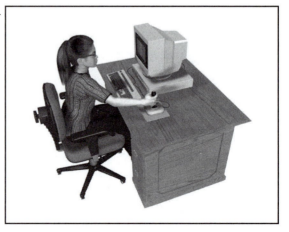

PROCEDURE

Simply follow the onscreen instructions for each of the three screening test (Worth 4 Dot, phoria, and fusional vergence).

EXPECTED FINDINGS AND POSSIBLE RESPONSES

The scoring on the BVA is automatic. The computer will indicate whether the patient has passed or failed the screening for each area tested.

Near Point of Convergence

EQUIPMENT NEEDED

- Thin pick-up stick or pencil with a sharp point
- Ruler

SETUP AND TESTING STRATEGY

Positioning is important, and the occupational therapist should try to find the best positioning that permits the patient to attend and concentrate on the task. For binocular vision testing, the patient's head will ideally be vertically erect.

PROCEDURE

1. Slowly move the pencil toward the patient at eye level and between the two eyes (Figure 6-4).
2. Ask the patient to keep the pencil tip single for as long as possible.
3. Ask the patient to tell you when he or she sees two pencil tips.
4. Once diplopia occurs, move the pencil in another inch or two and then begin to move it away from the patient.
5. Ask the patient to try to see "one" again.
6. Also watch the eyes carefully, and observe whether the eyes stop working together as a team. One eye will usually drift out (Figure 6-5).
7. Record the distance at which the patient reports double vision and when the patient reports recovery of single vision.

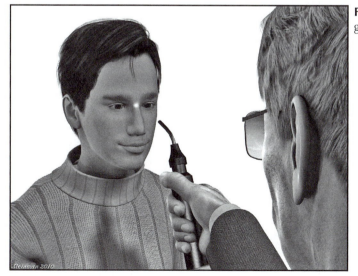

Figure 6-4. Near Point of Convergence Test.

Figure 6-5. The patient's left eye has turned out during the Near Point of Convergence Test.

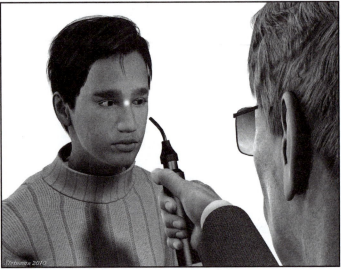

Expected Findings and Possible Responses

We expect the patient to report double vision or for the eyes to lose alignment when the pencil comes within 2 inches of his or her eyes. This is called the break, and a normal finding is between 2 and 4 inches. After the patient experiences double vision, we expect a recovery of fusion (single vision) from 4 to 6 inches. If a patient has a long-standing, significant binocular vision problem, he or she may not report double vision because he or she is suppressing the eye that turns out. That is why it is so important for the therapist to watch the patient's eyes to make an objective assessment of when the break and recovery occur. When a break occurs, you should be able to observe one eye drift out, and when the patient recovers fusion, you should be able to see the eyes move back into alignment.

Accommodative Testing

Accommodative problems are prevalent in school-aged children with learning problems and in patients with acquired brain injury. As discussed in Chapter Four, in a comprehensive evaluation, it is important to evaluate both accommodative amplitude and accommodative facility. In a screening, however, we generally only evaluate amplitude directly, and we try to gather information about facility from the symptom questionnaire. If we find a low amplitude of accommodation, we can predict that accommodative facility will also be abnormal. A normal amplitude of accommodation, however, does not necessarily mean that accommodative facility would be normal as well. The questionnaire in Appendix B can help you identify an accommodative facility problem. If the patient complains of several of the symptoms in the "Signs of Focusing Problems" section, a facility problem should be considered. One symptom that is particularly characteristic of a facility problem is that the patient complains of blurred vision when looking from far to near or near to far. If amplitude testing is normal and you are suspicious, it is best to refer for a comprehensive evaluation.

Amplitude of Accommodation
Equipment Needed
- 20/30 letter on the Gulden Fixation Stick ([Figure 6-6] see page 101 for contact information)
- An eye patch

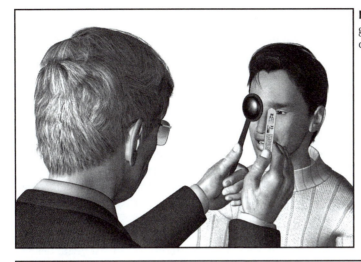

Figure 6-6. Tongue depressor target used to test amplitude of accommodation.

Table 6-4				
Expected Amplitude of Accommodation by Age				
Age	*Expected Number*		*Age*	*Expected Number*
3	17 D		30	8 D
6	16 D		33	7 D
9	15 D		36	6 D
12	14 D		39	5 D
15	13 D		42	4 D
18	12 D		45	3 D
21	11 D		48	2 D
24	10 D		51	1 D
27	9 D		54	0 D

SETUP AND TESTING STRATEGY

It is important to position the patient so that he or she is able to maximally attend and concentrate. Vertical positioning of the head is not as important with accommodation as it is with binocular vision testing. If the patient normally reads with glasses, they must be used for this task.

PROCEDURE

1. Patch the left eye.

2. It is important that the patient does not know the letter on the Gulden Fixation Stick before the test begins.

3. Hold the Gulden Fixation Stick with the 20/30 target about 1 inch in front of the right eye. The patient will be unable to identify the stimulus on the Gulden Fixation Stick at this distance.

4. Slowly move the target away from the patient's eye, and ask the patient to report as soon as he or she can identify the target.

5. Using a ruler, measure the distance from the eye to the Gulden Fixation Stick at which the patient was able to identify the stimulus. Record this measurement.

6. Divide 40 by the measurement found in Step 5 to determine the amplitude of accommodation. For example, say the patient is able to identify the target at 8 inches. To find the amplitude, divide 40 by 8, which equals 5 D.

7. Compare the patient's amplitude of accommodation to the expected amplitude for the patient's age (Table 6-4).

EXPECTED FINDINGS AND POSSIBLE RESPONSES

The amplitude of accommodation should be within 2 D of the expected finding to pass this screening test.

Ocular Motility (Saccades and Pursuits)

There are several methods of evaluating ocular motility function. These include direct observation, visual-verbal format tests, and objective tests. The objective tests require expensive equipment and are, therefore, not suitable for a screening. The first two methods, however, require only minimal equipment and are appropriate for a screening. The direct observation tests described below can be used for patients from the age of 5 years old through adulthood. Although there are several direct observation methods available, I have chosen a system that has received the most critical research scrutiny. The direct observation method described below was developed at the Northeastern State University College of Optometry (NSUCO).[5] Some experience is required to become comfortable with the test, and therapists should first perform the test with children and adults without vision problems before attempting to screen a patient with a potential problem. The advantage of direct observation tests is that only limited verbal interaction is required, and the examiner can make objective observations.

The other testing approach is called a visual-verbal format because the patient has to look at numbers and say the numbers out loud. This test is valuable with school-aged children and adults, and the results can be compared to normative data. This test is valuable when a child or adult is experiencing difficulty with reading, loss of place, skipping words, difficulty scanning the environment, and localizing objects. It requires good attention and expressive language skills. If there is an expressive language problem and difficulty with number recall, the test cannot be administered. A reliable and valid visual-verbal format test is only available for saccades, not pursuits.

Saccades: Direct Observation Method

EQUIPMENT NEEDED

- Two Gulden Fixation Sticks (see page 101 for contact information)
- Place a red circular sticker on one and a blue circular sticker on the other

SETUP AND TESTING STRATEGY

If possible, the patient should be standing with his or her feet shoulder-width apart directly in front of the examiner. If the patient cannot stand, try to position the patient so that the head is erect and not supported in any way. If this is not possible, it is best to position the head vertically erect with support. The test is performed binocularly and is appropriate for patients at least 5 years of age.

PROCEDURE

1. Hold two different Gulden Fixation Stick, 16 inches from the patient's face with each target about 4 inches from the patient's midline. The total horizontal separation of the targets should be about 8 inches (Figure 6-7).
2. No instructions are given to the patient to move or not to move his or her head.
3. Use the following instructional set: "When I say red, look at the red target. When I say blue, look at the blue target. Remember, do not look until I tell you."
4. Ask the patient to look from one target to the other for five round trips or a total of 10 fixations.
5. Determine if the patient can keep his or her attention under control to complete five round trips for saccades. Assign a score of 1 through 5 based on the scoring criteria in Table 6-5.

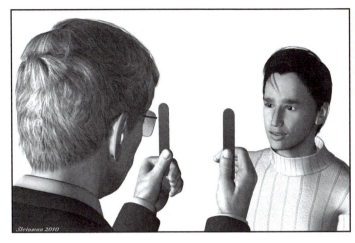

Figure 6-7. Saccades testing: Direct observation method using two different targets 16 inches from the patient's face with each target about 4 inches from the patient's midline.

6. Observe the accuracy of the eye movement. Does it take one eye movement to reach the target or multiple saccades? Assign a score of 1 through 5 based on the scoring criteria in Table 6-5.

7. Observe if the patient moves his or her head or body. Assign a score of 1 through 5 based on the scoring criteria in Table 6-5.

8. Compare the patient's score to the failure criteria in Table 6-6.

Expected Findings and Possible Responses

Table 6-5 lists the scoring criteria for direct observation of saccades, and Table 6-6 lists the failure criteria. Any score below the minimal levels listed in Table 6-6 would be reason for referral.

Pursuits: Direct Observation Method

Equipment Needed

- One Gulden Fixation Stick with a red circular sticker (see page 101 for contact information)

Setup and Testing Strategy

If possible, the patient should be standing with feet shoulder-width apart directly in front of the examiner. If the patient cannot stand, try to position the patient so that the head is erect and not supported in any way. If this is not possible, it is best to position the head vertically erect with support. The test is performed binocularly and is appropriate for patients who are at least 5 years of age.

Procedure

1. Hold one Gulden Fixation Stick 16 inches from the patient's face.

2. No instructions are given to the patient to move or not to move his or her head.

3. Use the following instructional set: "Watch the red circle as it goes around. Don't take your eyes off the red circle."

4. Move the target clockwise for two rotations and counter-clockwise for two rotations.

5. Determine if the patient can keep his or her attention under control to complete four rotations. Assign a score of 1 through 5 based on the scoring criteria in Table 6-7.

6. Observe the accuracy of the pursuit eye movements. Assign a score of 1 through 5 based on the scoring criteria in Table 6-7.

7. Observe if the patient moves his or her head or body. Assign a score of 1 through 5 based on the scoring criteria in Table 6-7.

Table 6-5

NSUCO Scoring Criteria for
Direct Observation of Saccades

Ability

POINTS	OBSERVATION
1	Completes less than two round trips
2	Completes two round trips
3	Completes three round trips
4	Completes four round trips
5	Completes five round trips

Accuracy

(Can the patient accurately and consistently fixate so that no noticeable correction is needed?)

POINTS	OBSERVATION
1	Large over- or undershooting is noted one or more times
2	Moderate over- or undershooting is noted one or more times
3	Constant slight over- or undershooting is noted (>50% of time)
4	Intermittent slight over- or undershooting is noted (<50% of time)
5	No over- or undershooting noted

Head and Body Movement

(Can the patient accomplish the saccade without moving his or her head?)

POINTS	OBSERVATION
1	Large movement of the head or body at any time
2	Moderate movement of the head or body at any time
3	Slight movement of the head or body (>50% of time)
4	Slight movement of the head or body (<50% of time)
5	No movement of the head or body

Table 6-6

NSUCO Saccade Test Referral Criteria by Age and Sex

Sex	Ability	Accuracy	Head Movement
Boys	Less than 5	Less than 3	5 to 6 years: less than 2 All other ages: less than 3
Girls	Less than 5	Less than 3	5 years: less than 2 6 to 9 years: less than 3 All other ages: less than 4

Table 6-7

NSUCO Oculomotor Test Scoring Criteria for Direct Observation of Pursuits

Ability

POINTS	OBSERVATION
1	Cannot complete half rotation in either clockwise or counterclockwise direction
2	Completes half rotation in either direction
3	Completes one rotation in either direction but not two rotations
4	Completes two rotations in one direction but less than two rotations in the other direction
5	Completes two rotations in each direction

Accuracy

(Can the patient accurately and consistently fixate so that no noticeable refixation is needed when doing pursuits?)

POINTS	OBSERVATION
1	No attempt to follow the target or requires greater than 10 refixations
2	Refixes five to 10 times
3	Refixes three to four times
4	Refixes two times or less
5	No refixations

Head and Body Movement

(Can the patient accomplish the pursuit without moving his or her head?)

POINTS	OBSERVATION
1	Large movement of the head or body at any time
2	Moderate movement of the head or body at any time
3	Slight movement of the head or body (>50% of time)
4	Slight movement of the head or body (<50% of time)
5	No movement of the head or body

Table 6-8

NSUCO Pursuit Test Referral Criteria by Age and Sex

Sex	Ability	Accuracy	Head Movement
Boys	Less than 5	5 to 6 years: less than 2 7 to 9 years: less than 3 10 years and older: less than 4	5 to 6 years: less than 2 7 to 9 years: less than 3 10 years and older: less than 4
Girls	Less than 5	5 to 8 years: less than 3 9 years and older: less than 4	5 to 9 years: less than 3 All other ages: less than 4

EXPECTED FINDINGS AND POSSIBLE RESPONSES

Table 6-7 lists the scoring criteria for direct observation of pursuits, and Table 6-8 lists the failure criteria findings.

Figure 6-8. The student must call out the numbers going down the columns on Test A (Developmental Eye Movement Test).

TEST A	
3	4
7	5
5	2
9	1
8	7
2	5
5	3
7	7
4	4
6	8
1	7
4	4
7	6
6	5
3	2
7	9
9	2
3	3
9	6
2	4

Saccades: Visual-Verbal Format

This test is less dependent on the skill of the examiner than the direct observation method of screening saccades. The test has also been normed for children 6 to 13 years old. After age 13, only limited additional improvement can be expected in performance on this test. Therefore, even though norms are only available for children, the test can be used with adults with acquired brain injury. In such cases, the expectation is that the patient should at least perform as well as the top level norms provided in the manual. Therapists interested in using this test should purchase the test and study the manual to gain maximum insight about administration and scoring.

EQUIPMENT NEEDED
• Developmental Eye Movement (DEM) Test

SETUP AND TESTING
The patient should be seated, and it is helpful to use a slantboard for the testplates. The test is performed binocularly.

PROCEDURE
1. Ask the patient to call out the numbers on Tests A and B as quickly as possible from top to bottom without using his or her finger (Figure 6-8).

2. Record time and any errors. There are a variety of errors the patient can make, including errors of addition, omission, and substitution. It is important to consult the testing manual about types of errors and recording procedures.

3. Ask the patient to call out the numbers on Test C (Figure 6-9) as quickly as possible without using his or her finger. This time, the patient must call out the numbers going across the page.

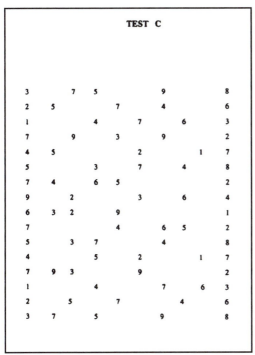

TEST C

Figure 6-9. This time, the patient must call out the numbers going across the page on Test C as quickly as possible (Developmental Eye Movement Test).

4. Record time and any errors. There are a variety of errors the patient can make including errors of addition, omission, and substitution. It is important to consult the testing manual about types of errors and recording procedures.

5. Determine the adjusted time by taking errors into consideration (consult manual for details).

6. Determine the ratio score (horizontal adjusted time/vertical adjusted time), and convert this raw score into a percentile based on the patient's age. This score gives us an assessment of the saccadic speed.

7. Determine the number of errors, and convert this raw score into a percentile based on the patient's age. This score gives us an assessment of accuracy.

EXPECTED FINDINGS AND POSSIBLE RESPONSES

A score at the 50th percentile is considered average. Both errors and ratio (speed) are scored separately. For screening purposes, a score below the 15th percentile on either errors or ratio is considered significantly low and requires a referral.

Visual Fields

Confrontation Fields

One of the more common vision problems associated with acquired brain injury is a visual field defect. Confrontation field testing is a method of screening for such deficits. It allows the therapist to screen for gross, peripheral vision field loss. It is important to realize that this screening procedure may be insensitive with some patients, and it is possible to miss a significant visual field loss using this procedure.[6,7] Therefore, it must be viewed as a screening test only. If the results of the screening are negative yet the patient displays behavior indicative of a field loss, a referral is still necessary.

EQUIPMENT NEEDED

• None

SETUP AND TESTING STRATEGY

Typically when an optometrist assesses visual fields, each eye is tested individually. In a routine optometric examination it is important to know if there is a difference between the two eyes. However, the purpose of visual field screening for an occupational therapist is different. The goal is to determine if there is a visual field problem with both eyes open that might be affecting the patient's ability to engage in various activities of daily living. It is not important to know if there is a significant visual field loss in just one eye. This will have minimal impact on activities of daily living. What is of primary importance is the visual field with both eyes together. Thus, the recommendation is to test with both eyes open.

The patient must be seated opposite the examiner, and it is important to position the patient so that the head is vertical. Confrontation field testing is not necessary in children who have not experienced head trauma. I suggest that it be reserved for adults and children with acquired brain injury. Although this is a significant test to attempt when dealing with such patients, it is important to remember that good fixation ability and a high level of concentration and attention are necessary. If these skills are not present, this testing will not be possible.

The underlying concept when doing confrontation field testing is that you compare your own visual field to the patient's visual field. Specifically, if you can see the target that you are presenting, then the patient should be able to see it.

PROCEDURE

1. Sit directly opposite the patient. You should be about 20 inches from the patient. It is preferable that the background for the patient be dark and uniform.
2. Explain that you will be moving the target from the side, and the patient should report as soon as he or she sees it while looking directly at your finger which you hold between your eyes.
3. Begin at the 12 o'clock position, and slowly move the target down until the patient first reports seeing it. Compare the patient's response to yours. If the patient cannot see the target as soon as you can, it is an indication of a possible problem.
4. Move clockwise to the 2, 4, 6, 8, and 10 o'clock positions, and repeat Step 3.
5. Record approximately where the patient reports seeing the target in each orientation tested.

Visual Inattention/Neglect

Confrontation field testing described above is designed to detect a left or right hemianopia or quadrant defect. However, it is also necessary to screen for visual inattention or visual neglect. A standardized test is available for this purpose called the Behavioural Inattention Test (BIT). The BIT is an objective behavioral test of everyday skills relevant to visual neglect, aimed at increasing the understanding of specific difficulties patients experience.

EQUIPMENT NEEDED

• Behavioural Inattention Test
Pearson
Phone: 800-328-5999
Fax: 888-556-2103
www.pearsonassessments.com

SETUP AND TESTING STRATEGY

Testing is performed with both eyes open. The patient and examiner are seated at a table.

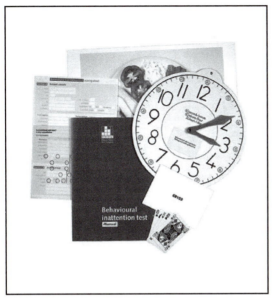

Figure 6-10. Behavioural Inattention Test (BIT).

Procedure

Follow the instructional set of the BIT. There are two parallel versions, each comprising six "conventional" subtests and nine behavioral subtests (Figure 6-10). Short and easy to understand and interpret, the BIT is applicable to a wide range of environmental settings. The BIT has been validated against conventional tests of neglect and therapists' reports. It also has excellent inter-rater, test retest, and alternate form reliability.

Visual Information Processing Screening

Visual Spatial Skills

The test described below evaluates the existence, nature, and frequency of occurrence of receptive letter and number reversals (reversals that the patient can recognize). In this test, the patient is asked to mark off those letters and numbers that are written backward or reversed (Figure 6-11). This test gives us information about the patient's development of normal internal and external spatial concepts.

Equipment Needed

- Gardner Reversal Frequent Test: Recognition Subtest
- A pencil

Setup and Testing Strategy

This test is appropriate for children 5 to 15 years old. After age 15, only limited additional improvement can be expected in performance on this test. Therefore, even though norms are only available for children 5 to 15 years old, the test can be used with adults with acquired brain injury. In such cases, the expectation is that the patient should at least perform as well as the top level norms provided in the manual. When administering this test, it is important to seat the patient so that he or she cannot observe books and other written material that may provide information about letter and number orientation. This is an untimed test, and patients who have difficulty in this area may become frustrated by this task and take excessively long periods of time to complete the test.

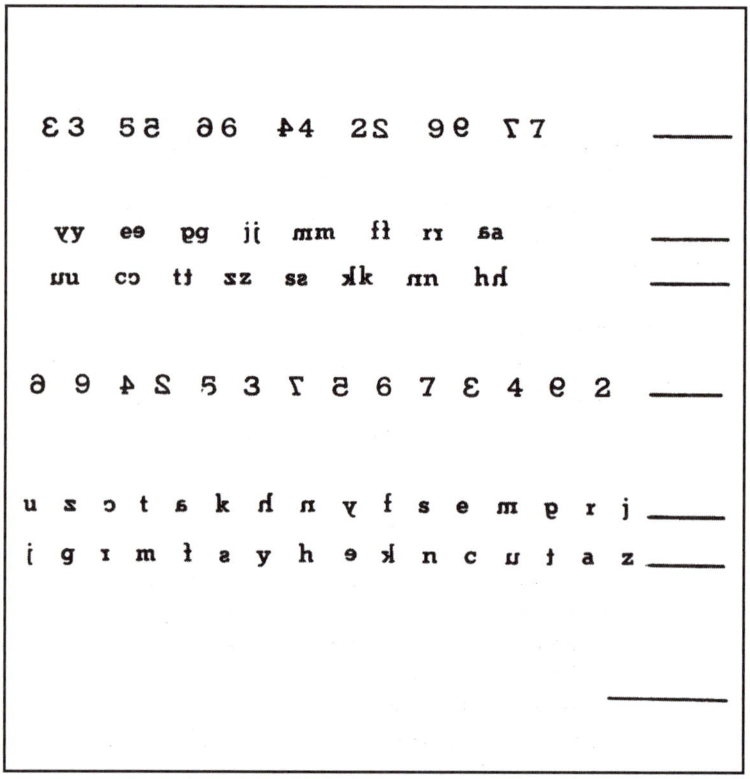

Figure 6-11. In the Gardner Reversal Frequent Test: Recognition Subtest, the child is asked to mark off those letters and numbers that are written backward or reversed.

Ɛ3   5Ƨ   ɘ6   ᴅ4   2Ƨ   9ɘ   ┌7   _____

ᴠy   ɘɘ   �   jï   mm   ꞁ1   rı   ᴀa   _____
ɹɹ   cɔ   t1   ꙅz   ꙅᴀ   ꓘk   nn   hꓒ   _____

ɘ   9   ᴅ   Ƨ   5   Ƨ   ┌   ꙅ   6   7   Ɛ   4   ɘ   Ƨ   _____

u   ꙅ   ɔ   t   ᴀ   k   ꓒ   ᴅ   ʏ   ꟻ   ꙅ   ɘ   m   ᴘ   r   j _____
ï   g   ɹ   m   ꞁ   ᴀ   y   h   ɘ   ꓘ   n   c   ᴜ   t   a   z _____

_____

Because we are performing this test as a screening, I recommend that you discontinue the test if it becomes clear after a short period of time that the patient is struggling.

PROCEDURE

1. Give the patient a pencil with an eraser and the examination sheet, and say the following: "In this first row, there are pairs of numbers. In each pair, one of the numbers is pointing in the right direction, and one is pointing in the wrong direction. Draw an X over the number pointing in the wrong direction."

2. Use similar instructions for the next two lines of letters.

3. For rows 4 through 6, use the following instructions: "In this row, some of the numbers are pointing in the right direction and some are pointing in the wrong direction. Put an X over all of the numbers pointing in the wrong direction."

4. The test is scored by counting the total number of errors. Two types of errors can occur: errors of omission and errors of commission. Errors of omission refer to mistakes in which the patient fails to cross out a letter or number that is printed backward. Errors of commission refer to errors in which the patient crosses out a letter or number that is actually correct.

5. The total of the two types of errors is the raw score, which can then be converted to a percentile score by using the tables supplied in the test manual.

EXPECTED FINDINGS AND POSSIBLE RESPONSES

For screening purposes, a score falling one standard deviation from normal (below the 15th percentile) is considered significant and requires referral or a complete visual information processing evaluation.

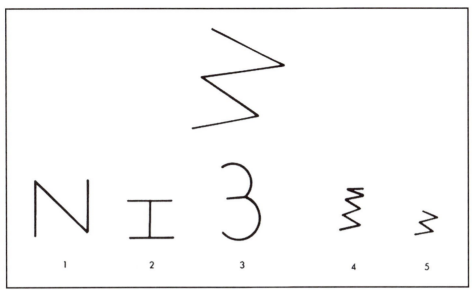

Figure 6-12. Test of Visual Perceptual Skills: Form Constancy Subtest. (Reprinted with permission from Psychological and Educational Publications Inc.)

Visual Analysis Skills

To screen this area, I suggest using the Test of Visual Perceptual Skills (TVPS): Form Constancy Subtest illustrated in Figure 6-12.

EQUIPMENT NEEDED

- Test of Visual Perceptual Skills: Form Constancy Subtest
  Bernell Corp
  Phone: 800-348-2225
  www.bernell.com

SETUP AND TESTING STRATEGY

This test probes the patient's ability to be aware of the distinctive features of forms including shape, orientation, and size without the need for motor involvement. It is made up of 16 different plates with stimuli that become more complex. It can be used between the ages of 4 to adult.

PROCEDURE

1. Introduce the test by telling the patient that he or she may not be able to answer all of the items correctly and that the pictures become more and more difficult.
2. Once you have the patient's attention, say the following: "Look at the picture" (point to the picture on top). "Now, find the one picture from these five that looks the same even though it may be bigger, smaller, darker, turned around, or upside down."
3. If the patient correctly determines the answer to plate A, continue with the rest of the items until the patient misses four of five consecutive items.
4. If the patient cannot determine the answer to plate A, point out and explain the correct response, then proceed once the patient seems to understand.
5. Discontinue when the patient fails four of five consecutive items.
6. It is important to prompt the patient to try even if he or she is unsure.
7. Record the patient's responses on the scoring sheet.

8. The raw score equals the number of correct responses up to the point where the patient misses four of five consecutive stimuli.

9. Refer to the test manual to convert the raw score to a percentile rank.

EXPECTED FINDINGS AND POSSIBLE RESPONSES

For screening purposes, a score falling one standard deviation from normal (below the 15th percentile) is considered significant and requires referral or a complete visual information processing evaluation.

Visual Motor Integration Skills

A well-known and accepted method of assessing visual motor integration skills is the Developmental Test of Visual Motor Integration. This test has well-developed normative data and can be used from age 3 years old through adulthood.

EQUIPMENT NEEDED

* Developmental Test of Visual Motor Integration (Beery and Buktenica)

SETUP AND TESTING STRATEGY

This test evaluates the patient's ability to integrate visual information processing and fine motor skills by assessing his or her ability to accurately copy a visual stimulus. The patient is presented with pictures of increasing complexity and is asked to reproduce the pictures as accurately as possible. Figure 6-13 is a sample of some of the forms used in this test.

When administering this test, it is important to have the test booklet and the patient's body centered with the desk and the booklet throughout the testing. Do not let the patient trace the picture, and erasures or second tries are not allowed.

PROCEDURE

1. Place the test form in front of the patient with the first three patterns to be copied and say, "These forms are to be copied in order. Give each space only one try."

2. Point to the first form and say, "Can you make one just like this? You make yours right here" (point to the space in which the patient is to draw the form). "Go ahead now and do the rest of them. There is no erasing allowed."

3. To score the test, use the very detailed scoring criteria included in the scoring manual.

4. Testing should be discontinued after three consecutive incorrect responses.

5. The raw score is the total of all correct forms, and this score can be converted to a percentile score using the tables in the scoring manual that comes with the test.

EXPECTED FINDINGS AND POSSIBLE RESPONSES

For screening purposes, a score falling one standard deviation from normal (below the 15th percentile) is considered significant and requires referral or a complete visual information processing evaluation.

Summary

The screening tests described in this chapter can be used by an occupational therapist to screen for vision problems in the three important areas of vision described earlier in this book. Tests that allow detection of problems in visual acuity, refraction, visual field, binocular vision, accommodation, ocular motility, and visual information processing are included. The screening form included in Appendix B can be used to record results and includes referral guidelines for each screening test.

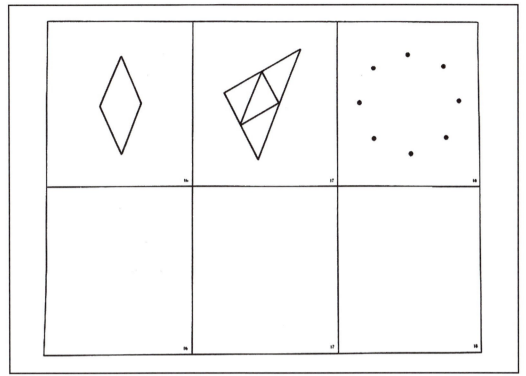

Figure 6-13. Developmental Test of Visual Motor Integration by Keith E. Beery and Norman A. Buktenica. © 1989 Modern Curriculum Press. (Reprinted with permission from Simon and Schuster Elementary.)

If a problem is detected, referral for a comprehensive vision examination is important. I have stressed the need to make sure that the professional to whom you refer the patient practices using the full model of vision described in this book. Otherwise, you will most likely be disappointed with the information you receive in return. The directories of optometrists who have achieved fellow status in the College of Optometrists in Vision Development and those who have achieved Diplomate status in the American Academy of Optometry are good resources for potential referral sources.

If the screening tests are inconclusive but you continue to observe behavior that suggests a vision problem, you should certainly refer the patient for a comprehensive vision examination.

References

1. Anderson DP, Ford RM. Visual abnormalities after severe head injuries. *Can J Surg*. 1980;23:163-165.
2. Gianutsos R, Ramsey G, Perlin RR. Rehabilitative optometric services for survivors of acquired brain injury. *Arch Phys Med Rehabil*. 1988;69:573-578.
3. Warren M. Identification of visual scanning deficits in adults after cerebrovascular accident. *Am J Occup Ther*. 1990;44:391-399.
4. Bouska MJ, Gallaway M. Primary visual deficits in adults with brain damage: management in occupational therapy. *Occup Ther Pract*. 1991;3:1-11.
5. Maples WC, Atchley J, Ficklin T. Northeastern State University College of Optometry's oculomotor norms. *J Beh Optometrist*. 1992;3:143-150.
6. Trobe JD, Acosta PC, Krischer JP, Trick GL. Confrontation visual field techniques in detection of anterior visual pathway lesions. *Ann Neurol*. 1981;10:28-34.
7. Harrington DO. *The Visual Fields: A Textbook and Atlas of Clinical Perimetry*. St. Louis, MO: CV Mosby; 1971:9.

Management of Refractive, Visual Efficiency, and Visual Information Processing Disorders

Mitchell Scheiman, OD, FCOVD, FAAO

Optometric Treatment Methods

This chapter is designed to describe various ways in which an occupational therapist can help in the management of patients with vision disorders. The first goal is to provide information about how optometrists treat various vision disorders using lenses, prism, occlusion, low vision aids, and vision therapy. The second objective is to provide detailed suggestions about how the occupational therapist can work along with the optometrist when managing children who are also being treated for a vision disorder. The final goal is to provide several treatment sequences that can be used by occupational therapists to supplement the vision therapy being performed by an optometrist in the areas of eye movements and visual information processing skills.

This chapter describes treatment for school-aged children and adults with normal cognitive ability. Children with learning disabilities or children and adults with mild cognitive and perceptual problems after acquired brain injury could also be treated according to the guidelines established in this chapter. Chapters Ten and Twelve deal specifically with treatment issues related to children functioning at a lower level and to children and adults with acquired brain injury with moderate to severe sequelae.

The tools that optometrists use to treat vision problems are lenses, prism, occlusion, low vision aids, and vision therapy. These treatment modalities can be used in isolation or in combination.

Use of Lenses

Lenses are effective for the treatment of various forms of refractive error including myopia, hyperopia, and astigmatism. Optometrists are often asked whether the child's nearsightedness or farsightedness will decrease as a result of wearing eyeglasses. The lenses that are prescribed are not intended to remediate or eliminate the refractive disorder. Rather, the eyeglasses are compensatory and allow the individual to see clearly while wearing the glasses.

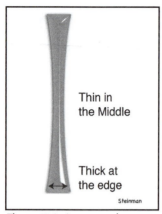

Thin in
the Middle

Thick at
the edge

Steinman

Figure 7-1. A concave lens or a "minus lens" used to treat myopia. (Reprinted with permission from Scheiman M, Scheiman M, Whittaker SG. *Low Vision Rehabilitation: A Practical Guide for Occupational Therapists*. Thorofare, NJ: SLACK Incorporated; 2007.)

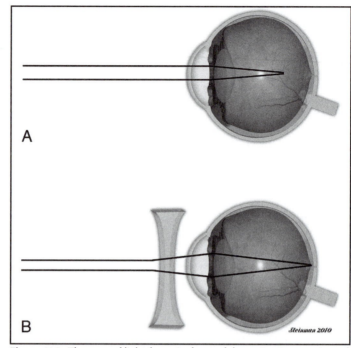

Figure 7-2. The rays of light focus in front of the retina in myopia and a concave or minus lens moves the point of focus to the plane of the retina.

Lenses for Myopia

Lenses have a very beneficial effect on myopia—immediately restoring clear vision. The type of lens that is used is called a concave lens or a "minus lens" (Figure 7-1). As described in Chapter Three, the rays of light focus in front of the retina in myopia, and a concave or minus lens moves the point of focus to the plane of the retina (Figure 7-2). Because myopia is a condition that generally causes reduced vision only at far, a decision has to be made about when the patient should wear the eyeglasses. Sometimes, it is only necessary to have the patient wear glasses for far tasks, such as driving and watching television and movies. When the degree of myopia is high or if in addition to myopia the patient has astigmatism, glasses may be prescribed for full-time wear. In some situations, the prescription that enables the patient to see at far is actually inappropriate for close work and tends to cause esophoria and accommodative problems that lead to eyestrain and discomfort. If this problem is detected during the examination, several options are available. In some cases, we simply ask the patient to remove the glasses for all reading tasks.

In certain situations, however, such as when treating a school-aged child, frequent removal of the glasses would be inconvenient and problematic. If the child is copying from the chalkboard and needs the glasses to see the board but needs to remove the glasses when he or she looks down at the desk, copying will be very difficult. A similar problem might occur with an adult working in an office setting. If this individual needs glasses to see across the room and to walk around but not for the computer terminal or deskwork, he or she will need to repeatedly remove the glasses. In both situations, we often prescribe a bifocal lens. With this type of lens, we can prescribe the best lens for distance and the best lens for near, allowing the patient to comfortably wear the eyeglasses at all times.

Myopia is a vision problem that in some cases can also be controlled or reduced using special intervention procedures. While some forms of myopia are based on hereditary factors, other forms may be environmental in nature.

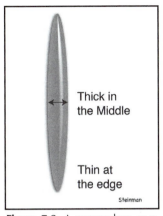

Figure 7-3. A convex lens or a "plus lens" used to treat hyperopia. (Reprinted with permission from Scheiman M, Scheiman M, Whittaker SG. *Low Vision Rehabilitation: A Practical Guide for Occupational Therapists.* Thorofare, NJ: SLACK Incorporated; 2007.)

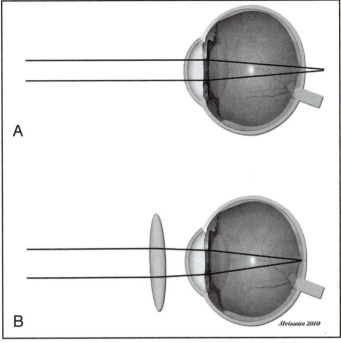

Figure 7-4. In hyperopia, the rays of light focus behind the retina. A convex or plus lens moves the point of focus to the plane of the retina.

LENSES FOR HYPEROPIA

The type of lens that is used for hyperopia is called a convex lens or a "plus lens" (Figure 7-3). In hyperopia, the rays of light focus behind the retina. A convex or plus lens moves the point of focus to the plane of the retina (Figure 7-4). Most people are slightly hyperopic, and glasses are not prescribed for all degrees of hyperopia. When the amount of hyperopia becomes clinically significant, however, glasses are prescribed because significant uncorrected hyperopia can lead to discomfort, eyestrain, blurred vision, and difficulty with attention and concentration when reading. Eyeglasses may be prescribed just for reading and close work, or if the amount of hyperopia is large enough, glasses may be necessary for full-time wear.

Esophoria, intermittent esotropia, and constant esotropia are conditions that are often associated with hyperopia, and the final eyeglass prescription must take these conditions into account as well. In most cases, prescribing for hyperopia has a beneficial effect on these binocular vision problems as well. Occupational therapists will often have to deal with an important issue when working with patients wearing glasses for hyperopia. If the patient is a child and unless the degree of hyperopia is very large, it is usually possible for the child to see just as clearly without as with the glasses. As discussed in Chapter Four, patients can overcome the blurred vision caused by hyperopia by accommodating. Because children can generally see as well without the glasses, we sometimes encounter problems with compliance. The occupational therapist will experience this when dealing with these children. It is important, therefore, to understand the importance of wearing glasses in cases of hyperopia and to reinforce this message. We usually tell parents that the glasses are not being prescribed to make the child's vision clear, rather the purpose of the glasses is to make vision comfortable and to allow the child to concentrate more effectively in school.

LENSES FOR ASTIGMATISM

Astigmatism is a condition that can cause reduced visual acuity at both far and close distances. It also has a differential effect, and rather than causing blurred vision of all aspects of the stimulus, it is selective for one orientation over others. For instance, one common type of astigmatism causes blurred vision of vertical lines but leaves horizontal lines unaffected. This is the reason why the lenses used to correct astigmatism are different from those used to treat hyperopia and myopia. The type of lens used to treat astigmatism is called a cylindrical lens and has different powers in different parts of the lens.

If a significant degree of astigmatism is left uncorrected, it can lead to eyestrain, headaches, and difficulty sustaining attention when reading. Thus, astigmatism is more similar to hyperopia than myopia. The human visual system is able to accommodate to overcome the blur caused by hyperopia and astigmatism. Accommodation has no beneficial effect with myopia. In astigmatism, accommodation is only partially effective, unlike in hyperopia in which accommodation can effectively eliminate the blur. Optometrists sometimes prescribe for mild to moderate degrees of astigmatism because the individual complains of discomfort and eyestrain, although the visual acuity may be adequate. The compliance problem mentioned above relative to hyperopia, therefore, applies to astigmatism as well. A young child may say that he or she sees just as well without as with the glasses and may object to wearing them. It is important that the occupational therapist reinforce the need to wear the glasses and that the purpose is not to make things clearer but to make the vision more comfortable.

LENSES FOR ACCOMMODATIVE PROBLEMS

In Chapter Four, I reviewed the four primary types of accommodative disorders: accommodative insufficiency, excess, infacility, and presbyopia. The treatment of choice for two of the four common accommodative problems (accommodative insufficiency and presbyopia) is lenses for reading. In both cases, the individual has lost the ability to effectively focus on objects that are brought close to him or her, such as reading from a book. The type of lens used is a convex or plus lens, and these lenses actually do some of the focusing for the individual, allowing him or her to use less effort. This tends to relieve the discomfort and blurred vision associated with accommodative insufficiency and presbyopia.

Because the eyeglasses used to treat these two conditions are only appropriate for close work, the individual will experience blurred vision when looking at a far object if the glasses are not removed. This can be an inconvenience in certain situations. For example, a school-aged child will need to remove and replace the glasses repeatedly during the day when copying from the board. An adult who works in an office setting requiring deskwork and movement throughout the office will have similar problems. To overcome these difficulties, we prescribe bifocal lenses. The top of the bifocal in many cases may have no prescription at all, but allows the individual to see clearly when he or she looks at an object located at a distance.

LENSES FOR BINOCULAR VISION PROBLEMS

A number of binocular vision disorders can be treated with eyeglasses. The two broad categories of binocular vision problems are esodeviations (eyes turn in) and exodeviations (eyes turn out). When the eyes turn in (esotropia) or have a tendency to turn in (esophoria), lenses tend to be very helpful. The use of a convex or plus lens will decrease the tendency for the eye to turn in and will have a beneficial effect on esodeviations. If the esodeviation is the same at distance and at far, a regular eyeglass prescription can be used. If the esodeviation is larger at near than at far, a bifocal may be necessary.

In cases of exodeviations in very young children or in children or adults who do not have the attention and cognitive ability necessary to benefit from vision therapy, minus lenses can sometimes help. Minus lenses tend to help the eyes turn inward and assist the patient in trying to use both eyes together. These lenses do not provide a long-term solution, however, and are usually used for short periods of time or as an aid in vision therapy.

LENSES FOR AMBLYOPIA

Two common forms of amblyopia called anisometropic and isometropic amblyopia are caused by a refractive condition of the eye. An essential part of the treatment program for these conditions is the use of eyeglasses. Eyeglasses are prescribed for full-time wear, and in many cases, additional treatment modalities such as occlusion therapy (patching) and vision therapy are required as well. Success in these cases is very dependent on the use of eyeglasses, and occupational therapists treating children with such problems can play an important role by reinforcing the need to wear the glasses.

LENSES FOR PREVENTION OF VISION PROBLEMS

Optometrists believe that some vision problems develop over time as a result of environmental factors. Myopia and some binocular vision and accommodative disorders fall into this category. In today's society, with the emphasis on reading and computer work, a great deal of stress is placed on the visual system. While some people can effectively deal with this stress, others experience great discomfort and interference with functional performance. Skeffington[1] refers to this as the socially compulsive, biologically unacceptable near point stress and believes this is the etiology of many of the visual problems people experience. According to Skeffington, refractive, binocular, and accommodative disorders are adaptations to the basic problem of excessive stress on the visual system. He developed an approach that includes the use of plus lenses and vision therapy to help prevent and reduce vision problems caused by environmental factors. The use of such lenses is an attempt to decrease the stress on the visual system and help restore the normal equilibrium that should be present. While there is some disagreement in the optometric profession about this theory, it is popular enough that occupational therapists will certainly see many patients who might be wearing lenses for this purpose. It is important, therefore, to understand that glasses may be prescribed for prevention of vision problems and to help reinforce compliance.

SUMMARY

Lenses are used very often in the treatment of refractive, accommodative, and binocular vision disorders, but they generally do not "correct" or eliminate the existing condition. Rather, in most cases, lenses allow the person to compensate and function visually in spite of the presence of an underlying vision disorder. In certain circumstances, optometrists may prescribe lenses to either try to prevent the development of vision problems or to try to reverse some of the adverse adaptations that may have occurred. Compliance with the doctor's wearing instructions is very important, and eye doctors need as much assistance from as many people as possible to ensure that eyeglasses are worn properly. In cases such as hyperopia, binocular vision, and accommodative disorders and amblyopia, poor compliance with the doctor's instructions can lead to decreased functional performance and lack of progress in treatment. Occupational therapists are in an ideal position to help in this way.

While most patients receive single vision lenses, some vision problems require the use of bifocals as described above. Bifocals are, therefore, not just for older adults; many children and young adults require bifocals as well. It is important for occupational therapists to have some insight into the reasons for bifocals to reinforce the need and importance of the eyeglasses in such cases. This means that communication between the optometrist and occupational therapist is important. You should certainly receive a complete report from any eye doctor who examines a patient who is under your care. It is wise to ask the patient or parent to request such a report as soon as you know such an examination will be taking place.

Figure 7-5. Two defining characteristics of any prism: the base and the apex. The base of a prism is the thicker portion.

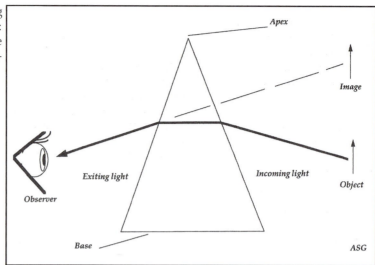

Use of Prism

A prism is a wedge-shaped lens that is thicker on one side than the other. Prisms, unlike lenses used to treat refractive error, do not have any optical power. Rather, the purpose of a prism is to deflect or bend the light rays in such a way so that the eyes can function more effectively as a team. Prism is used for three purposes in optometric care, 1) to treat some binocular vision disorders, 2) to expand visual field in patients with hemianopia, and 3) to modify posture and balance.

Figure 7-5 illustrates the two defining characteristics of any prism: the base and the apex. The base of a prism is the thicker portion. When prescribing prism to compensate for binocular vision problems, we prescribe base-in, base-out, base-down, or base-up prism. This refers to the location of the base of the prism relative to the patient's eye. In Figure 7-6a, the base-in prism is in front of the right eye, and in Figure 7-6b, the base-up prism is in front of the right eye. To treat exophoria, we prescribe base-in prism before both eyes; and for esophoria, we prescribe base-out before both eyes. For a vertical deviation, base-down prism is placed before one eye, and base-up in front of the other.

Figure 7-6a. Base-in prism in front of the right eye.

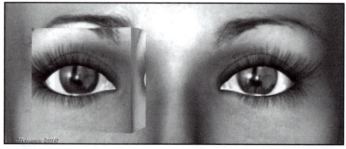

Figure 7-6b. Base-up prism in front of the right eye.

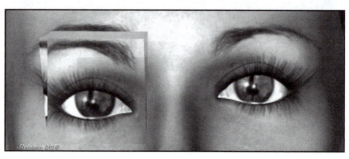

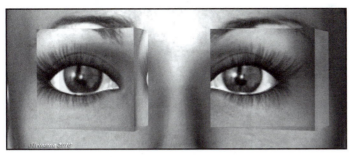

Figure 7-7. Example of yoked prism with the base of the prism to the left of the right eye and to the left of the left eye.

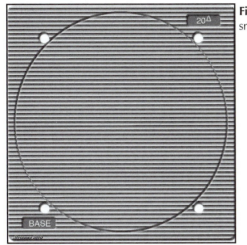

Figure 7-8. A Fresnel prism is a flexible, plastic sheet with small ridges.

A less commonly prescribed type of prism is called conjugate, or yoked, prism. A yoked prism prescription differs from the compensatory prism described above because the base of the prism will always be on the same side for each eye. For example, in Figure 7-7, the base of the prism is to the left of the right eye and to the left of the left eye. Compare this to Figure 7-6a, in which compensatory prism to correct for exophoria is placed with the base to the right of the right eye. Yoked prisms can be used to expand visual field and treat midline shift syndrome.

Prisms are available in a variety of forms. In most instances, prism is ground into the optical lens that is used to correct the patient's refractive error. One of the common forms that occupational therapists will see is the Fresnel prism. A Fresnel prism is a flexible, plastic sheet with small ridges (Figure 7-8). This plastic sheet can be cut to the shape of the patient's eyeglass lens and adheres to the back surface of the lens. Fresnel prisms have two advantages over traditional prisms. We are able to try Fresnel prism on a temporary basis, inexpensively, without changing the patient's permanent lenses. Another advantage is that when the amount of prism power required is high, the traditional optical prism becomes so thick and heavy that it cannot be comfortably worn and is cosmetically unacceptable. Fresnel prism is lighter and less apparent.

PRISMS FOR BINOCULAR VISION DISORDERS

Figure 7-9 illustrates how prism helps a patient with a binocular vision disorder. In Figure 7-9, the eyes turn in (esotropia) as a result of traumatic head injury. If this patient is an adult, he or she will experience double vision because the light rays are focused on the fovea of the left eye but on a nonfoveal area of the retina on the right eye. If the two foveas are not simultaneously stimulated by similar objects, the perception of double vision occurs. To solve this problem, a prism has been placed in front of the deviated eye. As you can see, the effect of the prism is to bend the light back onto the fovea, restoring single, binocular vision.

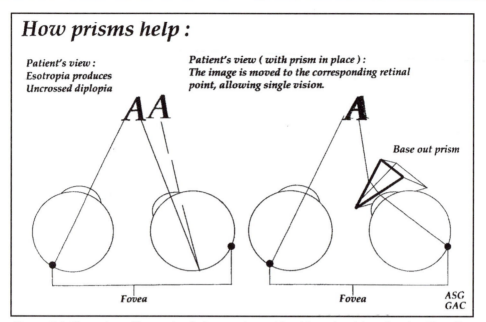

Figure 7-9. Illustration of how prism helps a patient with a binocular vision disorder. The effect of the prism is to bend the light back onto the fovea, restoring single, binocular vision.

Prisms are helpful for certain binocular vision problems because they decrease the demand of the neuromuscular components of the visual system. For example, if a child has an intermittent esotropia (the eyes turn in intermittently), the visual system will have to exert a great deal of neuromuscular effort to pull the eyes outward. This effort can lead to eyestrain, discomfort, and double vision when the effort cannot be sustained. The effect of prism is to simulate a decrease in the magnitude of the intermittent esotropia. This leads to a decrease in the amount of effort required to control the binocular problem. A reasonable analogy is to compare the use of prism for binocular disorders to the use of a cane for a muscle problem in the leg. Neither the prism nor the cane remediate the underlying problem, but while they are being used, the patient can function more effectively with less demand on the affected muscles.

Prisms are an important treatment modality for some binocular vision problems. As a general rule, prism tends to be more effective for esodeviations than for exodeviations.[2] In a recent randomized clinical trial, Scheiman et al[3] found that prism reading glasses were no more effective than placebo reading glasses for children with the most common exodeviation called convergence insufficiency. In adult patients, prism may be useful for convergence insufficiency based on another randomized clinical trial.[4] The most effective application of prism is in cases of vertical binocular vision disorders. In these cases, one eye drifts upward or downward. The capacity of the visual system to compensate for vertical deviation is very limited, and even the slightest tendency for this to occur is enough to make an individual uncomfortable and to cause significant functional problems in everyday life. The use of prism in such cases is highly effective. Prism is also used to treat certain types of constant strabismus in which the patient has developed very deeply ingrained adaptations, such as anomalous correspondence.

PRISMS FOR VISUAL FIELD DEFICITS

One of the most significant vision problems associated with traumatic brain injury and cerebrovascular accident is visual field loss. One of the treatment modalities available to help a patient compensate for this loss is prism. In recent years, studies[5,6] have demonstrated that a prism field

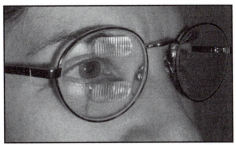

Figure 7-10. Peli Visual Field Expansion Device for Hemianopia is an effective treatment for patients with hemianopia.

expansion system called the Peli Visual Field Expansion Device for Hemianopia is an effective treatment for patients with hemianopia. As illustrated in Figure 7-10, a small horizontal segment of prism is placed above and below the patient's line of sight. This expands the visual field by as much as 30 to 40 degrees and allows the patient to be aware of potential obstacles in the periphery. A video simulation of this treatment method is available at www.eri.harvard.edu/faculty/peli/, and more information can be obtained from Chadwick Optical (White River Junction, VT), the company that produces the prism (http://chadwickoptical.com/hemianopia.htm).

PRISMS FOR MODIFICATION OF POSTURE AND BALANCE

In recent years, some optometrists have begun using prism to better posture and balance. This is referred to as the use of yoked prism. The two primary uses of yoked prism are to treat patients experiencing visual midline shift syndrome and to treat children with visual and behavioral problems associated with autism.

Focal and Ambient Visual Systems

The visual system is believed to be composed of two separate processes called the focal process and the ambient process. The focal process is related to the central visual function and the macula and provides information about objects at which the patient is looking. The ambient process provides information about location in space, balance, movement, coordination, and posture. After traumatic brain injury, the ambient visual process may lose its ability to match information with other sensory modalities causing difficulty with orientation in space, balance, movement, coordination, and posture.

Yoked or Ambient Prism Lenses for Visual Midline Shift Syndrome

When the prisms' bases face in the same direction in both eyes, they are called yoked. Designed to alter neural organization, yoked or ambient prisms may have an impact on the lives of those with autism and other delays or patients after acquired brain injury. Yoked or ambient prisms address a patient's ability to organize space and create a coherent body schema. These lenses are used therapeutically to change the neuromotor processing of the brain; after rehabilitation occurs, they are no longer needed.

Yoked prisms can cause the environment to appear to be curved up, down, left, or right. Objects may thus appear closer, farther away, or sloped. Prisms are employed in various magnitudes, which are measured in diopters. Altering both the magnitude and the direction of the prism can influence a patient's perception.

Kaplan[7] is the leading advocate of the use of yoked or ambient prism lenses to treat some of the visual and behavioral symptoms of autism. He suggests that yoked prisms deflect the light rays differently through the thin edge at the top and the thick edge at the base, influencing how the brain interprets where the body is in space. These prisms are designed to re-establish normal function of the ambient visual system. Kaplan et al[8] completed a double-blind crossover design study to assess the efficacy of wearing yoked or ambient lenses to reduce the behavioral symptoms of autism. Eighteen autistic individuals, ranging in age from 7 to 18 years, participated in the study. Behavior, attention, and orientation were evaluated at 1½, 2, 3, and 4 months. Compared to the placebo condition, the results showed a decrease in behavior problems at the 1½- and 2-month assessment periods and a slight loss of these benefits at the 3- and 4-month assessment periods. These findings support the prediction that ambient lenses have positive effects on autistic individuals. More study is necessary to demonstrate the effectiveness of these lenses. However, the treatment is relatively quick and inexpensive.

Visual Midline Shift Syndrome

Visual midline shift syndrome is a condition that is sometimes associated with acquired brain injury such as traumatic brain injury or stroke. In this condition the patient's midline shifts away from the center, usually away from the neurologically affected side of the body. Persons with a visual midline shift syndrome may walk as if the plane of the floor is tilted. Some patients report that the floor appears to be tilted. A potential treatment is to utilize yoked prisms before both eyes. The goal of the prism is to cause the midline to shift to a more centered position. This treatment has been popularized by Padula[9] in recent years, however, a randomized clinical trial is required to demonstrate its effectiveness. It is a relatively simple and inexpensive treatment option for such patients and, thus, worth an attempt even though there is limited research at this time.

Summary

Prisms have been used for many years for the treatment of binocular vision disorders. They do not "correct" or eliminate the existing binocular vision condition. Rather, prisms are used to allow the person to compensate and function visually in spite of the presence of an underlying vision disorder. More recent uses of prism have been introduced including expansion of visual field and attempts to modify visual behavior after acquired brain injury and in children with autism and other developmental delays. As with lenses, compliance with the doctor's wearing instructions is very important, and eye doctors need as much assistance from as many people as possible to ensure that eyeglasses are worn properly. Occupational therapists are ideal in helping in this way.

Use of Occlusion

Occlusion is used to actively treat amblyopia and strabismus, and as a last resort for patients with double vision who cannot be successfully treated using lenses, prism, vision therapy, or surgery. When prescribing occlusion, the clinician must make decisions about the type of occlusion, the amount of time to use occlusion, and which eye to occlude.

Types of Occlusion

The two types of occlusion are opaque and translucent. A variety of occlusion devices are illustrated in Figures 7-11a and 7-11b. The decision is based on the goal of the occlusion. If the objective is to force the patient to use the amblyopic type to achieve improvement in acuity, an opaque occluder is most desirable. Opaque occlusion completely eliminates all incoming visual stimulation and, therefore, tends to hasten progress. The disadvantage of opaque occlusion is that it has a poor cosmetic effect. When treating children with amblyopia, an opaque adhesive patch is generally recommended. Because this type of patch completely covers the eye, the child is unable to peek. A patch, such as the one illustrated in Figure 7-11b, although opaque, can easily be displaced by the child, and peeking could occur. This, of course, would prevent any progress.

Translucent occlusion is sometimes recommended if cosmesis is an issue. Another situation in which translucent occlusion is indicated for elimination of double vision is in an adult patient. A small, central circular patch using translucent tape is sometimes enough to help a patient avoid double vision (Figure 7-12).

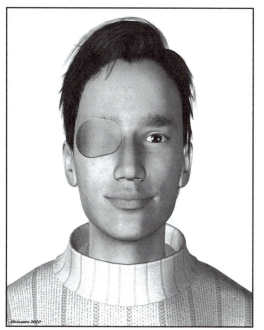

Figure 7-11a. Adhesive eye patch is an example of an opaque occlusion device.

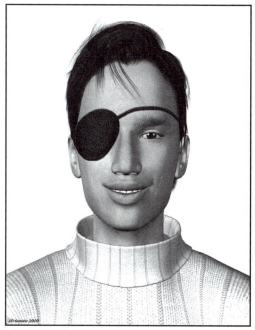

Figure 7-11b. Opaque occluder with elastic cord.

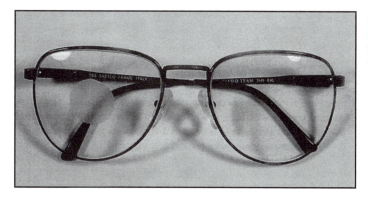

Figure 7-12. A small, central circular patch using translucent tape to help a patient avoid double vision.

THE AMOUNT OF TIME TO USE OCCLUSION

When treating amblyopia, the amount of time to occlude an eye is an important clinical decision. In children younger than 3 years of age, the visual system is still very plastic and susceptible to interference. Thus, long periods of constant, opaque occlusion can potentially lead to loss of vision in the dominant eye. Clinicians are very careful about the amount of time occlusion is used with infants and young children and re-evaluate often. As the child gets older, however, full-time or constant occlusion for strabismic amblyopia is commonly used.

When visual acuity is very poor, a child may have great difficulty functioning in school. In such cases, clinicians may initially decide to limit the amount of occlusion used. As visual acuity improves in the amblyopic eye, the amount of occlusion time can be increased.

OCCLUSION FOR AMBLYOPIA

Occlusion has been used for amblyopia treatment for more than 200 years. The rationale for using occlusion is that occluding the better eye stimulates the amblyopic eye. This stimulation allows the visual pathway of the amblyopic eye to develop, leading to improved visual acuity and function.

Full-time occlusion is generally recommended for constant strabismus, and part-time occlusion is recommended for intermittent strabismus. Part-time occlusion with an opaque patch is recommended for anisometropic amblyopia. Typically, about 2 to 6 hours of occlusion is recommended. The typical duration for occlusion therapy for strabismic or anisometropic amblyopia is 6 to 11 months with the maximum effect reached in the first 3 to 4 months.

OCCLUSION FOR STRABISMUS

In Chapter Four, I discussed the adaptations that occur in the visual system of a strabismic patient to eliminate double vision. Adaptations such as suppression and anomalous correspondence are common in patients with constant strabismus occurring before the age of 6 years. When both eyes are open, there is an active and constant need for these adaptations. If both eyes are allowed to remain open, these adaptations are constantly being reinforced and strengthened. If the goal of treatment is to restore normal binocular vision, it is important to use occlusion to prevent this reinforcement of suppression and anomalous correspondence. Therefore, even if a strabismic patient does not have amblyopia, occlusion may be used to eliminate binocular vision until the underlying problems are resolved.

OCCLUSION FOR ELIMINATION OF DIPLOPIA

Occlusion can also be used for patients experiencing annoying double vision. Double vision that cannot be eliminated with any form of treatment including lenses, prism, vision therapy, or surgery is referred to as intractable diplopia. This can occur in adults with acquired strabismus secondary to head trauma or with neurological disease. It is also a possible complication of strabismus surgery. When all other treatment modalities have failed, occlusion may be recommended as a last resort. When occlusion is used for intractable diplopia, the objective is to use a form of occlusion that has the least effect on cosmetic appearance. Small translucent patches are strategically placed on the patient's glasses. For example, if the double vision occurs when the patient looks down and to the right, the patch would be placed in the lower right-hand section of the right or left lens. In recent years, optometrists have also begun to use specially designed contact lenses that block the vision of one eye.

SUMMARY

Occlusion is an important optometric treatment modality. It is generally considered to be a passive form of therapy in contrast to vision therapy. Occlusion therapy is absolutely essential in the treatment of amblyopia and is an important auxiliary treatment method for strabismus.

Use of Low Vision Aids

Low vision is defined as reduced central visual acuity or visual field loss that even with the best optical correction provided by regular lenses results in visual impairment from a performance standpoint. Although the most important criterion is impairment of performance, for quantification purposes, visual acuity loss is usually used to help define whether a patient may benefit from low vision devices. Visual acuity of 20/70 or less (in the better eye) with best eyeglasses constitutes low vision.

The prevalence of low vision in the populations served by occupational therapists is significant. Visual field loss and decreased visual acuity are common problems associated with acquired brain injury. In the pediatric population, children with multiple impairments may also have either reduced visual acuity or visual field loss. It is likely that occupational therapists will encounter patients who require low vision aids.

TYPES OF AIDS

Low vision aids include a large variety of devices designed to help an individual function as well as possible in spite of visual loss. These aids are compensatory and do not resolve the underlying problem. Aids include specially designed eyeglasses, telescopes, microscopes, magnifiers, closed circuit television systems, contact lenses, reading stands, filters, large-print material, typoscopes, sunglasses, visors, and field expanders.

Telescopes

Telescopes are prescribed to improve performance for distance tasks of 10 feet or greater. Various designs are available, including telescopes that are hand-held and those that can be incorporated into the person's eyeglasses.

Microscopes

Microscopes are used for those tasks that require close work at distances from 2 to 20 cm. These devices usually are mounted in a frame, and various designs are available. Those that allow the largest field of view tend to interfere with mobility.

Magnifiers

Magnifiers are used to improve an individual's performance for near vision tasks. An advantage of a magnifier over a microscope is a longer working distance. As with all low vision devices, however, a longer working distance is achieved by sacrificing the size of the field of view. Many types of magnifiers are available including hand-held, standing, illuminated, and bar magnifiers.

Closed-Circuit Television System

This device provides an excellent field of view for performing close activities, and it provides high contrast and good magnification. Disadvantages are that most models are not portable and the equipment is expensive.

Field Expanders

A number of aids can help individuals with visual field loss. These include lenses, reverse telescopes, and Fresnel prism. Fresnel prism is often used to help people who experience visual field loss after acquired brain injury. This treatment approach is discussed in detail in Chapter Ten.

Other Aids

Other than the optical devices described previously, a number of nonoptical aids can be prescribed. Modification of illumination is very important for patients with low vision. Some patients require high, medium, or low levels of illumination. Large-print materials can be very helpful and include large-print books and large numbers for telephones and playing cards. Because low vision patients may need to hold a magnifier or other devices, stands are often helpful. These include reading stands, table easels, and music stands.

Chapters Thirteen through Fifteen cover the topics of low vision and low vision rehabilitation in detail.

SUMMARY

Individuals who have reduced visual acuity even with best correction or visual field loss may benefit from low vision aids. Prescribing low vision aids requires a great deal of experience. Often, the clinician must make a compromise between the best aid from an optical standpoint and the best aid from a cosmetic standpoint. There is no single aid that is optimal for all patients. Decisions about which aids are most appropriate require a full low vision evaluation by an experienced optometrist or ophthalmologist. Although the prescription of the most appropriate low vision aid is important, the second challenge is to help the patient learn how to use the aid successfully in activities of daily living. This is where the occupational therapist can play a very important role in the care of the patient with low vision. In many cases, co-management of patients with low vision by an optometrist and occupational therapist will lead to the best outcome.

Vision Therapy

WHAT IS VISION THERAPY?

Vision therapy, also known as orthoptics, vision training, visual training, and eye training, is an organized therapeutic regimen used to treat a number of neuromuscular, neurophysiological, and neurosensory conditions that interfere with visual function. Vision therapy encompasses a wide variety of procedures to improve a diagnosed neuromuscular or neurophysiological visual dysfunction. The treatment can be relatively simple, such as patching an eye as part of amblyopia therapy, or it may be complex, involving sophisticated instrumentation and computers.

Vision therapy usually involves a series of treatment visits during which carefully planned functional activities are carried out by the patient under close supervision in order to relieve the visual problem. The specific activities and instrumentation are determined by the nature and severity of the condition. The frequency and duration of treatments are dictated by the individual situation, although established guidelines, suggesting appropriate length of therapy for various diagnoses are available.

WHEN IS VISION THERAPY NECESSARY?

Most vision problems can be very easily corrected with eyeglasses. In fact, about 80% to 85% of the vision problems we detect can be treated with glasses or contact lenses. However, approximately 15% to 20% of the population with symptoms of blurred vision and eyestrain have vision problems that cannot be treated successfully using glasses alone. It is this group of people who need vision therapy. Vision therapy is generally required to treat problems of binocular vision, accommodation, eye movement, amblyopia, strabismus, and visual information processing disorders. Individuals with these problems experience eyestrain when reading or doing other close work, inability to work quickly, sleepiness, inability to attend and concentrate, double vision, and loss of vision. Even more significant, children with amblyopia and strabismus face the possible loss of vision if an appropriate vision therapy program is not initiated in a timely fashion. Children with visual information processing problems may have difficulty learning.

IS VISION THERAPY EFFECTIVE?

In recent years, evidence-based practice has become an important concept in all health care professions including optometry.[10,11] Evidence-based practice has been defined as the "integration of best research evidence with clinical expertise and patient values."[12] The best evidence is usually found in clinically relevant research that has been conducted using sound methodology.

Clinical research studies can be categorized based on the methodology used and is sometimes referred to as "levels of evidence" and is often portrayed as an evidence pyramid with case studies on the bottom and meta-analysis on top. A clinician may not always find the best level of evidence to answer a clinical question. The base of the pyramid is the weakest level of evidence and usually the most common type of study available. As you move up the pyramid the amount of available literature decreases, but increases in its relevance to the clinical setting. In the absence of the best evidence, the clinician needs to consider moving down the pyramid to other types of studies.

- A meta-analysis examines a number of valid studies on a topic and combines the results using accepted statistical methodology as if they were from one large study.

- Systematic reviews focus on a clinical topic and answer a specific question. An extensive literature search is conducted to identify all studies with sound methodology. The studies are reviewed, assessed, and the results summarized according to the predetermined criteria of the review question.

- Randomized controlled clinical trials are carefully planned projects that study the effect of a therapy on real patients. They include methodologies that reduce the potential for bias (randomization and masking) and that allow for comparison between intervention groups and control groups (no intervention).

- Cohort studies take a large population and follow patients who have a specific condition or receive a particular treatment over time and compare them with another group that has not been affected by the condition or treatment being studied. Cohort studies are observational and not as reliable as randomized controlled studies, since the two groups may differ in ways other than in the variable under study.

- Case series and case reports consist of collections of reports on the treatment of individual patients or a report on a single patient. Because they are reports of cases and use no control groups with which to compare outcomes, they have no statistical validity.

Studies have been performed to evaluate the methodological quality of journal articles in different medical specialties. Based on standardized criteria for the assessment of methodological rigor and clinical relevance of research articles, McKibbon et al demonstrated that only about 7% of articles published in the top 20 clinical journals in general internal medicine passed the prespecified criteria as having high methodological quality and clinical relevance.[13] A similar study in physical therapy found only 11% meeting the predefined standard.[14] Lai et al completed a similarly designed study for the ophthalmology literature and found that only 14.7% of the articles involving treatment passed the methodological assessment.[15]

Although a similar study has not been performed for the optometric literature on vision therapy, the results are likely to be comparable to other professions. Much of the literature on vision therapy effectiveness is based on case reports, case series, cohort studies, and literature reviews.[16-45] There have been some small placebo-controlled studies in the past[46-49] and recently a number of randomized clinical trials have been published.[50-53] The weight of the evidence supports the use of vision therapy for most nonstrabismic binocular vision, accommodative, and eye movement problems. Like all health care professions, optometry must strive to plan and implement more studies with rigorous design to investigate the effectiveness of commonly used treatments.

The prognosis for all accommodative and nonstrabismic binocular vision problems is good to excellent.[54] Studies investigating the clinical effectiveness of vision therapy for accommodative dysfunction have shown success in approximately 9 of 10 cases. In a retrospective study of 96 patients, Daum[29] found partial or total relief of both objective and subjective difficulties in 96% of the subjects studied. Hoffman et al[17] reported a vision therapy success rate of 87.5% in a sample of 80 patients with accommodative problems. Other studies, using objective assessment techniques, have investigated the actual physiological changes that occur due to vision therapy. Both Liu et al[24] and Bobier and Sivak[28] found that the speed and velocity of the accommodative response were significantly changed after therapy.

Numerous investigators have shown that vision therapy for nonstrabismic binocular vision disorders leads to improved physiological performance. In both prospective[26] and retrospective studies,[36] Daum showed that relatively short periods of vision therapy can provide long-lasting increases in fusional skills. Other studies have used both experimental and control groups to demonstrate the efficacy of binocular vision therapy.[46,47,49] Daum[49] investigated the effectiveness of vision therapy for improving fusional skills using a double-blind, placebo-controlled experimental design. He found statistically significant changes in the experimental group with no changes in the control group. Vaegan[46] also found large and stable improvement in his experimental group and no changes in the control group. Cooper et al[47] studied patients with convergence insufficiency using a matched subjects control group crossover design to reduce placebo effects. They found a significant reduction in symptoms and a significant increase in fusional skills after the treatment. During the control phase, significant changes in symptoms and vergence were not found.

Since 2005, the Convergence Insufficiency Treatment Trial Investigator Group has published the results of three randomized clinical trials demonstrating that office-based vision therapy is more effective than home-based vision therapy or a placebo control for the treatment of convergence insufficiency in both children and adults.[51-53]

In 2005, Scheiman et al[51] reported the results of a multi-center clinical trial of 47 children aged 9 to 18 years with symptomatic convergence insufficiency who were randomly assigned to receive a 12-week program of home-based pencil push-ups, office-based vision therapy, or office-based placebo therapy. Only patients in the office-based vision therapy group demonstrated both statistically and clinically significant changes in symptoms and clinical findings. In this study, office-based vision therapy was found to be more effective than home-based pencil push-ups or office-based placebo therapy in reducing symptoms and improving signs of convergence insufficiency. Moreover, it was the only treatment that resulted in normalization of convergence insufficiency-related symptoms and signs. Pencil push-up therapy was found to be no more effective than the placebo therapy. Similar results were reported by Scheiman et al in a study of 46 adult patients (19 to 30 years old) with convergence insufficiency.[52]

Most recently the same group of investigators reported the results of a large scale multi-center, randomized clinical trial of 221 children aged 9 to 17 years with symptomatic convergence insufficiency who were randomly assigned to receive a 12-week program of home-based pencil push-ups, home-based computer vision therapy and pencil push-ups, office-based vision therapy with home reinforcement, and office-based placebo therapy.[53] The results showed that 12 weeks of office-based vision therapy resulted in a greater percentage of patients reaching predetermined success criteria when compared with home-based pencil push-ups, home-based computer vision therapy and pencil push-ups, and office-based placebo therapy.

These recent high quality studies of the effectiveness of vision therapy for convergence insufficiency indicate that office-based vision therapy is the most effective treatment for the condition and should be the first-line treatment for convergence insufficiency.

Clinical studies have also been performed to investigate the efficacy of treating eye movement dysfunction. Wold et al[55] reported on a sample of 100 patients who had completed a vision therapy program for a variety of problems including accommodation, binocular vision, pursuits, and saccades. Saccadic and pursuit function was determined using subjective clinical performance scales like those described in Chapter Six. Pre- and post-testing revealed statistically significant changes in both saccadic and pursuit function.

In a more recent clinical study, Rounds et al[56] used an objective eye movement recording system to assess reading eye movements before and after vision therapy. Although no statistically significant changes were found, the experimental group showed trends toward improving reading eye movement efficiency (less regressions and number of fixations and increased span of recognition) compared to the control group.

Young et al[57] also used an objective eye movement recording instrument to assess reading eye movements before and after therapy. They studied 13 school children who had failed a vision screening. The children each had three 5-minute vision therapy sessions per day for 6 weeks. They received a total of 6 hours of eye movement vision therapy. Post-testing revealed a significant decrease in the number of fixations, an increase in reading speed, and a decrease in fixation duration.

Fujimoto et al[58] investigated the potential for using vision therapy procedures prerecorded on videocassettes for eye movement vision therapy. They had three groups of subjects. The first group of nine subjects received standard eye movement vision therapy. The second group received videocassette-based eye movement therapy, while the third group received no treatment. The results showed that both standard eye movement vision therapy and videocassette-based therapy were equally effective in improving saccadic ability.

When evaluating the efficacy of optometric vision therapy as a treatment tool for improving visual information processing skills, it is important to address two separate issues.[59] First, how effective is vision therapy at improving visual information processing skills? For example, when providing a therapy program for visual motor skills, is it likely that this ability will improve? Second, if there are improvements in visual information processing skills, is the child more available or responsive to educational instruction? That is, after remediation of specific visual deficits, will the child respond more appropriately to academic intervention for specific educational deficits?

In addressing the first issue, most studies evaluating the effectiveness of visual therapy have used a broad variety of training procedures in all three areas of visual information processing (visual spatial, visual analysis, and visual motor) at the same time. Academic performance was then re-evaluated following the treatment. Several of these studies have found significant improvements in visual information processing skills following therapy.[60,61] Studies that have concentrated on the treatment of isolated visual perceptual skills have also supported the effectiveness of therapy for visual spatial,[62,63] visual analysis,[64,65] and visual motor skills.[66] For example, Greenspan[63] administered a program of perceptual motor therapy that included therapy for bilaterality and body image development to a group of underachieving children and measured the frequency of reversal errors. The control group received only standard orthoptic therapy. The experimental group showed a statistically significant improvement in directionality and a reduction in the total number of reversal errors following the perceptual therapy. These studies indicate that the level of performance of individual visual information processing skills can be enhanced through an optometric vision therapy program designed to address specific visual information processing deficits.

Improving the ability of the child to benefit from academic instruction has been supported by similar research.[61,65,67-69] These studies have demonstrated statistically significant improvements in standardized tests of academic skills compared to a control group. For example, Seiderman[61] provided visual and perceptual therapy to 18 learning-disabled children who were matched with a control group. The experimental group showed an improvement on the Word Reading and Paragraph Meaning subtests of the Stanford Achievement Test.

These studies taken from an interdisciplinary group of researchers provide positive evidence that therapy for visual information processing can be expected to improve specific skills and help the child benefit from academic instruction. In reviewing the literature that addresses therapy for perceptual skills, Solan and Ciner[70] cite several factors that are important for a successful therapy program. First, the patient should have a documented perceptual deficit that is associated with the reading or learning disorder. Broad-based therapy programs to improve readiness skills in normal patients may not be effective. Second, therapy programs should be individualized to address the specific deficits that the patient manifests. Therapy programs should address specific problem areas while taking into account the patient's developmental level, auditory processing, and visual attention and cognitive style. Finally, therapy should complement and not replace reading and other educational instruction. The role of the optometrist in the management of visual information processing deficits is to improve visual spatial, visual analysis, and visual motor skills in those patients who manifest these problems. This should enable the patient to participate more effectively in the classroom and to benefit from other educational therapies.

This research indicates that significant scientific support exists for the effectiveness of vision therapy in modifying and improving ocular motor, accommodative, binocular, and visual information processing disorders.

Influence of Vision Deficits on Occupational Therapy

In Chapters Three through Five, we discussed visual acuity, refractive, eye disease, visual efficiency, and visual information processing problems. In these chapters, we also demonstrated that vision problems can interfere with a person's ability to participate in activities of daily living, such as caring for one's self, working, going to school, playing, and living independently. For occupational therapists to be maximally effective in rehabilitation, they must understand the complexity and importance of vision and take these problems into consideration when planning and implementing occupational therapy.

Occupational Therapy Intervention

Occupational therapy intervention for the various vision problems discussed in this book can take one of three forms: Supportive intervention, compensatory intervention, and direct remediation.

Supportive Intervention

First, the therapist can be supportive of the optometric treatment recommendations and help ensure that the patient follows the treatment recommendations at least during occupational therapy. In most cases, this would involve making sure that the patient wears the prescribed glasses, prisms, or eye patch in the appropriate manner. It is helpful to suggest different frame colors or some other identifying feature for patients who need different glasses for distance and for near.

Compensatory Intervention

The therapist may also be able to modify the task or the environment or help the patient compensate for the vision disorder in question in some other way. The goal should be to manipulate and organize the patient's visual environment so that he or she receives the highest level of visual processing possible in spite of the deficits. For instance, in situations in which visual acuity is not correctable with lenses, environmental adaptations may be helpful. Examples include enlarging targets, controlling contrast, and lighting. Limitations in eye movements may result in an inability to move the eyes up or down. Management in such cases involves raising or lowering the target or working area to accommodate the patient's needs. Tables 7-1 through 7-5 list the recommended supportive and compensatory interventions for each vision problem discussed in this book.

Direct Remediation

A third option in some cases is to attempt to actually eliminate or remediate the underlying vision problem and restore normal visual function. The remainder of this chapter provides detailed information and guidelines for direct remediation in the areas of ocular motor dysfunction and visual information processing disorders and describes a select group of therapy procedures. These procedures are not designed to be used by therapists in isolation of, or instead of, optometric intervention. My goal in this section is to address an issue that occurs virtually every time I co-manage a patient with an occupational therapist. In my clinical experience, the occupational therapist has a number of questions he or she wants me to answer when he or she refers a patient to me to rule out vision problems that could be affecting occupational therapy. Of course, he or she wants to know if any vision problems are present. If they are present, he or she wants to know how they may be affecting the patient's performance in a variety of functional activities and activities of daily living. Finally, the occupational therapist invariably would like to know how he or she can intervene to limit the negative effects of the vision problems on performance. He or she wants to know how to

Table 7-1

Vision Problems: Symptoms, Effect on Function, Occupational Therapy Management Suggestions—Visual Acuity, Refractive Conditions, and Eye Health Problems

Vision Problem	Symptoms and Effect on Function	Supportive and Compensatory Intervention	Direct Remediation
Reduced visual acuity (correctable with lenses)	• Blurred vision • Squinting • Holds objects close or must get close to objects • Avoids visual tasks	• Refer to an optometrist • If glasses are prescribed, support this recommendation and ensure compliance during OT procedures	• If treated early, visual acuity problems generally do not require direct remediation
Low vision: Reduced visual acuity (uncorrectable with lenses)	• Blurred vision • Squinting • Holds objects close or must get close to objects • Avoids visual tasks • Difficulty recognizing faces • Difficulty with mobility • Difficulty with activities of daily living with significant visual requirements (driving, reading, writing, grooming, finances, cooking, cleaning)	• Refer to an optometrist • If glasses or low vision devices are prescribed, support this recommendation and ensure compliance during occupational therapy procedures • Modify working distances for all tasks • Increase lighting • Increase contrast (white plates on dark placemats) • Reduce complexity of task • Enlarge all targets and print • Use visual markers to help patient keep place	• Direct remediation is not effective, only supportive and compensatory procedures are useful
Refractive conditions	• Blurred vision • Excessive effort • Discomfort when involved with any visual task • Squinting • Holds objects close or must get close to objects • Avoids visual tasks	• Refer to an optometrist • Glasses will be necessary • Encourage proper use of glasses • If loss of acuity has occurred, decrease the working distance • If patching is recommended, encourage proper use of the patch	• If treated early, refractive conditions generally do not require direct remediation

Table 7-2

Vision Problems: Symptoms, Effect on Function, Occupational Therapy Management Suggestions—Visual Field Deficits

Symptoms and
Effect on Function

- Walking: Inferior field loss causes difficulty with mobility; trouble seeing steps or curb; shortened and uncertain stride when walking; poor balance; tendency to trail behind others when walking; walks next to wall and holds onto wall with hands; uncomfortable in middle of room; anchored to ground; does not turn head as much; bumps into things frequently; disoriented when moving whether in car or walking
- Trouble identifying visual landmarks
- Superior field deficit causes difficulty seeing signs, worse if in wheelchair
- Leaves food on half of plate
- Misidentification of details; misreading of long words
- Difficulty with reading; misreads words; poor accuracy; slow reading rate; difficulty with page navigation; cannot stay on line
- Difficulty with writing; cannot stay on line; inaccurate with serious effects on check writing
- Self-grooming: Cannot find necessary items
- Dressing: Cannot find necessary items
- Telephone: Cannot take accurate messages
- Driving: Cannot drive usually
- Shopping: Cannot drive; cannot find items
- Emotional problems: Anxiety; reduced self-confidence; increased passivity; social isolation

Supportive and
Compensatory Intervention

- Referral for full vision examination
- Ensure use of appropriate glasses, which may incorporate lenses and prism
- Make patient aware of how visual defect interferes with various activities
- Emphasize conscious attention to detail
- Teach organized scanning techniques into deficient field
- Increase speed and accuracy of eye movements
- Use occlusion to force patient to look into deficient field
- Engage patient in as many real-life activities as possible
- Use ambulation as much as possible
- Use letter tracking and symbol tracking
- Provide markers to help reading
- When patient is writing, encourage him or her to look at pen or pencil tip

Direct Remediation

- Visual field defects cannot be improved through therapy although supportive and compensatory procedures can have great benefit

Table 7-3

Vision Problems: Symptoms, Effect on Function, Occupational Therapy Management Suggestions—Visual Efficiency Problems: Binocular Disorders

Vision Problem	Symptoms and Effect on Function	Supportive and Compensatory Intervention	Direct Remediation
Binocular vision disorders: Strabismic	• Cosmetic problem, the eyes looked crossed or "wall-eyed" • If intermittent, may cause double vision that can interfere with eye-hand and mobility tasks • If intermittent, may cause eyestrain • Loss of vision if left untreated and the strabismus is unilateral	• If strabismus is present, refer to an optometrist • Use eye patch to eliminate double vision during OT activities • Encourage use of an eye patch during OT, if prescribed by the optometrist	• Discuss issue of use of patch during OT procedures • Incorporate motility activities into OT program
Binocular vision disorders: Nonstrabismic	• Intermittent double vision • Discomfort and eyestrain for all visual tasks • Tires easily during occupational therapy session • Inattentive during occupational therapy session • Poor concentration • Loss of place when reading • Difficulty with eye-hand tasks • Difficulty with ADL that require stereopsis (driving, near tasks involving reaching for objects, pouring liquids)	• If symptoms present, refer to optometrist Glasses and prisms may be necessary—encourage compliance • If bifocals have been prescribed, ensure that the patient does close work while using the bottom of the bifocal • Use of patch may provide relief of symptoms until treatment is complete (consult with optometrist) • Use of guide on page may help decrease loss of place • Take frequent breaks • Reduce emphasis on tasks requiring intense visual attention • Reduce emphasis on tasks requiring stereopsis	• OTs who work with an optometrist in a rehabilitation hospital may be able to perform vision therapy procedures • Under all other conditions, only supportive and compensatory treatment is available
Amblyopia	• If unilateral, generally no symptoms • If bilateral, symptoms will be identical to low vision category although less severe	• Refer to optometrist • If patching is prescribed, ensure that the child uses the patch during OT procedures • During course of active amblyopia treatment, use compensatory approaches listed under "Low Vision" section	• The OT can have the child wear a patch while engaged in any OT procedure • OT may be able to incorporate ocular motility techniques while one eye is patched

Table 7-4

Vision Problems: Symptoms, Effects on Function, Occupational Therapy Management Suggestions—Visual Efficiency Problems: Accommodative and Ocular Motility Disorders

Vision Problem	Symptoms and Effect on Function	Supportive and Compensatory Intervention	Direct Remediation
Accommodative	• Discomfort and eyestrain for all visual tasks • Blurred vision • Rubs eyes • Tires easily during OT session • Inattentive during OT session • Poor concentration • Difficulty with ADL that require sustained close work	• If symptoms present, refer to optometrist • If glasses are prescribed, ensure compliance • If bifocals have been prescribed, ensure that patient does close work while using bottom of bifocal • Use of larger print may help provide relief of symptoms until treatment is complete • Take frequent breaks	• OTs who work with an optometrist in a rehabilitation hospital may be able to perform vision therapy procedures • Under all other conditions, only supportive and compensatory treatment is available
Ocular motility disorders	• Excessive head movement • Frequent loss of place • Skips lines • Poor attention span • Copying is slow and results poor with coloring and drawing • Difficulty with ADL that require frequent change in fixation and accurate eye movements (driving, reading, writing)	• Refer to optometrist for evaluation and treatment recommendations • Use of guide or finger is helpful while treatment is ongoing • De-emphasize tasks requiring precise and frequent eye movement skills	• OTs who work with an optometrist in a rehabilitation hospital may be able to perform vision therapy procedures • OTs in other settings can incorporate eye movement tasks into OT plan with supervision from optometrists; vision therapy suggestions in this book can provide basic guidelines

(continued)

Table 7-4

Vision Problems: Symptoms, Effects on Function, Occupational Therapy Management Suggestions—Visual Efficiency Problems: Accommodative and Ocular Motility Disorders (continued)

Vision Problem	Symptoms and Effect on Function	Supportive and Compensatory Intervention	Direct Remediation
Nystagmus	• Blurred vision • Squinting • Holds objects close or must get close to objects • Avoids visual tasks • Difficulty recognizing faces • Difficulty with mobility • Difficulty with ADL with significant visual requirements (driving, reading, writing, grooming, finances, cooking, cleaning)	• Refer to optometrist • If glasses are prescribed, support this recommendation and ensure compliance during OT procedures • Modify working distances for all tasks • Increase lighting • Increase contrast (white plates on dark placemats) • Reduce complexity of tasks • Enlarge all targets and print • Use visual markers to help patient keep his or her place	• Direct remediation is not effective; only supportive and compensatory procedures are useful

Table 7-5

Vision Problems: Symptoms, Effect on Function, Occupational Therapy Management Suggestions—Visual Information Processing Problems

Vision Problem	Symptoms and Effect on Function	Supportive and Compensatory Intervention	Direct Remediation
Visual perception disorders	• Confusion of left and right • Confusion of likenesses and differences • Tends to use other senses to make what should be visual discriminations • Unable to selectively attend to appropriate visual stimulus • Performs tasks slowly • Ignores details during visual tasks • Poor recall of visually presented material • Sloppy drawing skills • Difficulty with copying and getting thoughts down on paper • Difficulty with most ADL that have a high demand on visual information processing (driving, reading, writing, sports, mobility)	• Refer to optometrist for consultation to rule out visual acuity, refractive, eye health, and visual efficiency problems • Simplify visual tasks • Careful design of OT program to take attention factors into consideration • Eliminate extraneous distractions • Limit amount of visual stimuli • Use high-contrast stimuli	• OT uses approaches such as sensory motor integration or NDT • OT may prescribe visual perceptual therapy or work together with an optometrist

---

Table 7-6

General Guidelines and Principles for Vision Therapy

- Determine a level at which the patient can perform easily.
- Be aware of the patient's frustration level.
- Use positive reinforcement.
- Maintain an effective training level.
- Make the patient aware of the goals of vision therapy.
- Set realistic therapy objectives and maintain flexibility with these objectives or endpoints.

---

be supportive and help the patient compensate and if there is anything he or she can possibly do to help in the direct remediation of the vision problem.

My approach has always been to encourage therapists to help me with the direct intervention. I believe these patients require as much reinforcement and therapy as possible. If I am seeing the child once or twice a week and vision therapy is reinforced by the occupational therapist at other times, progress is enhanced. It is important to understand that the procedures described below are not a substitute for optometric vision therapy. Rather, the occupational therapist can supplement the work being done in vision therapy. The techniques I describe below can be used by therapists to supplement optometric vision therapy being done in the optometric office. If an occupational therapist uses these procedures, then a very close working relationship with the optometrist and a coordination of techniques are critical.

Another situation in which an occupational therapist may perform vision therapy techniques under the supervision of an optometrist is in a rehabilitation setting. A trend that is becoming more common is that optometrists are becoming more directly involved in the care of patients with acquired brain injury within rehabilitation hospitals. In most cases, the optometrist examines the patient within the hospital and prescribes appropriate treatment that may include lenses, prism, occlusion, and vision therapy. The vision therapy is carried out in the hospital by occupational therapists under the supervision of the optometrist (see Chapters Nine and Ten for more detail).

General Principles and Guidelines for Vision Therapy

Before discussing specific vision therapy procedures, it is important to understand that there are general principles and guidelines that apply to all vision therapy techniques. Vision therapy is similar in many ways to other types of therapy that involve learning and education. If we look at other types of learning, it becomes clear that there are specific guidelines to facilitate learning and success. Because vision therapy can be considered a form of learning and education, similar principles and guidelines must be used to achieve success.

The following guidelines have been derived from basic learning theory (Table 7-6):

- Determine a level at which the patient can perform easily. Working on this level makes it easier for the patient to become aware of the important feedback cues, strategies, and objectives involved in vision therapy and also builds confidence and motivation.
- Be aware of the patient's frustration level. Signs of frustration include general nervous and muscular tension, hesitating performance, and possibly a desire to avoid the task.
- Use positive reinforcement. The patient should be rewarded for attempting a task, even if it is not successfully completed. Reinforcers can be verbal praise, tokens that can be exchanged for prizes, or participation in a task that the patient enjoys.
- Maintain an effective training level. Start at the initial level at which the task is easy, and gradually increase the level of difficulty, being very careful to watch for signs of frustration.

Vision therapy should be success oriented (ie, built on what the patient can do successfully as opposed to giving tasks that are too difficult).

- Make the patient aware of the goals of vision therapy. The patient must know why he or she is in vision therapy. He or she should be able to explain what his or her problem is, how it affects performance, and the goals of vision therapy. This is true for children as well as adults. Even with a young child, the therapist should try to establish some understanding on the part of the child about what is wrong with his or her eyes and why vision therapy is necessary. For each therapy technique, the child should be able to explain what he or she needs to do to accomplish the desired task.

- Set realistic therapy objectives and maintain flexibility with these objectives or endpoints. With all therapy techniques, we expect to achieve certain general objectives before we proceed to the next procedure. In this text, we call these objectives endpoints. It is important to understand that these endpoints are only guidelines and that flexibility and clinical judgment are ultimately just as important in deciding when to move on to another procedure. The objective of vision therapy is to solve the patient's problems as quickly as possible.

Computer-Based Versus Non-Computer-Based Vision Therapy

Computers and computer software have become an important component of vision therapy in recent years. Vision therapy can certainly be performed without any computer software and I have included many non-computer-based techniques in this chapter. However, just as computer software has enhanced many aspects of our lives and the way we function, computer software has become an important element of vision therapy. Today our patients are very comfortable and familiar with computers and almost expect the use of computers in all aspects of their lives.

There are a number of excellent vision therapy software programs available, but most can only be purchased by a licensed optometrist. Occupational therapists do have one vision therapy software program available to them that can be used for both eye movement and visual processing therapy. It is called Tracking and Perceptual Skills for Occupational Therapists (TPOT).

TPOT is a software program designed to be used by occupational therapists and other therapists for vision rehabilitation of eye movement and visual processing problems. The software can be used with both children (as young as 6 years old) and adults. TPOT contains 14 different programs that can be used for remediation of eye movement and visual processing problems.

TPOT has procedures for the remediation of the following vision problems:

- Eye movement problems
- Saccadic dysfunction (tracking)
- Visual processing problems
- Visual spatial dysfunction
- Visual analysis dysfunction

The TPOT software can be used with children with developmentally based eye movement and visual processing disorders and adults and children after acquired brian injury with acquired eye movement and visual processing disorders. In both cases the TPOT software can be a useful tool to supplement other therapeutic activites.

The TPOT software can be used in an office or clinic setting as part of an overall therapy program, or the software can be sent home so that the patient can supplement the office-based vision rehabilitation with home-based treatment. We suggest that patients work 5 days per week, 20 minutes per day working with the TPOT software at home.

The TPOT software can be ordered at www.visionedseminars.com.

Ocular Motor Therapy: Specific Guidelines

- In all cases of ocular motility dysfunction, consider optical correction of refractive problems before beginning vision therapy. These problems should always be managed in conjunction with an optometrist.
- In all cases of ocular motility dysfunction, consider treatment of accommodative and binocular vision disorders before beginning vision therapy for ocular motor problems.
- Begin working with a technique that is within the capabilities of the patient.
- It is important to achieve some early success.
- Emphasize accuracy first and then speed of either the saccadic or pursuit eye movement.
- Many children with ocular motor dysfunction also have attention problems and impulsive cognitive styles. In fact, sometimes it is not clear if the impulsivity and inattention are the etiology for the poor fixation and ocular motility or whether the motility problems are the basis for the attention and impulsivity problems. To try to slow the child down and work toward encouraging a more reflective, thoughtful, analytical style, we recommend stressing accuracy of the response at first. As accuracy improves during therapy, speed can then be incorporated as a variable.
- For saccades, go from gross (large) to fine (small) eye movements. For pursuits, the sequence is the opposite, from fine (small) to gross (large) eye movements.
- Begin motility therapy monocularly, and continue until both eyes are approximately equal in ability. Once monocular skills are equal, accurate, and fast, begin binocular ocular motility activities.
- Eliminate head movements during both pursuit and saccadic eye movements that can be reasonably accomplished without head movement.
- Increase the complexity of the task to develop more reflexive, automated pursuits and saccades. This can be accomplished by adding a metronome, a balance board, or simple cognitive tasks during any ocular motility task.

Vision Therapy Techniques for Saccades and Pursuits

The techniques described below should be effective for children and adults functioning at a 5- to 6-year-old level and above (Table 7-7). For patients performing below this level, refer to Chapters Ten and Twelve.

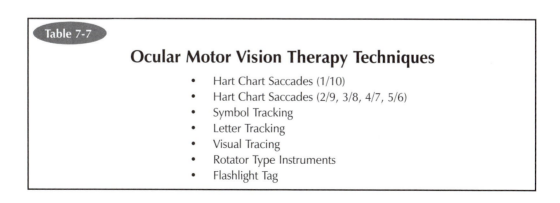

Table 7-7

Ocular Motor Vision Therapy Techniques

- Hart Chart Saccades (1/10)
- Hart Chart Saccades (2/9, 3/8, 4/7, 5/6)
- Symbol Tracking
- Letter Tracking
- Visual Tracing
- Rotator Type Instruments
- Flashlight Tag

Non-Computer-Based Therapy Techniques
HART CHART: SACCADIC THERAPY
Objective
The objective of the Hart Chart for saccadic therapy is to increase the speed and accuracy of saccadic fixation.

Equipment Needed
*   Large Hart Chart for distance viewing
*   Eye patch

Description and Setup
Place the Hart Chart (Figure 7-13) about 5 to 10 feet from the patient. Occlude the patient's left eye with an eye patch, and instruct the patient to call out the first letter in column 1 and then the first letter in column 10, the second letter from the top in column 1 and the second letter from the top in column 10, the third letter from the top in column 1 and the third letter from the top in column 10, and so on. Continue until the patient has called out all letters from columns 1 and 10. As the patient calls out the letters, write down his or her responses, and when the task is completed, have the patient check his or her accuracy. Requiring the patient to check for errors is in itself another saccadic therapy technique. Now, the patient will have to make saccades from far to near to check for errors.

Once this task can be completed in about 15 seconds without any errors, you can increase the level of difficulty in several ways. Ask the patient to continue calling out letters in the other columns. Specifically, after completing columns 1 and 10, have the patient call out columns 2 and 9, 3 and 8, 4 and 7, and 5 and 6. The inner columns are more difficult because they are surrounded by other targets.

An even greater level of difficulty can be achieved by requiring saccades from the top of one column to the bottom of another. Instead of a left to right and right to left saccade, the patient will have to make an oblique saccade. For example, ask the patient to call out the top letter in column 1 and then the bottom letter in column 10, the second letter from the top in column 1 and the second letter from the bottom in column 10. Continue this pattern through the entire chart.

Other variations to increase the level of difficulty are possible, including incorporating the beat of a metronome and requiring the patient to maintain balance on a balance board while engaged in the task.

Endpoint
Discontinue this technique when the patient can complete columns 1 and 10 in 15 seconds with no errors, and all of the internal columns in 2 minutes with no errors.

ANN ARBOR LETTER AND SYMBOL TRACKING
Objective
The objective of the Letter and Symbol Tracking is to increase the speed and accuracy of saccadic fixation.

Equipment Needed
*   Ann Arbor Letter and Symbol Tracking workbooks
*   Plastic sheet, 8½ x 11 inches
*   Paper clip
*   Pen used for overhead transparencies (washable type)
*   Eye patch

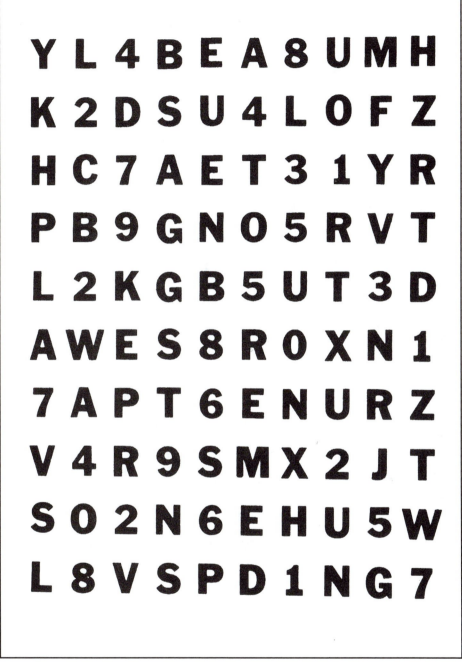

Figure 7-13. The Hart Chart used to increase the speed and accuracy of saccadic fixation.

Description and Setup

Figures 7-14 and 7-15 illustrate the two workbooks. Both are designed to improve saccadic accuracy and speed. To permit the repeated use of the workbooks, I suggest that you cover the page being used with a plastic sheet and secure the plastic with a paper clip. I use overhead transparency sheets for this purpose.

A B C D E F G H I J K L M N O P Q R S T U V W X Y Z
a b c d e f g h i j k l m n o p q r s t u v w x y z

19

Iln chako evi nomd zeby thipg nare.
Zuth pirm nuroc dif stok. Nileg myt
lolf. Tixs nom raus zab tuin lugah.
Marb sewt rotsir puje. Yonak nesud
voz alee. Xart chod bugm turh sref
trea gen foru. Vab reps tique kowj.
Dagh meulb fwer ilg sida. Ubc they
bouf yed neoph vaik. Wolen kig peab
nad tenc xerb. Rait rebey fal zibt

_____ Min. _____ Sec.

Kog dalp stey molb ihn zurc taiwf
pim noxod. Prus myl wof kipet ghul.
Zalv ubx pufo cirk ghons taw. Quos
mey lairp sut vaej obk tund zoelec
pech. Tym surg aben burz. Dof terav
tecib ulaw kars fups. Irt quech adg
doif vok nebel ach laurt. Goxe misd
chitk queal doj neav libef tagow.
Ligeh axd yabel fom nepok ratzin

_____ Min. _____ Sec.

Figure 7-14. Ann Arbor Letter Tracking workbook designed to improve saccadic accuracy and speed.

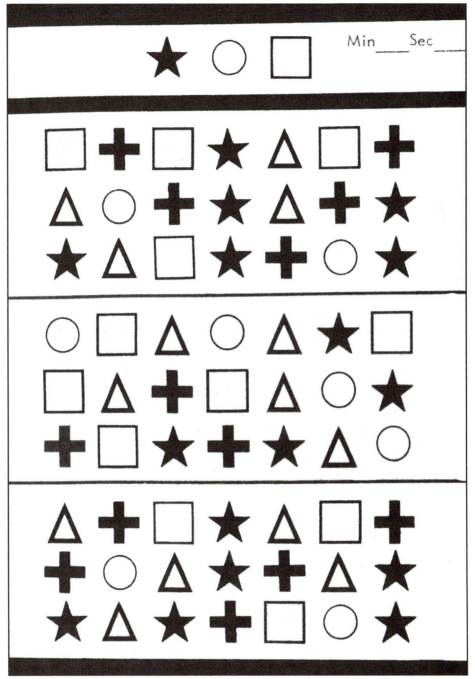

Figure 7-15. Ann Arbor Symbol Tracking workbook designed to improve saccadic accuracy and speed.

As you can see in Figure 7-14, each page of Letter Tracking has two or more paragraphs of what appears to be random letters. Occlude one of the patient's eyes, and tell the patient to begin at the upper right and scan from left to right to find the first letter "A" and then make a line through it. Ask the patient to then find the very first "B" and cross it out, and continue through the entire paragraph finding the letters of the alphabet in order. The goal is to complete this task as quickly as possible. The therapist should time the therapy procedure. The patient's accuracy can also be evaluated. If the patient is scanning for the very first letter "D" for instance and inadvertently misses it and finds a "D" later in the paragraph, he or she will be unable to find the entire alphabet sequence in the paragraph. The workbook has five different size letters, creating another level of difficulty.

I suggest that after the patient finds and marks a specific letter, the pen be lifted off the page so that the patient will have to use saccades to find the next letter.

If the patient experiences difficulty with this task, Symbol Tracking (see Figure 7-15) can be used. Children in first grade will sometimes have difficulty because of lack of familiarity with the alphabet. This can cause great frustration and make the therapy technique very unpleasant for the patient. In such cases, use Symbol Tracking, which uses large pictures, symbols, numbers, and fewer letters. The task is, therefore, considerably easier and is very useful with younger children or those with very severe ocular motility disorders.

Endpoint

Discontinue this technique when the performance in each eye is approximately equal and when the patient can successfully complete the paragraphs in about 1 minute.

VISUAL TRACING

Objective

The objective of this technique is to improve the accuracy and speed of pursuit eye movements.

Equipment Needed

- Visual tracing workbooks
- Plastic sheet, 8½ x 11 inches
- Paper clip
- Pen used for overhead transparencies (washable type)
- Eye patch

Description and Setup

Figure 7-16 provides an illustration of the visual tracing workbooks. The workbook contains tracing tasks that gradually increase in level of difficulty from the beginning to the end of the book. Two therapy methods can be used. The easiest procedure is to occlude one of the patient's eyes and ask the patient to place the pen on the letter "A" and trace along the line until the end of the line. The objective is for the patient to determine the number at the end of the line beginning with the letter "A." Instruct the patient to then continue until he or she has found the answer for each line.

As the patient's accuracy and speed improve, the next level of difficulty can be added. In this technique, the patient must perform the same task using just his or her eyes. The patient must make a pursuit eye movement without the support of following the line with the pencil.

Endpoint

There are no specific clinical guidelines for this procedure. Continue this technique until the patient can perform with a reasonable degree of accuracy and speed.

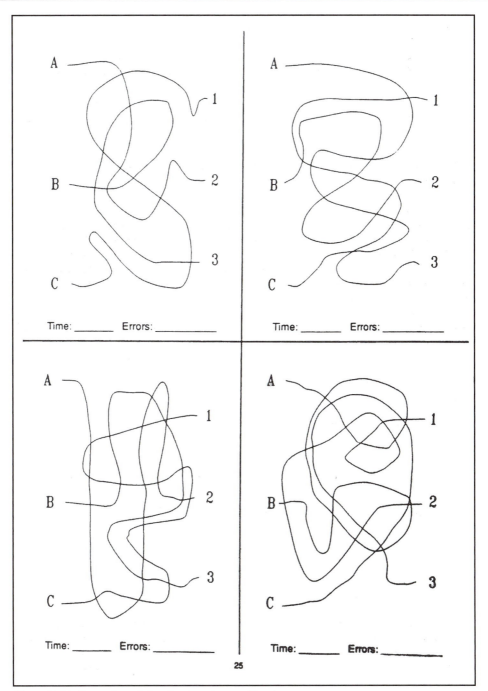

Figure 7-16. Illustration of the visual tracing workbooks.

Figure 7-17. An automatic rotating pegboard that can be used to treat pursuit eye movement disorders.

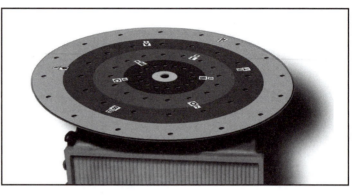

ROTATOR TYPE INSTRUMENTS
Objective
The objective of this technique is to improve the accuracy and speed of pursuit eye movements.

Equipment Needed
* Rotating pegboard
* Golf tees
* Eye patch

Description and Setup
Figure 7-17 illustrates an automatic rotating device that can be used to treat pursuit eye movement disorders. The instrument in Figure 7-17 is called a rotating pegboard. Many different procedures can be performed with this instrument. After occluding one of the patient's eyes, instruct the patient to place a golf tee into a hole in the pegboard. Stress that you want the patient to first find the specific hole he or she will be using, and then in one motion place the peg in the hole. Once the patient can accomplish this, turn on the rotating pegboard. Now, instruct the patient to locate the first hole and hold the golf tee directly over the hole (although not touching it) for one full rotation. After the patient can successfully match the speed of the rotating pegboard for one revolution, instruct him or her to insert the peg in the hole with one motion. Have the patient continue this until all of the holes are filled with golf tees. Of course, the holes on the innermost part of the rotating pegboard are the easiest to work with, and the outer holes are the most difficult.

To combine saccadic eye movements with pursuit eye movements, you can draw a pattern for the patient to follow on a wall directly behind the rotating pegboard. A typical pattern might require the patient to only place a peg in every third hole. The code itself can be simple or complex depending on the capability of the patient. This device can be constructed using a record player and pegboard, or it can be purchased from the vendor listed in Appendix A.

Endpoint
Discontinue this procedure when the patient can accurately complete the entire pegboard following a peg placement code.

FLASHLIGHT TAG
Objective
The objective of this procedure is to improve the speed and accuracy of pursuit eye movements.

Equipment Needed
- Two flashlights
- An eye patch

Description and Setup

This is a simple technique in which the therapist holds one flashlight and the patient holds the other. The technique is performed monocularly. Using your flashlight, simply create a pattern on the wall, and instruct the patient to follow your pattern, keeping his or her flashlight superimposed on yours. Begin with predictable, repeatable patterns and gradually introduce random, unpredictable patterns.

Computer-Based Therapy Techniques
TPOT—EYE ROTATIONS

This procedure develops large angle, rhythmic eye movements.

Description

Randomly colored, circle targets with a single random character in the center are sequentially presented on the Therapy Screen in predefined locations (Figure 7-18). Four target location patterns can be defined by the Rotation Pattern Option. Since each target is displayed at a constant, predefined location on the screen and the distance between each target is about the same, a sense of rhythm and timing can be developed as the patient moves his or her eyes from target to target. Using the pre-target beep for auditory clues can help to develop eye tracking timing.

The patient should try to move his or her eyes to accurately look at (fixate) and focus each target as it is flashed. Each time the patient sees the Target Character he or she should press the <SPACE BAR> key to score. The patient must respond while the target is displayed to receive a correct score. Multiple clicks or presses during longer display times may result in overscoring and poor performance statistics.

To make this procedure more difficult:
- Decrease the display speed.
- Decrease the font size.
- Decrease the circle size.
- Decrease the pattern separation.
- Use random for rotation direction and rotation pattern.
- Turn the pre-display beep off (eliminated the auditory timing clues).

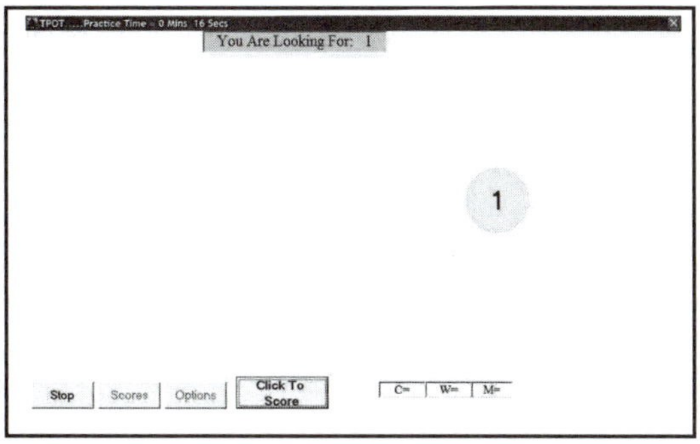

Figure 7-18. TPOT software: Eye Rotations.

TPOT—Tracking Numbers

Description

A green Information Box appears displaying the Target Character for which the patient will be searching. The Target Character will continue to be displayed in the green box in the lower right hand corner of the Therapy Screen.

The patient should try to move his or her eyes to accurately look at (fixate) and focus each character as it is displayed. The patient presses the <SPACE BAR> key to score.

To make this procedure more difficult:

- Set characters per line to either 2 or 8.
- Decrease the display time.
- Decrease the font size.
- Turn the display borders off.
- Use double digit numbers or lowercase letters.

TPOT—Tracking Sequences

Description

This procedure is similar to the Tracking Numbers program. Eye tracking movements in this procedure are developed using targets that require pattern recognition and visual sequential memory skills. Instead of single character targets, however, the program randomly generates a two- to five-character target sequence that must be recognized as random sequences are flashed across the screen. This requires a higher level of cognitive processing since you must track and fixate each displayed sequence and decide whether it matches the target sequence.

The patient should try to move his or her eyes to accurately look at (fixate) and focus each sequence as it is displayed. The patient presses the <SPACE BAR> key to score.

To make this procedure more difficult:

- Set characters per line to either 2 or 6.
- Decrease the display time.
- Decrease the font size.
- Turn the display borders off.

TPOT—Character Searching

Description

A grid of random characters (Letters, Numbers, or Both) is presented on the screen (Figure 7-19). A target character is displayed at the bottom of the screen. The patient should visually scan the grid from left to right and count the number of characters in the grid that match the target letter or number. The patient enters his or her answer using the computer keyboard. If the count is incorrect, the patient is prompted to try again. This is a timed procedure, so try the goal is to answer as quickly as possible.

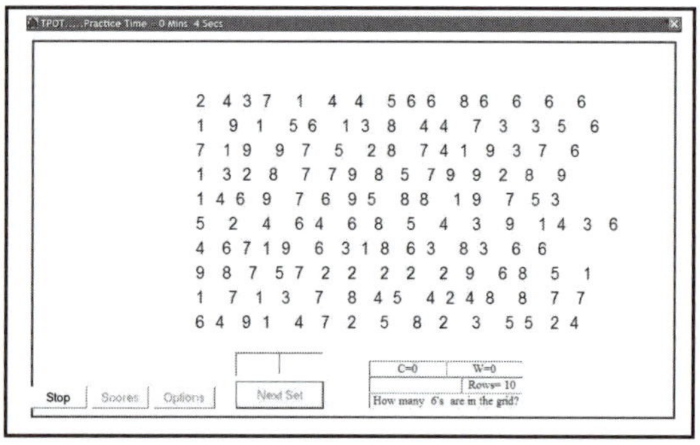

Figure 7-19. TPOT software: Character Searching.

To make this procedure more difficult:

- Increase the number of rows.

- Increase the characters per row.

- Decrease the font size.

- Use lowercase letters.

Intervention for
Visual Information Processing Disorders

Before dealing with visual information processing problems, it is important to first treat any refractive error or visual efficiency problems. We believe that refractive, binocular, ocular motility, and accommodative problems should be resolved first because they can have a negative effect on visual information processing. The concept is that before we begin to deal with the individual's ability to process information accurately, we must ensure that the input into the system is stable, clear, accurate, and efficient.

The treatment of visual perceptual and visual information processing problems is shared by several professions today. Optometrists, occupational therapists, psychologists, and cognitive therapists are some of the professionals who provide such services. We believe, however, that in many cases, professionals who do not evaluate and test for refractive and visual efficiency problems will not be as effective as possible and may prolong therapy if these more basic conditions are not treated first. Several studies have shown that, after treatment of visual efficiency problems alone, visual information processing skills also show some improvement. This concept is particularly important for brain injury patients because of the prevalence of acuity, binocular, accommodative, and visual field deficits. The presence of these problems makes it difficult to even interpret the results of visual information processing testing.

Visual information processing therapy is designed to remediate deficits in three general areas: visual spatial, visual analysis, and visual motor integration skills. The Visual Information Processing Test Battery described in Chapter Five is designed to identify specific weaknesses in each of these areas and to allow a differential diagnosis. I suggest remediation of only those areas that are deficient.

In this chapter, I will describe a sequence of therapy procedures that can be used to treat visual spatial and visual motor integration problems. For a more complete discussion and a description of procedures for the area of visual analysis skills, I suggest referring to *Optometric Management of Learning-Related Vision Problems*.[71]

Patient Factors

Several patient factors should be considered when planning a visual information processing therapy program for a patient. These include the relative strength of visual and auditory/language skills, cognitive style, and past history of success or failure.

If auditory and language skills are deficient, modifications must be made in therapy. Verbal directions should be simplified, and the therapist should present activities in a sequence of small steps. In contrast, when verbal skills are average to above average, the therapist can use verbal mediation to aid the weaker visual processing skills.

Cognitive style must also be taken into consideration. The impulsive patient will make a fast decision without considering all possible options. The reflective patient will get lost in the details of the task and will hesitate to make a decision. Of course, the optimal style is to be fast and accurate. A patient who is impulsive should be allowed to make mistakes, but the therapist should stress how the patient's strategy for solving the problem was effective or ineffective. In addition,

---

Table 7-8

Strategies to Be Used During
Visual Information Processing Therapy

- Present techniques and stimuli that guarantee initial success.
- Do not stress speed initially (except for reflective children).
- Question child about strategy.
- Have child verbalize strategy.
- Impulsive children should be encouraged to perform with maximum accuracy rather than maximum speed.
- Reflective children should be encouraged to work at maximum speed even if it results in some errors.

---

the therapist should try to slow the patient down by using some of the following strategies: Have the patient verbally describe what he or she is doing, thinking, or planning or have the patient point to each choice before making a decision. In contrast, with the reflective patient, the therapist can encourage the patient to respond rapidly and work toward automaticity in all skills.

The last area of concern is providing the patient in visual information processing therapy with a success-oriented environment. The vast majority of children with visual information processing problems reach your office with a history of school failure. Because of this failure, they tend to develop certain adaptive behaviors to avoid situations that result in a lack of success. They may be hesitant to perform certain activities, or they may just try to rush through things.

It is vital, therefore, that the initial stages of visual information processing therapy be a positive experience for the patient. Often, the first several sessions are used just to develop the right environment. The patient should be given techniques that are all within his or her capability to perform. If you give home vision therapy, use only procedures that will not create any additional frustration at home for the child and parent.

Role of the Therapist in Visual Information Processing Therapy

In order to be successful in visual information processing therapy, the therapist and patient must function in an interactive way. The role of the therapist is to help the patient learn a strategy or process to achieve an intended goal. This is a critical concept. The specific therapy procedure used is not as important as the goal of the task and the strategy necessary to achieve the goal.

The role of the therapist is to interact with the patient by asking questions, making the patient check his or her answer, and providing alternative strategies. Table 7-8 lists strategies to be used during visual information processing therapy.

Intervention for Visual Spatial Skills

Visual spatial skills refer to the patient's awareness of internal and external spatial concepts and are used to organize the environment. The two subskills in this category are laterality and directionality. Table 7-9 lists the various techniques I recommend for improving visual spatial skills.

Non-Computer-Based Techniques

LATERALITY

This is the ability to identify right and left on one's self using verbal labels.

Table 7-9

Therapy Procedures for Visual Spatial Skills

Laterality	*Endpoint*
Identification of dominant hand	Understands differences between hands
Simon Says	Complete with limited errors
Floor Map	Complete with limited errors

Directionality	*Endpoint*
Floor Map	Complete with limited errors
Road Maps	Complete with limited errors
Directional Arrows	Complete sheet with limited errors
Visual Motor Sheets	Complete with limited errors
Letter Reversal Sheets	Complete grid with limited errors
Flip Flops	Complete with limited errors
Reversal Flash Cards	Complete with limited errors

Overall Objective of Therapy

The objective of this therapy is to have the patient understand how the right side is different from the left side of his or her body.

Subgoal 1

To make the patient aware of the right and left side of the body. Therapy techniques include Discussion of Right/Left Hands, Simon Says, and Floor Map.

Discussion of Right/Left Hands

Equipment Needed. None

Description. The easiest way to teach laterality skills is identifying the dominant hand and illustrating the differential function of the two hands. The first task is to identify the dominant hand. This can be done by asking the following series of questions:

- Show me how you brush your teeth.
- Show me how you hammer a nail.
- How do you cut with scissors?
- How do you write with a pencil?
- How do you throw a ball?

The dominant hand is the hand used for most of these tasks. If a dominant hand exists, proceed to engage the patient in motor activities in which the two hands are used differently, such as throwing a ball, writing, or cutting. The goal of this entire procedure is simply to discuss and demonstrate the differences in skill between the two hands so that the patient has a way of differentiating between the two.

Initially, if there is no clear dominant hand, you may have to mark one or the other with a rubber band, ring, or some similar device. Generally, the hand marked should be the one that appears to perform better during motor tasks.

At the end of this procedure, we want the patient to be able to think about and visualize a motor act in which he or she knows one hand performs better than the other. By doing so, he or she will be able to differentiate between the two and know which is right and which is left.

Endpoint. The patient can consistently identify right and left on his or her own body.

Simon Says

Equipment Needed. None

Description. This well-known children's game can be used effectively to work on laterality. The therapist can play this game in the office with one or more children. In most cases, after introducing this game in the office, the therapist should assign this as a home therapy procedure.

Endpoint. The patient can consistently identify right and left on his or her own body.

Floor Map

Equipment Needed. Masking tape

Description. Create a road on the floor by placing masking tape on the floor. Create many turns in the road so that the patient must decide which direction to turn at each intersection. It is helpful at the beginning of this exercise to place a string or rubber band on the dominant hand of the patient to assist him or her initially. Ask the patient to negotiate the floor map and at each intersection to tell you whether he or she has to turn right or left. When the patient is indecisive, it is important for you to help him or her generate a strategy. For example, the therapist can ask the patient what hand he or she throws with and to try to transfer this information to the floor map task.

As therapy progresses, the patient should be able to verbalize his or her strategy: "I throw and write with my left hand so I need to turn left now." Finally, the patient should be able to guide him- or herself through the floor map without the need to stop and think about the difference between the right and left sides of his or her body.

As a variation, give the patient a map on paper or a chalkboard, and have the patient write down whether he or she would turn left or right at each intersection.

Endpoint. The patient can consistently, and without a great deal of thought, identify right and left and can describe his or her strategy.

DIRECTIONALITY

This is the ability to interpret left and right directions in space.

Overall Objective of Therapy

The objective of this therapy is to have the patient transfer his or her understanding of right and left on his or her own body to objects in space.

Subgoal 1

The patient should be able to identify right and left on animate objects. Therapy techniques include Floor Map and Road Maps.

Floor Map

Equipment Needed. Masking tape

Description. Use the same floor map that was created previously. Instead of the patient walking through the map, he or she now has to guide the therapist through the floor map. The goal is for the patient to realize that if the object can turn by itself in space, then right and left will appear to be opposite to his or her own right and left. This requires interpretation of right and left from a different perspective (usually this concept cannot be achieved until the patient is 7 years old).

Initially, the patient may need motor support to perform this task. He or she may have to turn him- or herself to begin to understand this concept. Eventually, the patient should be able to guide another person through the floor map without motor support. In addition, we want the patient to be able to verbalize his or her strategy.

Endpoint. The patient can consistently, and without a great deal of thought, identify right and left and can describe his or her strategy.

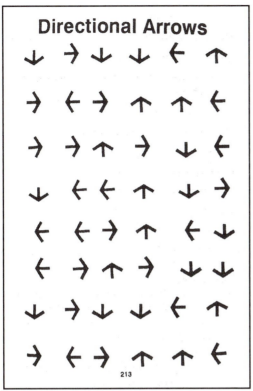

Figure 7-20. Directional arrow worksheet used to treat directionality problems. (Reprinted with permission from Learning Potentials Publishers.)

Road Maps
Equipment Needed. Hand-drawn road maps

Description. The therapist pushes a small toy car through a hand-drawn road. The patient is asked to call out the direction the car must turn at each intersection.

Endpoint. The patient can consistently, and without a great deal of thought, identify right and left and can describe his or her strategy.

Subgoal 2
The patient should be able to identify right and left on inanimate objects facing him or her. The patient should understand that if the object cannot turn in space by itself, the right and left will appear on the same side as those of the patient. This concept is easier to grasp than right and left on an animate object. Children should be able to achieve this by age 5 or 6. Therapy techniques include Directional Arrows and Visual Motor Sheets.

Directional Arrows
Equipment Needed. Directional arrow worksheet (Figure 7-20)

Description. I suggest four levels to this task:

- Level One. Ask the patient to move his or her hand in the direction of the arrow. The patient does not have to call out the correct direction at this level.
- Level Two. Ask the patient to call out the direction of the arrows beginning from the upper left and going left to right across the rows. It is important to periodically stop the patient and ask how he or she knows the arrow is pointing to the right or left. He or she should be able to say, "Because this is my right hand and the arrow is pointing to this side, it must be pointing to the right."

Figure 7-21. Visual Motor Activity Sheet A used to treat directionality problems. (Reprinted with permission from Learning Potentials Publishers.)

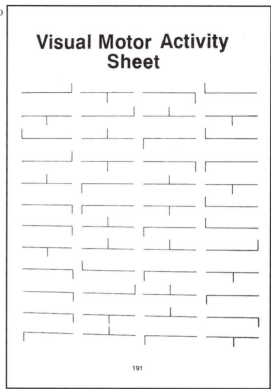

- Level Three. To work on automaticity, have the patient call out the direction of the arrows to the beat of a metronome.
- Level Four. Another method for working on automaticity is to have the patient move his or her hand in the direction the arrow is pointing but call out the opposite direction.

Endpoint. The patient can consistently, and without a great deal of thought, identify right and left and can describe his or her strategy.

Visual Motor Sheets—Sheet A

Equipment Needed. Visual Motor Activity Sheet A (Figure 7-21)

- Level One. Have the patient sit next to you at a table. Tell him or her to call out the position of the vertical line relative to the horizontal line. For example, the top row going left to right on the worksheet would be right up, middle down, right down, left up.
- Level Two. Have the patient do the same activity as in Level One except now use a metronome. At the beat of the metronome, the patient must call out the direction. Using the metronome increases the level of difficulty because the patient now has to respond to the beat and with greater automaticity.

Visual Motor Sheets—Sheet B

Equipment Needed. Visual Motor Activity Sheet B (Figure 7-22)

- Level One. For this worksheet, the hands and feet are coded to symbols as indicated in Figure 7-23. The circle is coded to the hand, the triangle to the foot. If the circle is to the right of the line, the patient is to raise his or her right hand. If the triangle is to the left of the line, the patient is to stomp his or her left foot. If the line passes directly through the middle of the circle, the patient is to raise both hands.

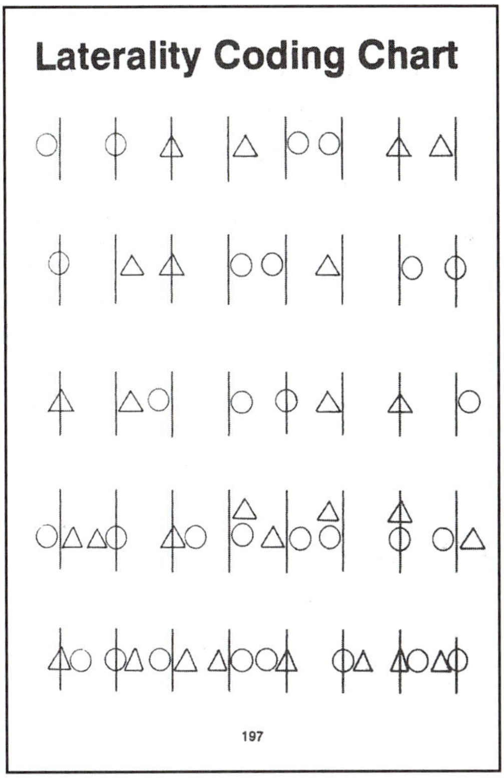

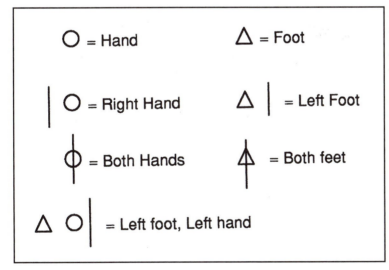

Figure 7-22. Visual Motor Activity Sheet B used to treat directionality problems. (Reprinted with permission from Learning Potentials Publishers.)

Figure 7-23. For Visual Motor Activity Sheet B, the hands and feet are coded to symbols as indicated in the figure. (Reprinted with permission from Learning Potentials Publishers.)

- Level Two. Have the patient do the same activity as in Level One except now use a metronome. At the beat of the metronome, the patient must call out the direction. Using the metronome increases the level of difficulty because the patient now has to respond to the beat and with greater automaticity.

Endpoint. The patient can consistently, and without a great deal of thought, identify right and left and can describe his or her strategy.

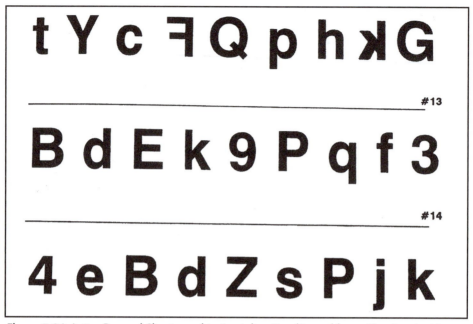

Figure 7-24. Letter Reversal Sheets used to treat directionality problems. (Reprinted with permission from Learning Potentials Publishers.)

Subgoal 3

The final goal of directionality therapy is to apply these concepts to spatial orientation of forms and letters. In this stage, the patient must be able to describe distinctive features of these letters and forms. For example, the only difference between a lower case "b" and a lower case "d" is the location of the semicircle.

It is important for the patient to use the concepts learned earlier to develop a strategy for distinguishing easily reversible letters. The patient should develop a verbal strategy using directional concepts to identify each letter. Therapy techniques include Letter Reversal Sheets, Flip Flops, and Reversal Flash Cards.

Letter Reversal Sheets

Equipment Needed. Letter Reversal Sheets (Figure 7-24)

Description. Place the Letter Reversal Sheet (see Figure 7-24) on a desk. Ask the patient to cross out all of the letters that appear backward. The patient must identify any reversal errors.

Endpoint. The patient can consistently, and without a great deal of thought, identify the reversed letters.

Flip Flops

Equipment Needed. Plastic transparency, transparency pen, and flip-flop patterns (enclosed with materials)

Description. The patient is asked to look at a stimulus (Figure 7-25). The therapist instructs the patient to visualize the stimulus rotated in several possible positions, including rotated 90 degrees to the right, rotated 90 degrees to the left, flipped sideways, flipped upside down, or any combination of these. The patient must then draw the stimulus, taking the transformation into consideration.

In the beginning, it is helpful to draw the stimulus on a clear plastic sheet. Using this sheet, you can demonstrate what the form would look like after the various transformations.

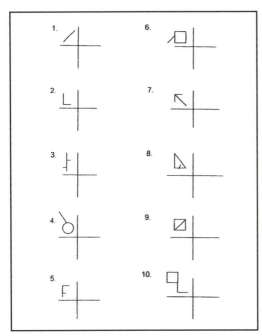

Figure 7-25. Flip-Flop Patterns.

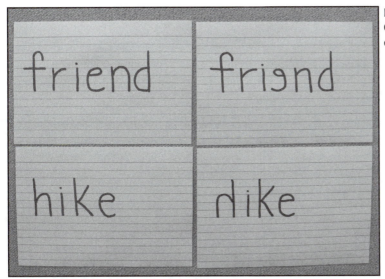

Figure 7-26. Reversal Flash Cards used to treat directionality.

Endpoint. The patient can consistently, and without a great deal of thought, make the various transformations and describe his or her strategy.

Reversal Flash Cards

Equipment Needed. Reversal flash cards (Figure 7-26)

Description. This procedure uses traditional flash cards used by children to study vocabulary and spelling words. The only difference is that two cards are made for each word. On one card, all letters are written correctly. On the second card, one or more letters are purposefully reversed.

- Level One. The patient must find all the cards with reversals and then copy them correctly.
- Level Two. Flash each card for about 3 seconds. Have the patient tell you if any of the letters were reversed or not. Have him or her correctly print the word that had letters reversed.

This procedure can be performed at home with the parent making up a set of cards using the patient's school words.

Endpoint. The patient should be able to achieve 90% correct with one transformation.

Computer-Based Techniques
TPOT—RIGHT OR LEFT
Description

In this activity, a character named Mr. Stickman is facing either toward the patient or looking away from the patient holding a balloon in his right or left hand (Figure 7-27). Or, he might be facing front or back kicking a ball with his right or left foot. As each new character is presented, the patient should try to determine as quickly as possible which hand Mr. Stickman is using to hold the balloon or which foot he is using to kick the ball. The Reaction Time Score displayed on the Therapy Screen measures the average response time for each Stickman. The Average Time Score displayed on the Score Screen and Score Printout calculates the average response time for all Stickmen tried during the therapy sessions.

To make this procedure more difficult:
- Begin therapy with the Display Speed OFF. As skill is gained, use progressively faster Display Speeds.

TPOT—FLIPPER
Description

In this activity, a target image is presented in the picture box at the top of the Therapy Screen. Four answer image boxes are placed at the bottom of the Therapy Screen (Figure 7-28). The images

Figure 7-27. TPOT software: Right or Left.

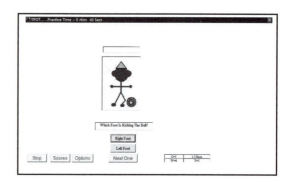

Figure 7-28. TPOT software: Flipper.

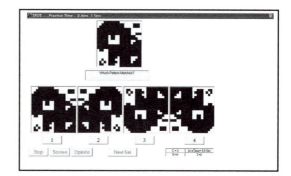

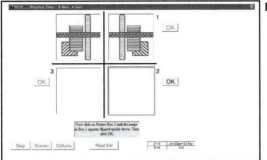

Figure 7-29. TPOT software: Flip Forms.

in the answer boxes will be the target picture flipped, turned, or rotated. One of the answer boxes might even match the target picture in the top picture box. A question about the target picture will be presented below the top image. For example, "Which of the answer pictures matches the target?" Or, "Which of the answer images is flipped right to left?" Or, "Which of the four answer images is flipped upside down?" The patient should try to respond as quickly as possible. Performance is measured by both correct answers and how fast you respond.

To make this procedure more difficult:
- Use higher numbered images.

TPOT—FLIP FORMS

In this exercise, there are four picture boxes. The target image is displayed in the upper left box. The patient should click on box 1 until the target image appears flipped right to left (Figure 7-29). When the patient feels the answer is correct, he or she should click on the OK button. The patient then does the same with picture boxes 2, 3, and 4. Performance will be measured not only by correct answers but also speed of the response.

To make this procedure more difficult:
- Select images with higher numbers.

Intervention for Visual Analysis Skills

Visual analysis skills refer to the ability to analyze and interpret visual information. This aspect of visual information processing is sometimes referred to as motor-free visual perception. Subcategories include, visual discrimination, visual figure ground, visual closure, and visual memory.

Computer-Based Therapy for Visual Analysis Skills

VISUAL DISCRIMINATION

TPOT—Discriminating Color Grids

Description. This procedure creates four grids containing patterns of randomly colored squares. Grid size can be varied from 2 to 16 squares (Figure 7-30). Three of the patterns are identical, one is different. The patient should visually compare each of the four patterns and determine which pattern is different using visual discrimination skills. The correct answer will be highlighted in green.

To make the procedure more difficult:
- Increase grid size.
- Turn the grid borders off.
- Decrease the different colors to two.
- Use harder colors.

Figure 7-30. TPOT software: Discriminating Color.

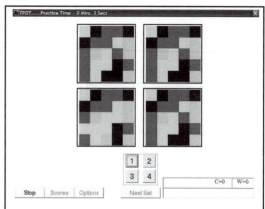

Figure 7-31. TPOT software: Pattern Duplicator.

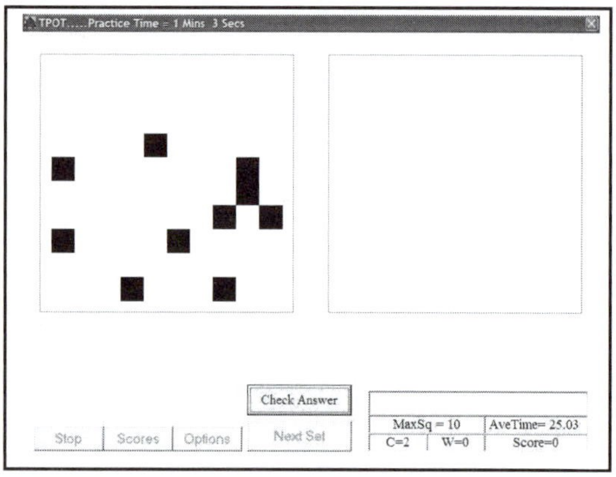

TPOT—Pattern Duplicator

Description. This procedure develops visual spatial relationships utilizing a 25 or 100 square pattern that must be duplicated. When therapy begins, a random pattern is generated in the left hand grid (Figure 7-31). The goal is reproduce that same pattern on the right-hand grid. The patient does so by clicking on the squares in the grid. The computer will check the answer and score it as correct or incorrect. If wrong, the number of incorrect squares in the pattern will be displayed.

To make this procedure more difficult:

• Turning the GRID BORDERS off makes the pattern duplication more difficult.

VISUAL FIGURE GROUND

TPOT—Shape Counting

Description. A number of shapes appear on the screen and the patient must count the number of shapes (Figure 7-32). As the program becomes harder, the shapes begin to become superimposed on one another and figure ground discrimination skills are required to count the shapes. The patient should count and enter the number of foreground targets seen. This is a timed procedure.

To make this procedure more difficult:

• Increase the maximum number of shapes.

• Increase the background complexity.

• Decrease the border size.

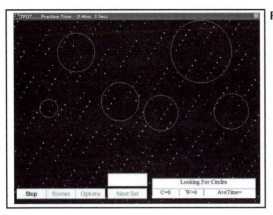

Figure 7-32. TPOT software: Shape Counting.

VISUAL CLOSURE
TPOT—Closing Lines and Boxes
Description. Two target options are available:

With the CONVERGING LINES option, two lines are flashed on the screen. The patient should visualize the lines and try to determine where the lines would meet if they were extended to their meeting point. Visual closure skills are required to visualize the extension of the lines to their crossing point.

In the BOX mode, three corners (indicated by three circles) of a randomly sized rectangle are flashed on the screen. The patient should visualize the rectangle that would be formed by these three circles (corners) and determine where the fourth corner of the rectangle would be.

To make this procedure more difficult:
- Decrease the display speed.
- Turn visual confusion on.

TPOT—Closing Letters
Description. In this exercise, a target letter, hidden under the gray cover, is presented in the picture box at the top of the Therapy Screen (Figure 7-33). The patient should click on the <ERASE TILES> button. A few of the gray blocks will disappear revealing part of the hidden letter. The patient should try and can guess the letter. If not yet possible he should erase a few more tiles. The goal is to determine the answer as quickly as possible and by erasing as few of the blocks as

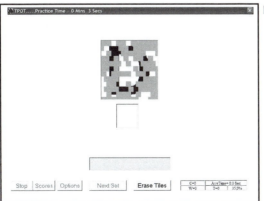

Figure 7-33. TPOT software: Closing Letters.

Figure 7-34. TPOT software: Tic Tac Toe Rotations.

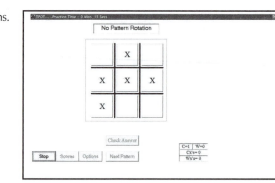

possible. Performance is measured by correct answers, and how fast the patient responds, and by how many blocks were erased.

VISUAL MEMORY

TPOT—Tic Tac Toe Rotations

Description. This procedure requires both visual memory and visual spatial skills. The familiar Tic Tac Toe grid is utilized in this procedure to flash patterns of X's on the grid (Figure 7-34). When the X's are flashed, the patient should try to visualize the pattern on the grid. The patient uses the left mouse key to click on the squares in the grid to recreate the flashed pattern. If the patient makes a mistake, he or she should click on the square again to remove the X. When the patient is ready to check the answer, he or she should click on the <CHECK ANSWER> button. A small grid will appear on the right side of the screen displaying the correct Tic Tac Toe pattern. As skill is gained, PATTERN ROTATION should be introduced. Visualization becomes even more important for these procedures since the patient must mentally manipulate the spatial relationships in the pattern. After the X pattern is presented on the Tic Tac Toe grid, the patient must enter the pattern rotated either clockwise or counter clockwise.

To make this procedure more difficult:
- Decrease the display time.
- Increase the maximum number of X's that are presented.
- Use a small font size.
- Rotate the answer.

TPOT—Visual Sequencing

Description. This procedure develops visual sequencing, visual sequential memory, and visual spatial relationships utilizing the Tic Tac Toe grid to sequentially present colored squares in various patterns on the grid. Each square in the pattern is presented sequentially rather than simultaneously as the X's in the Tic Tac Toe procedure. The patient should try and visualize and remember both the location and sequence of colored square as they are flashed on the grid. After the sequence has been presented, the patient clicks on the appropriate squares in the grid to reproduce the sequence. Once the correct number of squares has been pressed, the answer will be checked and scored automatically.

To make this procedure more difficult:
- Decrease the display time.
- Turn the pre-display beep off.
- Increase the sequence length.
- Use increasing sequence length.

Table 7-10
Therapy Procedures for Visual Motor Integration Skills

Visual Motor Integration	Endpoint
Visual tracing workbook	Accurate performance
Visual fine motor integration workbook	Accurate performance
Geoboard and dot maps	Accurate performance
Parquetry	Complete all patterns with accuracy
Pegboard designs	Complete all patterns with accuracy
Design blocks and patterns	Complete all patterns with accuracy

Intervention for Visual Motor Integration Skills

Visual motor integration skills refer to the patient's ability to integrate visual information processing skills with fine motor movement. If there are problems in both fine motor and visual motor integration based on the test battery, I suggest a sequential approach in which remediation proceeds in two phases: fine motor and then visual motor integration. In my experience as an optometrist, I have found that when a patient has an obvious fine motor problem and difficulty with fine motor skills, a referral to an occupational therapist with experience and knowledge of handwriting difficulties and fine motor problems is warranted. I often work together with occupational therapists with such children. The occupational therapist will work on the fine motor coordination difficulty and handwriting skills while I will work on the underlying visual motor integration problems.

In the discussion that follows, I have chosen to describe two examples of fine motor techniques and one visual motor integration procedure in great detail. The concepts and principles described relative to this procedure are important and represent the essence of how to succeed in remediating these difficulties. These concepts and principles can be readily applied to numerous other techniques for working with visual motor integration problems. Table 7-10 lists the techniques that I recommend for improving visual motor integration skills.

Overall Goal of Visual Motor Integration Therapy

The goal is to allow the patient to become aware of the importance of the eye leading the hand, the relationships of parts of figures to each other and to the total background, and to place these relationships on paper using a pencil.

Subgoal 1

Teach the patient to have the eye lead the hand. Therapy techniques include Visual Tracing Workbooks and Visual Fine Motor Integration Workbooks.

VISUAL TRACING WORKBOOK
Equipment Needed
- Visual tracing workbook

Description
This 34-page workbook contains a series of tracing activities arranged in order of increasing difficulty (Figure 7-35).

Figure 7-35. Visual Tracing Workbook used to treat fine motor problems.

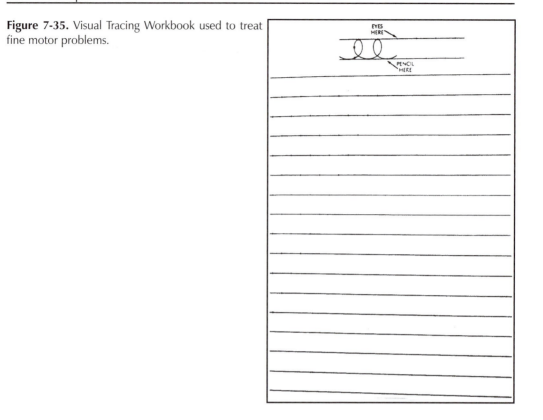

- Level One. The patient uses a pointer and attempts to follow the line with the pointer on the line at all times. After tracing the line with the pointer, have the patient follow the line only with his or her eyes.
- Level Two. Same as level one but now the patient is timed.

Endpoint
The patient should be able to accurately trace lines with and without a pointer. He or she should be able to complete the most difficult tracings within 75 seconds.

Subgoal 2

Have the patient be aware of the relationship of parts of figures to each other and to the background as he or she copies the figures. Therapy techniques include Geoboard and Dot Maps, Parquetry, Pegboard Designs, and Design Blocks.

GEOBOARD AND DOT MAPS
Equipment Needed
- 25-pin geoboard
- Plastic transparencies
- Transparency pen

Description
In this technique, the patient is asked to copy a design from a map to a geoboard or from a map to a map. The map is simply a 5- x 5-inch matrix of dots (Figure 7-36).

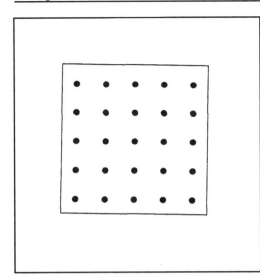

Figure 7-36. Geoboard and Dot Maps. In this technique, the child is asked to copy a design from a map to a geoboard, or from a map to a map. The map is simply a 5- x 5-inch matrix of dots.

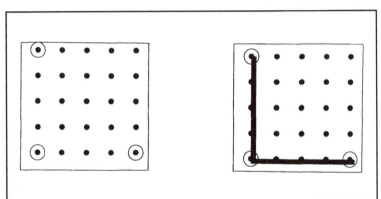

Figure 7-37. The child is asked to copy the pattern from the 25-dot map on the left. This figure demonstrates the specific procedure that should be used.

- Level One. Begin this therapy procedure using a 25-pin geoboard and a 25-dot map. The therapist uses rubber bands to copy Pattern 49 onto the 25-pin geoboard. The patient is asked to look at this pattern and copy it using the overhead transparency pen on the 25-dot map.

In most cases, this will be a good starting point for the patient. If it seems too difficult, you have two options. The first is to use a second 25-pin geoboard and have the patient copy the pattern on your geoboard onto his or her geoboard with rubber bands. This is easier than copying onto a 25-dot map because the geoboard is a concrete, physical item the patient can touch and manipulate. If this is still too difficult, use a five- or nine-dot geoboard or map along with the easier patterns (Patterns 1 to 48). In this very simple first stage, the patient is asked to copy your design onto his or her geoboard or map.

It is critical to remember that there must be interaction between the therapist and patient. Simply asking the patient to copy these patterns will probably have little positive effect. From the very beginning, it is important to establish that the patient must work with some strategy and analyze the pattern carefully before attempting to reproduce the pattern. For example, in Figure 7-37, the patient is asked to copy the pattern from the 25-dot map on the left. Instead of just copying it, we want the patient to verbalize and demonstrate his or her strategy. The following is the procedure we recommend. The therapist should instruct the patient as follows:

1. Identify the line you will copy first from my map.
2. Place a circle around the first dot of the line you will copy.

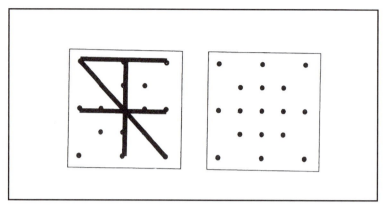

Figure 7-38. Copying from 25-dot map to a 17-dot map.

3.   Now find the same dot on your map and place a circle around it.

4.   Go back to the pattern on my map and find the last dot of the line you will draw.

5.   Now find this same dot on your map and place a circle around it.

6.   Place your pencil on the first circle on your map, look at the second circle, and now slowly draw the line between the two circles.

7.   Find the next line you are going to draw and circle the first dot; continue with numbers 3 to 6.

Although this process may seem time consuming and too easy for the patient initially, it is important to establish this strategy early in therapy so that when the patterns do become hard, the patient will have an approach for overcoming obstacles.

Continue working in this manner until you reach Pattern 200.

•   Level Two. Once the patient can successfully perform Patterns 49 to 200 according to the instructions in Level One, begin from Pattern 100, and this time after you copy your Pattern onto your 25-dot map, instruct the patient to copy his or her onto a 17-dot map (Figure 7-38).

In this case, you have removed some of the detail and structure. The patient is instructed to copy his or hers and pretend that all of the dots are present.

•   Level Three. Once the patient can successfully perform Patterns 49 to 200 according to the instructions in Level Two, begin from Pattern 100, and this time after you copy your pattern onto your 25-dot map, instruct the patient to copy his or hers onto a nine-dot map.

In this case, you have removed more of the detail and structure. The patient is instructed to copy his or hers and pretend that all of the dots are present.

•   Level Four. Once the patient can successfully perform Patterns 49 to 200 according to the instructions in Level Three, begin from Pattern 100, and this time after you copy your pattern onto your 25-dot map, instruct the patient to copy his or hers onto a five-dot map.

•   Level Five. Once the patient can successfully perform Patterns 49 to 200 according to the instructions in Level Four, begin from Pattern 100, and this time after you copy your pattern onto your 25-dot map, instruct the patient to copy his or hers onto a zero-dot map.

•   Level Six. The patient is asked to copy patterns as quickly as possible. When you introduce this level, the patient no longer must verbalize his or her strategy or use the circle method described above. We simply want to have him or her perform quickly and accurately.

In addition to these six levels, several variations can be introduced at any of the levels to add variation, challenge, and complexity to the task.

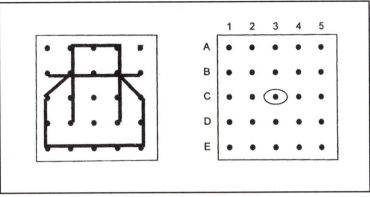

Figure 7-39. Advanced procedure using the map technique.

- Variation One. To vary the task and to increase the level of difficulty at any point, you can modify the instructions in levels one through six as follows:

  Instead of asking the patient to copy the design you construct, ask the patient to make a design of his or her choice on his or her 25-dot map. Have him or her hide this from you so that only he or she can see the design. Ask the patient to give you verbal instructions so that you can make your pattern look the same as his or hers without you seeing it.

  This allows you to determine if he or she has really developed a strategy. For example, the patient may use the following language: "Place your pencil on the first dot in the upper right hand corner and draw a line straight down to the dot in the lower right hand corner."

- Variation Two. Another variation and a level that is considered more difficult is to ask the patient to identify each dot on the map using a coordinate system. This variation can be introduced periodically whenever you think the patient may be ready.

  An example of this is illustrated in Figure 7-39. In this example, the dot circled on the right-hand map would be called C3. Instead of using the procedure suggested in Level One, in which the patient was instructed to circle the first and last dots of the line before drawing, he or she must now identify the dots using coordinates.

  To copy the top line in Figure 7-39 he or she would say: "I will begin with dot A2 and move my pencil right until I reach dot A4."

- Variation Three. The patient is asked to copy your pattern onto his or her map, but she is only given a short period of time to view the pattern and must draw his or hers from memory.

Endpoint
The patient should be able to complete all patterns with limited errors and should be able to achieve this success with speed and automaticity.

Summary
The procedure described above, with its increasingly more difficult levels and variations can be applied to virtually any other visual motor integration task. Some of the common techniques used include parquetry, pegboard designs, and design blocks. The important point is that it is necessary to force the patient to analyze the stimulus and develop a plan or strategy to reproduce it. The various levels and variations described above help accomplish these goals. They also encourage verbalization, a reflective cognitive style early on, and at the end of the sequence, an increase in the speed of the patient's response.

References

1. Skeffington AM. *Introduction to Clinical Optometry.* Santa Ana, CA: Optometric Extension Program Foundation, Optometric Extension Program Postgraduate Courses. Vol 37, Oct. 1964-Sept 1965.

2. Scheiman M, Wick B. *Clinical Management of Binocular Vision Disorders: Heterophoric, Accommodative, and Eye Movement Disorders.* 3rd ed. Philadelphia, PA: Lippincott Williams and Wilkins; 2008.

3. Scheiman M, Mitchell GL, Cotter S, et al. A randomized clinical trial of base-in prism for convergence insufficiency in children 9-17 years. *Br J Ophthalmol.* 2005;89:113-123.

4. Teitelbaum B, Pang Y, Krall J. Effectiveness of base in prism for presbyopes with convergence insufficiency. *Optom Vis Sci.* 2009;86(2):153-156.

5. Bowers AR, Keeney K, Peli E. Community-based trial of a peripheral prism visual field expansion device for hemianopia. *Arch Ophthalmol.* 2008;126(5):657-664.

6. Giorgi RG, Woods RL, Peli E. Clinical and laboratory evaluation of peripheral prism glasses for hemianopia. *Optom Vis Sci.* 2009;86:492-502.

7. Kaplan M. *Seeing Through New Eyes.* Philadelphia, PA: Jessica Kingsley Publishers; 2006.

8. Kaplan M, Edelson SM, Seip JL. Behavioral changes in autistic individuals as a result of wearing ambient transitional prism lenses. *Child Psychiatry and Human Development.* 1998;29:65-76.

9. Padula WV, Argyris S. Post trauma vision syndrome and visual midline shift syndrome. *NeuroRehabilitation.* 1996;6:165-171.

10. McBrien N. Optometry: an evidence-based clinical discipline. *Clin Exp Optom.* 1998:81:234-235.

11. Mozlin R. Evidence-based medicine. *J Am Optom Assoc.* 2000;71:490-500.

12. Straus SE, Richardson WS, Glasziou P, Haynes RB. *Evidence-Based Medicine: How to Practice and Teach EBM.* 3rd ed. New York, NY: Elsevier Churchill Livingstone; 2005.

13. McKibbon KA, Wilczynski NL, Haynes RD. What do evidence-based secondary journals tell us about the publication of clinically important articles in primary healthcare journals? *BMC Medicine.* 2004;2:33.

14. Miller PA, McKibbon KA, Haynes RB. A quantitative analysis of research publications in physical therapy journals. *Phys Ther.* 2003;83:123-131.

15. Lai TYY, Leung GM, Wong VWY, et al. How evidence-based are publications in clinical ophthalmic journals? *Inv Ophthalmol Vis Sci.* 2006;47:1831-1838.

16. Sanfilippo S, Clahane AC. The effectiveness of orthoptics alone in selected cases of exodeviation: the immediate results and several years later. *Am Orthoptic J.* 1970;20:104-117.

17. Hoffman L, Cohen A, Feuer G. Effectiveness of non-strabismic optometric vision training in a private practice. *Am J Optom Arch Am Acad Opt.* 1973;50:813-816.

18. Cornsweet TN, Crane HD. Training the visual accommodative system. *Vision Res.* 1973;13:713-715.

19. Provine RR, Enoch JM. On voluntary ocular accommodation. *Percept Psychophysiol.* 1975;17:209-212.

20. Cooper EL, Leyman IA. The management of intermittent exotropia: a comparison of the results of surgical and non-surgical treatment. *Am Orthoptic J.* 1977;27:61-67.

21. Wick B. Binocular vision therapy for general practice. *J Am Optom Assoc.* 1977;48:461-466.

22. Wick B. Vision therapy for presbyopic nonstrabismic patients. *Am J Optom Physiol Opt.* 1977;54:24-247.

23. Wold RM, Pierce JR, Keddington J. Effectiveness of optometric vision therapy. *J Am Optom Assoc.* 1978;49:1047-1054.

24. Liu JS, Lee M, Jang J, et al. Objective assessment of accommodative orthoptics. I. Dynamic insufficiency. *Am J Optom Physiol Opt.* 1979;56:285-291.

25. Weisz CL. Clinical therapy for accommodative responses: transfer effects upon performance. *J Am Optom Assoc.* 1979;50:209-216.

26. Grisham JD. The dynamics of fusional vergence eye movements in binocular dysfunction. *Am J Optom Physiol Opt.* 1980;57:205-213.

27. Daum K. The course and effect of visual training on the vergence system. *Am J Optom Physiol Opt.* 1982;59:223-227.

28. Bobier WR, Sivak JG. Orthoptic treatment of subjects showing slow accommodative responses. *Am J Optom Physiol Opt.* 1983;60:678-687.

29. Daum KM. Accommodative insufficiency. *Am J Optom Physiol Opt.* 1983;60:352-359.

30. Daum KM. Accommodative dysfunction. *Doc Ophthalmol.* 1983;55:177-198.

31. Daum K. A comparison of results of tonic and phasic training on the vergence system. *Am J Optom Physiol Opt.* 1983;60:769-775.

32. Daum KM. Predicting the results in the orthoptic treatment of accommodative dysfunction. *Am J Optom Physiol Opt.* 1984;61:184-189.

33. Cohen AH, Soden R. Effectiveness of visual therapy for convergence insufficiencies for an adult population. *J Am Optom Assoc.* 1984;55:491-494.

34. Daum KM. Equal exodeviations: characteristics and results of treatment with orthoptics. *Aust J Optom.* 1984;67:53-59.

35. Daum KM. Divergence excess: characteristics and results of treatment with orthoptics. *Ophthalmol Physiol Opt.* 1984;4:15-24.

36. Daum K. Convergence insufficiency. *Am J Optom Physiol Opt.* 1984;61:16-22.

37. Rouse MW. Management of binocular anomalies: efficacy of vision therapy in the treatment of accommodative deficiencies. *Am J Optom Physiol Opt.* 1987;64:415-420.

38. Grisham JD, Bowman MC, Owyang LA, Chan CL. Vergence orthoptics: validity and persistence of the training effect. *Optom Vis Sci.* 1991;68:441-451.

39. Cooper J, Medow N. Intermittent exotropia of the divergence excess type: basic and divergence excess type. *Bin Vis Eye Mus Surg Qtly.* 1993;8:187-222.

40. Shorter AD, Hatch SW. Vision therapy for convergence excess. *N Engl J Optom.* 1993;45:51-53.

41. Ficcara AP, Berman J, Rosenfield M, et al. Vision therapy: predictive factors for success in visual therapy for patients with convergence excess. *J Optom Vis Dev.* 1996;27:213-219.

42. Gallaway M, Scheiman M. The efficacy of vision therapy for convergence excess. *J Am Optom Assoc.* 1997;68:81-86.

43. Adler P. Efficacy of treatment for convergence insufficiency using vision therapy. *Ophthalmol Physiol Opt.* 2002;22:565-571.

44. Abdi S, Rydberg A. Asthenopia in schoolchildren, orthoptics and ophthalmological findings and treatment. *Doc Ophthalmol.* 2005;111:65-72.

45. Aziz S, Cleary M, Stewart HK, Weir CR, Are orthoptic exercises an effective treatment for convergence and fusion deficiencies? *Strabismus.* 2006;14:183-189.

46. Vaegan JL. Convergence and divergence show longer and sustained improvement after short isometric exercise. *Am J Optom Physiol Opt.* 1979;56:23-33.

47. Cooper J, Selenow A, Ciuffreda KJ, et al. Reduction of asthenopia in patients with convergence insufficiency after fusional vergence training. *Am J Optom Physiol Opt.* 1983;60:982-989.

48. Cooper J, Feldman J, Selenow A, et al. Reduction of asthenopia after accommodative facility training. *Am J Optom Physiol Opt.* 1987;64:430-436.

49. Daum K. Double blind placebo-controlled examination of timing effects in the training of positive vergences. *Am J Optom Physiol Opt.* 1986;63:807-812.

50. Birnbaum MH, Soden R, Cohen AH. Efficacy of vision therapy for convergence insufficiency in an adult male population. *J Am Optom Assoc.* 1999;70:225-232.

51. Scheiman M, Mitchell GL, Cotter S, et al. A randomized trial of the effectiveness of treatments for convergence insufficiency in children. *Arch Ophthalmol.* 2005;123:14-24.

52. Scheiman M, Mitchell GL, Cotter S, et al. A randomized clinical trial of vision therapy/orthoptics versus pencil push-ups for the treatment of convergence insufficiency in young adults. *Optom Vis Sci.* 2005;82:583-595.

53. Convergence Insufficiency Treatment Trial Investigator Group. Randomized clinical trial of treatments for symptomatic convergence insufficiency in children. *Arch Ophthalmol.* 2008;126:1336-1349.

54. Ciuffreda K. The scientific basis for and efficacy of optometric vision therapy in nonstrabismic accommodative and binocular vision disorders. *Optometry.* 2002;73:735-762.

55. Wold RM, Pierce JR, Keddington J. Effectiveness of optometric vision therapy. *J Am Optom Assoc.* 1978;49:1047-1053.

56. Rounds BB, Manley CW, Norris RH. The effect of oculomotor training on reading efficiency. *J Am Optom Assoc.* 1991;62:92-99.

57. Young BS, Pollard T, Paynter S, Cox R. Effect of eye exercises in improving control of eye movements during reading. *J Optom Vis Dev.* 1982;13:4-7.

58. Fujimoto DH, Christensen EA, Griffin JR. An investigation in use of videocassette techniques for enhancement of saccadic movements. *J Am Optom Assoc.* 1985;56:304-308.

59. Rouse MW, Borsting E. Management of visual information processing problems. In: Scheiman M, Rouse MW, eds. *Optometric Management of Learning-Related Vision Problems.* 2nd ed. St. Louis, MO: CV Mosby; 2006:432-433.

60. Farr J, Leibowitz HW. An experimental study of the efficacy of perceptual-motor training. *Am J Optom Physiol Opt.* 1976;53:451-455.

61. Seiderman AS. Optometric vision therapy results of a demonstration project with a learning disabled population. *J Am Optom Assoc.* 1980;51:489-493.

62. Hendrickson LN, Muehl S. The effect of attention and motor response pretraining on learning to discriminate B and D in kindergarten children. *J Ed Psych.* 1962;53:236-241.

63. Greenspan SB. Effectiveness of therapy for children's reversal confusions. *Acad Ther.* 1975-76;11:169-178.

64. Walsh JF, D'Angelo R. Effectiveness of the Frostig program for visual perceptual training with headstart children. *Percept Mot Skills.* 1971;32:944-946.

65. Brown RT, Alford N. Ameliorating, attentional deficits and concomitant academic deficiencies in learning disabled children through cognitive training. *J Learn Disabil*. 1984;17:20-26.

66. Rosner J. The development of a perceptual skills program. *J Am Optom Assoc*. 1973;44:698-707.

67. Getz DJ. Learning enhancement through visual training. *Acad Ther*. 1980;15:457-466.

68. Halliwell JW, Solan HA. The effects of a supplemental perceptual training program in reading achievement. *Except Child*. 1972;38:613-621.

69. Rowell RB. *The effect of tachistoscope and visual tracking program on the improvement of reading at the second grade level*. Doctoral thesis. Ann Arbor, MI: University Microfilms; 1976.

70. Solan HA, Ciner EB. Visual perception and learning: issues and answers. *J Am Optom Assoc*. 1989;60:457-460.

71. Scheiman M, Rouse MW. *Optometric Management of Learning-Related Vision Problems*. 2nd ed. St. Louis, MO: CV Mosby; 2006.

Chapter Eight

Visual Problems Associated With Learning Disorders

Mitchell Scheiman, OD, FCOVD, FAAO

Overview

Pediatric optometrists, pediatric occupational therapists, and school-based occupational therapists all spend a considerable amount of their professional time testing and treating children with learning disorders. Public Law (PL) 94-142 was passed in 1975 and has made available a free, appropriate public education that emphasizes special education and related services to children with a wide range of handicapping conditions. Because occupational therapy is included as one of the related services, the profession has become deeply involved in the care of learning disabled children. In fact, school systems are listed as the second most common work setting for occupational therapists.[1]

Optometry also has a long history of involvement in this area. Much of the interest has been generated by the concern of parents and by the referrals of teachers, psychologists, occupational therapists, and other professionals who turn to optometrists for answers about whether a child has a vision problem that could be contributing to or responsible for poor school performance. Optometrists believe that vision can contribute to learning difficulties, but that it is generally not the primary etiological factor. Rather, vision disorders may interfere with a child's school performance and may make it difficult for a child to perform up to potential. Optometrists believe that there is a strong relationship between vision and learning and that every child who is experiencing problems in school requires an appropriate optometric evaluation.

Controversy exists, however, about the relationship between vision and learning. Some professionals, primarily ophthalmologists, claim that there is no significant relationship between vision and learning.[2] They suggest that as long as a child can see clearly and has healthy eyes, vision can be ruled out as an issue. Based on the material presented in Chapters One, Three, Four, and Five, it should be evident that this controversy is based on differences in the definition of vision. Ophthalmology's definition of vision is a very limited one and generally only requires good visual acuity and normal eye health. Most research would, in fact, support the statement that visual acuity and eye health have no relationship to learning. It is easy to understand, therefore, why an individual or a profession using such a definition would believe that there is no significant relationship between vision and learning. Optometry, however, believes that vision is more complex than visual acuity and eye health. We use the Three Component Model of Vision described in Chapters Three through Five. Strong research demonstrates that, using this comprehensive definition, there is indeed a strong relationship between vision and learning.

There is also controversy about whether vision therapy is an effective treatment approach for children with learning disorders. This second area of contention is again based on misconceptions and disagreement about definitions. Ophthalmology claims that vision therapy is an ineffective approach for the treatment of learning disabilities.[2] In fact, this is not an unreasonable statement, and optometry has never claimed that vision therapy is a cure for learning disabilities. Rather, optometrists believe that vision therapy is an effective approach for the treatment of visual efficiency and visual information processing problems. The effect of vision therapy on a child's learning ability is most comparable to the effect of medication for attention deficit disorder. Ritalin (methylphenidate), for instance, is not expected to directly improve reading performance. Rather, as a result of improved concentration and attention, the child is able to benefit from educational intervention. Similarly, improvements in visual skills can result in better attention, concentration, and learning efficiency and can enable the child to benefit from standard or remedial education. Thus, the key concept is that optometrists evaluate and treat vision problems that may be interfering with school performance. Optometry's position is that vision problems should not be treated in isolation but rather as part of a multidisciplinary approach designed to supplement rather than substitute for classroom or resource room instruction.[3-6]

Why is vision such an important factor in learning? If you think about the activities that a child has to perform on a daily basis in school to learn effectively, it is evident that vision is the sensory system through which a significant percentage of learning must occur. A study by Ritty et al[7] demonstrated how important visual acuity, accommodation, binocular vision, and ocular motor abilities are in the typical elementary school classroom. They found that 75% of the academically related task time in the classroom is spent on reading and writing at near distance and on tasks that require near-to-distance-to-near alternate viewing. To perform well at these tasks, a child requires normal visual acuity, accommodation, binocular vision, and ocular motor skills.

Prevalence of Vision Disorders in Children With Learning Disabilities

General Studies

Studies have shown a very high prevalence of visual efficiency problems in learning disabled children. Sherman[8] found a very high prevalence of accommodative (76%), binocular (92%), and ocular motility (96%) disorders in a population of learning disabled children. In a similar type study, Hoffman[9] examined 107 learning disabled children and also found a high prevalence of binocular vision (87%), accommodative (83%), and ocular motility (95%) disorders. In an extensive review of the literature, Grisham and Simons[10] concluded that there is a relationship between refractive status and binocular vision and reading. This was further supported by a meta-analysis of the same literature.[11] O'Grady explored the relationship between vision and educational performance by studying a random sample of 227 second-grade children. Of the sample, 16.2% were found to have significant vision disorders.[12] The children with vision problems were found to perform significantly poorer on the educational tests than the other children.

Visual information processing problems have also been found to be prevalent in learning disabled children. Hoffman[9] found problems in bilateral integration (46%), directionality (74%), visual discrimination (50%), and visual motor integration problems (81%), while Sherman[8] found form reproduction disorders in 72% of the population he studied. Groffman[13] recently reviewed the literature relating visual perceptual problems to learning and found that meta-analysis of single-factor studies showed that reading achievement was significantly related to visual perceptual performance. Kavale reviewed 161 studies and used meta-analysis to statistically integrate the results from these studies.[14] His results suggested that visual perception is an important correlate of reading achievement and that visual perceptual skills should be included in the complex of factors predictive of reading achievement.

Refractive Error

Eames[15] compared the refractive distribution of 114 reading disabled children selected from a private practice and a university clinic with 143 controls. He found a significant difference (P = 0.001) in the prevalence of hyperopia between the reading disabled and the control group (43% compared to 27%). In another report, Eames[16] compared 1000 reading disabled children with 150 controls. The prevalence of hyperopia was much greater among disabled readers (43%) than the control group (13%).

Other studies reported interactions between refractive status and visual-perceptual motor development.[17,18] Although these studies were not investigations of reading per se, children with visual-perceptual motor delays are at risk for reading underachievement. In the first study of a sample of 712 children ages 6 to 12 years, only 18% of the children with significant hyperopia displayed age-appropriate visual motor skills, in contrast to 74% of the emmetropic and myopic children.[17] In a second and related study of 48 6- to 12-year-old hyperopes, those children who were corrected prior to their fourth birthday manifested fewer visual-motor delays than those who were corrected later.[18] In a more recent study of 32 children, 4 to 7 years old, the authors found that those with uncorrected hyperopia showed reduced performance on tests of letter and word recognition, receptive vocabulary compared to the children with no refractive error.[19]

Binocular Vision

Eames[20] found the prevalence of exophoria to be nearly four times greater in the nominal reading disabled group than in the control group. In his latter, large sample study, Eames[16] found a somewhat greater prevalence of near point exophoria in the reading disabled group (33% compared to 22%; P = 0.007). In a generally well-constructed research study, Good[21] used a case-control paradigm and found that none of the control group had a significant phoria, whereas 40% of the reading disabled did. Evans, Efron, and Hodge[22] found the prevalence of significant phoria was nearly twice as frequent in a sample of reading disabled than in a sample of second- to fifth-grade normal readers.

Ocular Motor

Because eye movement deficiencies intuitively seem to be so closely linked with reading, numerous studies have investigated this relationship. When reading age-appropriate text, the eye movements of poor readers are characterized by an increased number of forward fixations per line of text, an increased number of regressions, longer fixation durations, and a greater prevalence of intraword scanning when compared to normal readers.[23] In children with reading and other learning difficulties, several studies have found a very high prevalence of eye movement anomalies.[8,9,24] In a sample of 50 children with learning disabilities between the ages of 6 and 13 years, Sherman[8] found that 96% had problems with ocular motor inefficiency (saccadic and pursuit problems). Hoffman[9] reported on a larger sample of 107 children with learning problems. His results revealed that 24% of the sample had ocular motor problems. He also reported on the results of 25 children without learning problems and found that 24% had ocular motor problems. It is interesting to note that both Sherman and Hoffman found that ocular motor dysfunction was the most prevalent vision disorder in their samples of learning disabled children.

Effect of Vision Problems on Occupational Therapy Intervention

Table 8-1 lists the signs and symptoms associated with visual efficiency and visual information processing problems. Many of these symptoms interfere with a child's ability to attend and concentrate when engaged in any visual task and occur when the child is working on near tasks such as reading, writing, cutting, coloring, and other types of desk work. Children also will sometimes avoid such activities rather than experience eyestrain, headaches, and double vision.

Vision problems can hinder the occupational therapy process in a variety of ways, and Flax[25] has stressed the importance of performing a task analysis when assessing the impact of a vision problem on performance. It is not sufficient to simply ask if vision is impacting on a child's performance. Rather, the occupational therapist should try to define the visual demands of a task and determine if there is a relationship. Tables 8-2 and 8-3 provide guidance for this task analysis.

Flax[25] uses the following example to demonstrate the value of task analysis relative to vision and reading performance. Two children are brought to an optometrist to determine if vision might be interfering with reading performance. Both have the same general complaint of poor comprehension. In case one, it is established that there is no difficulty with pronouncing each word correctly regardless of the grade level or difficulty of the word. There are no indications of fatigue; the child works for hours quite diligently but does not seem to understand what is being read. He can pronounce words but not define them. He does no better when the passage is read aloud to him. When attempting to explain what has just been read, he repeats the very same words that were in the text but does not offer synonyms, alternative phrases, or anything suggesting insight despite the fact that the mechanics of reading seem to be intact. Given this history, visual factors are unlikely to be major contributors to this youngster's reading problem. Language factors or even low intelligence are more apt to be the cause of the child's problem. His ability to repeat almost verbatim suggests that there is no problem with visual intake of the reading material.

The second child can decode unfamiliar words. But, this child shows a decline in efficiency on longer assignments, and reading comprehension becomes even worse on smaller type. This child frequently omits words, rereads the same line, and skips lines. This youngster loves being read to and can discuss and recall effectively when material is read aloud to him. This child can define words and give synonyms, and he has good understanding of anything that he hears. His problem occurs when he has to read several pages of text. It is at this point that reading comprehension suffers. In this case, vision is likely to be related to the reading comprehension difficulty. This child shows good language ability, and, importantly, when the material is heard rather than seen, there is no comprehension problem. This history suggests the possibility of difficulty with ocular motility, binocular vision, or accommodation. There may even be contribution because of uncorrected refractive conditions.

The same type of task analysis is important for the occupational therapist. Problems are likely to cause the symptoms listed in Table 8-1 if the therapy procedure requires fine detail and prolonged attention and concentration, and then ocular motility, accommodation, and binocular vision. If, however, the material used in occupational therapy has large type and few details, ocular motility, accommodation, and binocular vision are not taxed greatly.

Given the high prevalence of vision problems in learning disabled children, occupational therapists should always consider the possibility that a vision problem could be present, particularly if progress is slower than expected and if some of the symptoms or signs described in Table 8-1 are present.

Table 8-1

Effect of Vision Problems on Occupational Therapy

Visual Problem	*Effect on Function*
Refractive conditions	• Decreased visual acuity • Excessive effort to perform visual tasks • Discomfort when involved with any visual task • Intermittent blurred vision • Loss of vision • Need to hold things close
Binocular vision disorders: strabismic	• Cosmetic problem, eyes look crossed or turned out • If strabismus is intermittent, it can cause double vision that can interfere with eye-hand and mobility tasks • If strabismus is intermittent, it can lead to eyestrain • Loss of visual acuity (amblyopia) if left untreated and if the strabismus is unilateral
Binocular vision disorders: nonstrabismic	• Intermittent double vision • Discomfort and eyestrain for all visual tasks • Tires easily • Inattentive • Poor concentration • Loss of place when playing or reading • Difficulty with eye-hand tasks
Accommodative disorders	• Discomfort and eyestrain for all visual tasks • Tires easily • Inattentive • Poor concentration • Blurred vision • Rubs eyes
Ocular motility disorders	• Excessive head movement when engaged in visual tasks • Frequent loss of place • Skips lines • Poor attention span • Copying is slow and inaccurate • Results poor with coloring and drawing
Visual information processing disorders	• Confusion of left and right • Confusion of likenesses and differences • Tends to use other senses to make what should be visual discriminations • Unaware of what should be attended to • Performs slowly • Ignores detail during visual tasks • Poor recall of visually presented material • Sloppy drawing skills • Difficulty with copying and getting thoughts on paper

---

> ### Table 8-2

Task Characteristics Placing a
High Demand on Visual Efficiency Skills

The Occupational Therapy Task Requires
- Attention to small internal details of visual stimuli such as words and pictures
- Precise ocular motor control
- Accurate sequential inspection of words, visual stimuli
- Sustained attention on a visual task
- Extensive use of dittos which may be of poor print quality
- Speed and accuracy
- Emphasis on speed and comprehension
- Movement during a visual task

Tasks with the above requirements are likely to cause the symptoms listed in Table 8-1 under the sections of non-strabismic binocular vision disorders, accommodation, and ocular motility.

> ### Table 8-3

Task Characteristics Placing a
High Demand on Visual Information Processing Skills

The Occupational Therapy Task Requires
- Decisions about directional orientation
- Symbol and word recognition
- Matching of shapes
- Visual memory
- Visualization
- Copying of visual stimuli

Tasks with the above requirements are likely to cause the symptoms listed in Table 8-1 under the section of visual information processing.

Case Studies

Case One
CASE HISTORY

Paul, a 12-year-old seventh-grader, was brought in for an examination because his school performance had decreased significantly this school year. Until this year, Paul had been an outstanding student, achieving excellent grades in all subjects. The specific problem revolved around Paul's inability to read comfortably. He complained that after 10 to 15 minutes of reading, his eyes felt tired and ached. If he continued to read, he eventually experienced headaches, and, finally, the words would blur and move on the page. Because of his inability to read comfortably, he was falling behind in his assignments. He felt that the amount of required reading had increased significantly this year.

His medical history was negative, and he was not taking any medication. He had passed a visual screening at the pediatrician and in school earlier in the school year. He never had a full vision evaluation. There was no significant family history of learning problems. Both parents were college graduates with high expectations for Paul's education.

VISUAL ACUITY, REFRACTION, EYE HEALTH

This part of the examination revealed normal 20/20 visual acuity in both the right and left eyes. The eye health evaluation was normal. Paul was found to have a very low degree of hyperopia (farsightedness), which is considered normal for his age.

VISUAL EFFICIENCY TESTING

This testing was designed to evaluate accommodation, binocular vision, and ocular motility skills. The near point of convergence was receded, a high degree of exophoria (eyes turn out) was found at the reading distance, and his ability to compensate for the exophoria was found to be very poor. Accommodation was also found to be inadequate. Specifically, he had a great deal of difficulty relaxing the accommodative system. Ocular motility was found to be normal.

VISUAL INFORMATION PROCESSING EVALUATION

Because Paul had an excellent academic record for the first 6 years of school, we felt that if a vision problem was a contributing factor to his current problems, it would be a visual efficiency disorder or a refractive error. Because significant visual efficiency problems were detected, we did not feel that visual information processing testing was necessary.

ASSESSMENT AND DIAGNOSIS

The history in this case was clearly characteristic of a learning problem associated with a visual efficiency disorder. Analysis of the optometric findings revealed a receded near point of convergence, high exophoria at near, decreased compensatory ability, and poor accommodative facility. Based on these data, we reached a diagnosis of convergence insufficiency and accommodative excess.

We felt that these visual efficiency problems were clearly related to Paul's presenting complaints. Given Paul's history of excellent academic performance in grades 1 through 6, we felt that if we could eliminate the visual efficiency problems along with the associated symptoms, there would be a positive effect on academic performance.

TREATMENT PLAN

We recommended a program of vision therapy. Eighteen 45-minute office visits were necessary. The patient was seen twice a week, and after 9 weeks, Paul reported elimination of all of his initial complaints and was able to read comfortably as long as desired. As Paul's comfort improved, his ability to study was enhanced, leading to better academic performance.

SUMMARY

This is an important case because it demonstrates the importance of using a comprehensive model of vision. If this child had been examined by an eye care professional who only performed testing to probe the areas of visual acuity, refractive error, and eye health, no vision problem would have been detected. Unfortunately, this is a common occurrence. The child is referred for an eye examination and is returned with a statement that there is no vision or eye problem. The binocular and accommodative disorders were only detected in this case after visual efficiency testing was performed.

It is critical that when an occupational therapist is concerned about a vision problem, a referral is made to an eye care professional who will perform a comprehensive examination based on the type of model presented in this book. The eye care professional most likely to be able to deliver this type of care is an optometrist. However, it is important to realize that not all optometrists will provide this level of vision care. It is wise to contact the College of Optometrists in Vision Development and the American Academy of Optometry. These organizations can provide a list of optometrists in your area who can provide this type of care (see Chapter One).

Case Two
CASE HISTORY

Jimmy, a 7½-year-old first-grader, was referred for a vision evaluation by a psychologist who had just completed a psycho-educational evaluation. Jimmy learned to speak very early and was always a very verbal child. Although his parents' expectations had been very high for him, Jimmy had a history of school-related problems since kindergarten. In kindergarten, he experienced difficulty with letter and number recognition and fine motor coordination. He had great difficulty in first grade with handwriting and copying from the board. He reversed letters and numbers excessively and had difficulty with his sight word vocabulary. His parents noted that when they read to him, his comprehension was excellent. Because of these reported difficulties, he was retained in first grade. In spite of this retention, he continued to experience problems, and his parents finally brought him to a psychologist for psycho-educational testing.

The parents brought a copy of the psycho-educational evaluation report. This report indicated that there were no significant emotional issues, and the Weschler Intelligence Scale for Children results included a verbal IQ of 128 and a performance IQ of 104. The weakest scores were in coding (scaled score 5) and block design (scaled score 6). Jimmy scored almost 2 years behind his chronological age on the Bender Gestalt Test, a test of visual motor integration. Auditory processing and language skills were strengths for Jimmy.

Achievement testing was also done as part of the psycho-educational testing. This testing suggested a 1-year lag in reading with weaknesses in sight word vocabulary, comprehension, and age-appropriate math skills.

In the patient summary, the psychologist reached a diagnosis of a learning disability with primary weaknesses in visual processing and strengths in language function. He recommended part-time placement in a resource room and reading tutoring. In addition, he suggested a comprehensive optometric evaluation and an occupational therapy evaluation.

Jimmy's medical history revealed a normal gestation, but a very long and difficult labor and delivery by cesarean section. Otherwise, there was no significant medical history. Developmental milestones showed a variable pattern. Language skills developed faster than average. For instance, Jimmy used two-word sentences by 18 months of age and was always a very verbal child. Fine motor skills, however, developed more slowly than expected. He always had difficulty holding a crayon and did not enjoy cutting, coloring, or playing with puzzles. He could not copy a circle until about 4 years of age. Jimmy had difficulty with most sports and tended to avoid such activity. There did not seem to be any family history of learning problems, and there had been no other testing.

VISUAL ACUITY, REFRACTION, EYE HEALTH

Visual acuity was 20/20 in both eyes, eye health was normal, and a moderate degree of hyperopia was found in both eyes.

VISUAL EFFICIENCY TESTING

Binocular vision testing revealed a moderate degree of esophoria (eyes turned in), and his ability to compensate for this tendency was inadequate. The accommodative system was normal, but ocular motility testing revealed very poor performance in the area of saccades and pursuits. On the Developmental Test of Eye Movements, Jimmy scored at only the first percentile in both accuracy and speed.

Table 8-4

Visual Information Processing Results for Case Two

Visual Spatial Skills	Test	Score
Directionality	Gardner Reversal Frequency Test:	
	Recognition Subtest	5%
	Execution Subtest	40%
Visual Analysis Dysfunction	Test	Score
Visual form constancy	TVPS: Visual Form Constancy	37%
Visual memory	TVPS: Visual Memory	25%
	TVPS: Visual Sequential Memory	37%
Visual Motor Integration	Test	Score
Visual motor integration	Visual Motor Integration Tests	10%
Fine motor skills	Grooved Pegboard	10%
	Wold Sentence Copy Test	First grade

VISUAL INFORMATION PROCESSING EVALUATION

Table 8-4 lists the tests administered and the results. Key weaknesses were in directionality (fifth percentile), visual memory (25th percentile), visual motor integration (10th percentile), and fine motor skills (10th percentile).

ASSESSMENT AND DIAGNOSIS

The optometric evaluation revealed difficulties in both visual efficiency and visual information processing. There was a significant amount of hyperopia, and his eyes were found to have a significant tendency to cross inward (esophoria). His tracking ability (saccadic fixation) was significantly below age level. Based on this information, we reached a diagnosis of hyperopia, convergence excess, and ocular motor dysfunction.

In addition, the visual information processing evaluation indicated problems in visual spatial, visual analysis, visual motor integration, and fine motor skills.

These findings can be related to many of the problems that Jimmy was experiencing in school. His difficulty with reversals, letter and number recognition, fine motor coordination, and copying from the board are characteristic of children with problems in directionality, visual memory, visual motor integration, fine motor skills, and saccadic fixation problems (see Table 8-1).

Even though he was not complaining of any of the common signs or symptoms associated with hyperopia and esophoria, we felt these were significant issues that would need to be addressed in the treatment plan because of their potential to cause eyestrain and difficulty with attention and concentration.

OCCUPATIONAL THERAPY EVALUATION

The school occupational therapist received the testing from both the psychologist and the optometrist and performed an evaluation primarily designed to determine why Jimmy was having trouble with handwriting and sports. Using the Bruininks-Oseretsky Test of Motor Proficiency, the therapist found that Jimmy scored about 1½ years below age level on bilateral integration, strength, upper limb coordination, and fine motor control. On the Peabody Developmental Scales, he scored at the age level of a 6 year old. Based on clinical observation of a handwriting sample, the therapist found problems with letter and size formation, spacing of letter and words, and overall spatial organization. Clinical observation of spontaneous activity suggested problems with postural security and low muscle tone.

TREATMENT PLAN

The optometrist and occupational therapist worked together to plan the most appropriate treatment program for this child. The optometrist prescribed eyeglasses to be worn at all times in school. He prescribed a vision therapy program with a primary emphasis on binocular vision and ocular motility. He also designed therapy to deal with the problems in directionality, visual memory, and visual motor integration. This therapy was carefully programmed to coincide with the occupational therapist's treatment plan. The therapist designed a program to work with his fine motor, handwriting, and sensory integration difficulties. Jimmy also received help at school and had private reading tutoring. We asked the teachers to temporarily de-emphasize written work, particularly copying from the board.

After 12 months of combined educational, occupational therapy, and optometric intervention, Jimmy made outstanding progress. He now found it easier to get his thoughts down in writing, copying from the board was considerably better, he was no longer reversing excessively, and he was willing to engage in sports. His reading level increased about 6 to 9 months, and he was no longer as frustrated in school.

Summary

These two cases underscore the complexity and the challenge of managing learning-related vision disorders. Through these cases, we have tried to emphasize the importance of an interdisciplinary approach. In Case One, the vision problem was the primary cause of the child's academic difficulty, and treatment of the visual efficiency problem transferred directly to improved school performance. However, this type of case is not the most common presentation. In most instances, even if a vision problem is present, it will be only one of several factors contributing to the child's problems. Case Two is an illustration of a child who required intervention from several professionals including occupational therapy and optometry.

References

1. American Occupational Therapy Association. *Guidelines for Occupational Therapy Services in School Systems.* Rockville, MD: Author; 1987.
2. Joint Statement. Learning disabilities, dyslexia, and vision. *Pediatrics.* 2009;124(2):837-844.
3. Scheiman M, Rouse MW. *Optometric Management of Learning Related Vision Problems.* 2nd ed. St. Louis, MO: CV Mosby; 2006.
4. Hoffman LG, Rouse MW. Vision therapy revisited: a restatement. *J Am Optom Assoc.* 1987;58:536-541.
5. Kastenbaum SM. In defense of training. *Optom Wkly.* 1974;65:1120-1122.
6. Pitcher-Baker G. Does perceptual training improve reading? *J Optom Vis Training.* 1974;5:40-45.
7. Ritty MJ, Solan HA, Cool SJ. Visual and sensory-motor functioning in the classroom: a preliminary report of ergonomic demands. *J Am Optom Assoc.* 1993;64:238-244.
8. Sherman A. Relating vision disorders to learning disability. *J Am Optom Assoc.* 1973;44:140-141.
9. Hoffman LG. Incidence of vision difficulties in children with learning disabilities. *J Am Optom Assoc.* 1980;51:447-450.
10. Grisham JD, Simons HD. Refractive error and the reading process: a literature analysis. *J Am Optom Assoc.* 1986;57:44-55.
11. Simons HD, Gassler PA. Vision anomalies and reading skill: a meta-analysis of the literature. *Am J Optom Physiol Opt.* 1988;65:893-904.
12. O'Grady J. The relationship between vision and educational performance: a study of year 2 children in Tasmania. *Aust J Optom.* 1984;67:126-140.
13. Groffman S. The relationship between visual perception and learning. In: Scheiman M, Rouse MW, eds. *Optometric Management of Learning Related Vision Problems.* 2nd ed. St. Louis, MO: CV Mosby; 2006:179-214.

14. Kavale K. Meta-analysis of the relationship between visual perceptual skills and reading achievement. *J Learning Disabilities*. 1982;15:42-51.

15. Eames TH. A comparison of the ocular characteristics of unselected and reading disability groups. *J Educ Res*. 1932;25:211-215.

16. Eames TH. Comparison of eye conditions among 1,000 reading failures, 500 ophthalmic patients, and 150 unselected children. *Am J Ophthalmol*. 1948;31:713-717.

17. Rosner J, Rosner J. Comparison of visual characteristics in children with and without learning difficulties. *Am J Optom Physiol Opt*. 1987;64:531-533.

18. Rosner J, Rosner J. Some observations of the relationship between the visual perceptual skills development of young hyperopes and age of first lens correction. *Clin Exp Optom*. 1986;69:166-168.

19. Shankar S, Evans MA, Vobier WR. Hyperopia and emergent literacy of young children: pilot study. *Optom Vis Sci*. 2007;84:1031-1038.

20. Eames TH. A frequency of physical handicaps in reading in reading disability and unselected groups. *J Educ Res*. 1935;29:1-5.

21. Good GH. Relationship of fusion weakness to reading disability. *J Exp Educ*. 1939;8:115-121.

22. Evans JR, Efron M, Hodge C. Incidence of lateral phoria among SLD children. *Acad Ther*. 1976;11:431-433.

23. Pirozzolo FJ. Eye movements and reading disability. In: Rayner K, ed. *Eye Movements in Reading*. New York, NY: Academic Press; 1983.

24. Lieberman S. The prevalence of visual disorders in a school for emotionally disturbed children. *J Am Optom Assoc*. 1985;56:800-803.

25. Flax N. General issues. In: Scheiman M, Rouse MW, eds. *Optometric Management of Learning Related Vision Problems*. 2nd ed. St. Louis, MO: CV Mosby; 2006:127-152.

Chapter Nine

Visual Problems Associated With Acquired Brain Injury

Lynn Fishman Hellerstein, OD, FCOVD, FAAO and
Mitchell Scheiman, OD, FCOVD, FAAO

Overview

When a acquired brain injury (ABI) occurs, the effects on the visual process and the integration of vision with other sensory modalities can be devastating. ABI may lead to impairment in one or more functions, including vision, arousal, attention, language, memory, reasoning, abstract thinking, judgment, problem solving, sensory abilities, perceptual abilities, motor abilities, psychosocial behavior, information processing, and speech.[1] Visual-perceptual dysfunction is one of the most common and devastating residual impairments of brain injury.[2] Perceptual deficits may affect the skills necessary for activities of daily living, including dressing, eating, reading, and working. Most activities of daily living require effective and optimal visual efficiency, visual processing, and visual motor performance. The deficit may be anywhere from a visual efficiency problem of "seeing clearly" to a problem of form perception, eye-hand coordination, or visual attending. Visual dysfunctions caused by brain injury can have a devastating effect on performance and quality of life.

Activities used in rehabilitation programs typically require or depend on both the visual efficiency and visual information processing system. It is, therefore, essential for occupational therapists to know visual status and function before initiating rehabilitation. Because of the high prevalence of vision disorders in the ABI population and the importance of vision in rehabilitation, optometrists should play a role as a member of the rehabilitation team. Optometrists can help co-manage the overall rehabilitation of a patient who has been neurologically compromised by minimizing any deficit of the visual system and by providing consultation and guidance to members of the rehabilitative team.[3] This chapter will discuss the visual problems associated with brain injury, and Chapter Ten will discuss visual rehabilitation for this population.

ABI is generally used to refer to both traumatic brain injury (TBI) and stroke or cerebrovascular accident (CVA).

Traumatic Brain Injury

Thurman et al[4] define TBI as an occurrence of injury to the head that is documented in a medical record, with one or more of the following conditions attributed to head injury:

- Observed or self-reported decreased level of consciousness

- Amnesia

- Skull fracture

- Objective neurological or neuropsychological abnormality

- Diagnosed intracranial lesion

TBI may result in significant impairment of an individual's physical, cognitive, and psychosocial functioning.

The reported incidence of TBI in the United States is about 175 to 200 per 100,000 population or about 2 million head injuries each year.[5] Over 1.5 million Americans suffer nonfatal traumatic brain injuries each year that do not require hospitalization.[4,6] Another 300,000 individuals suffer brain injuries severe enough to require hospitalization, with 99,000 resulting in a lasting disability. A total of 56,000 people die each year as a result of TBI.[4] The prevalence of TBI is estimated to be 2.5 to 6.5 million individuals.[7]

The number of people surviving TBI has increased significantly in recent years, which is attributed to faster and more effective emergency care, quicker and safer transportation to specialized treatment facilities, and advances in acute medical management. TBI affects people of all ages and is the leading cause of long-term disability among children and young adults.

Individuals aged 15 to 24 have the highest risk of TBI,[4] and TBI affects males at twice the rate of females. In addition, the mortality rate is higher among males, suggesting that males are more likely than females to suffer severe injuries.[4]

Although the largest group of TBI survivors are young adults in their prime working years, many survivors, particularly those with a severe TBI, do not return to work. Estimates vary widely, ranging from a low of 12.5% to as high as 80%, of those who do not return to work. The ability to return to work is highly correlated to the post-acute functional limitations of the survivor.[8,9] Of those who survive each year, approximately 70,000 to 90,000 endure life-long debilitating loss of function. A survivor of a severe brain injury typically faces 5 to 10 years of intensive services at an estimated cost in excess of $4 million. Two thousand survivors exist in a vegetative state. Motor vehicle crashes cause half of all TBIs, with falls accounting for 2%, assaults and violence 12%, and sports and recreation 10%. The economic loss from TBI has been estimated to be about $4 billion per year.

The severity of TBI has been classified as mild, moderate, and severe.[10] Mild TBI is a very common injury, resulting in about 300,000 hospital admissions each year.[11] Many more people are believed to sustain mild TBI, but they do not require hospitalization. As a result, an accurate estimation of the number of mild TBI cases per year is not available. About 80% of people admitted to a hospital with the diagnosis of TBI have mild TBI.[12] Hellerstein et al[13] studied the vision characteristics of patients with mild TBI and found significant differences between the group with TBI group and age-matched patients without TBI. They concluded that the term *mild TBI* is very misleading and does not necessarily translate to "mild functional loss." The more severe injuries require hospitalization and various types of rehabilitative therapy.

Vision Problems and Traumatic Brain Injury

A number of studies have been published in recent years reporting the prevalence of vision problems after TBI in both the civilian[14,15] and military populations.[16-18] Suchoff et al[14] completed a prospective study of 62 consecutively (mean age 49, 19 to 70 years) admitted patients into a rehabilitation hospital. Although there were patients with both TBI and CVA in the sample, they did not report the results for the two groups separately. They found a high prevalence of binocular vision (42%), eye movement (40%), visual field (23%), and accommodative disorders (10%).

In a larger, retrospective study of the civilian population, Ciuffreda et al[15] reported on 160 patients with TBI. They found that 56% had binocular vision disorders and convergence insufficiency was the most common binocular vision problem (42.5%). Fifty-one percent had eye movement problems (saccadic and pursuit deficits and nystagmus), and 41% had accommodative disorders.

Investigation of the prevalence of vision problems after TBI in the military has become a priority in recent years because over 30,000 US soldiers have been wounded in Iraq and Afghanistan, and TBI is the "signature wound" of these wars. Studies have shown that 30% of troops engaged in combat greater than 4 months are at risk for disabling neurologic disorders from blast waves of improvised explosive devices; 60% of injuries are due to roadside bombs and improvised explosive devices.

Goodrich et al[16] studied 50 patients admitted to the polytrauma rehabilitation center from December 2004 to November 2006. The mean age of subjects was 28.1 years, and all had experienced a TBI, with blast injuries accounting for half of all injuries. Seventy-four percent of the subjects complained about the following: Blurred distance vision, sensitivity to light, missing a part of their vision, bumping into objects or walls, blurred near reading vision, and inability to comfortably read continuous text. The most common vision disorders were convergence insufficiency (30%), visual field deficits (30%), accommodative dysfunction (22%), and eye movement problems (20%). Over 60% of the subjects reported reading difficulties as well. The authors concluded that visual impairments are both frequent and severe in a population of patients with polytrauma and, therefore, all patients with polytrauma should have routine comprehensive vision examinations.

Brahm et al[17] studied frequency of visual impairment in combat-injured polytrauma rehabilitation center inpatient and polytrauma network site outpatient military personnel with TBI. Subjects included 68 inpatients and 124 outpatients with a mean age of 28 years old. They found that 84% of polytrauma rehabilitation center patients and 90% of polytrauma network site patients had TBI associated with blast event. The prevalent conditions were convergence insufficiency (42%), accommodative insufficiency (42%), pursuit/saccadic dysfunction (33%), and visual field defects (32%). As in the previous study, many patients complained about reading difficulties (64%). The authors concluded that combat troops exposed to blast with associated TBI are at risk for visual dysfunction, and that the results of the study support a policy of vision examination for all service-members who screen positive for TBI.

Finally, Stelmack et al[18] reported on a retrospective medical record review of 103 patients with polytrauma. Seventy-five percent of the patients with TBI reported visual symptoms and the most prevalent vision disorders were accommodative disorder (47%), convergence disorders (28%), and visual field loss (14%).

It is interesting to note that the results of studies in both the civilian and military population are similar and suggest that convergence insufficiency, accommodative dysfunction, eye movement problems, and visual field problems are the vision disorders occupational therapists are most likely to encounter in patients after TBI.

Stroke/Cerebrovascular Accident

Stroke or CVA is a clinically defined syndrome of rapidly developing symptoms or signs of focal loss of cerebral function with no apparent cause other than that of vascular origin, but the loss of function can at times be global.[19] Symptoms last more than 24 hours or lead to death. The syndrome varies in severity from recovery in a day, to incomplete recovery, to severe disability, to death.[19] Stroke cases can now be classified in epidemiology studies by type. Wolf et al[20] reported that, in the Framingham study, 45% of strokes were classified as atherosclerotic, 19% as cerebral embolism, 19% as transient ischemic attacks, 5% as intracerebral hemorrhage, 4% as subarachnoid hemorrhage, and 2% as other, for men aged 55 to 84 years.

Stroke is the third leading cause of death and the leading cause of chronic disability in the adult population of the United States.[21] About 750,000 individuals sustain strokes each year, and there is a prevalence of about 3.5 to 4 million survivors of stroke.[20] Of these survivors, about one-third have mild impairments, another one-third are moderately impaired, and the remainder are severely impaired. CVA can occur at any age, but it is much more common in the elderly. The death rate doubles every 10 years between the ages of 55 and 85.[13] The incidence of stroke varies with location. For example, the incidence has been reported to be as low as 238 per 100,000 in Dijon, France, to 362 per 100,000 in Rochester, Minnesota, to 627 per 100,000 in Novosibirsk, Russia.[19] In the United States, there have been consistently higher rates of stroke in the southeastern states since the 1930s.[22] With the aging of the population, it is likely that CVA will become even more common in the future. Given the high prevalence of vision problems after CVA, optometrists have an important role to play in the vision care of this population.

Vision Problems Associated With Stroke

There are fewer studies investigating the prevalence of vision problems after CVA. In the Suchoff et al[14] study described earlier, 25 of the 62 patients had CVA, rather than TBI. However, the authors did not report the results for the two groups separately. They found a high prevalence of binocular vision (42%), eye movement (40%), visual field (23%), and accommodative (10%) disorders.

The only study that reported on the CVA population separately is the study by Ciuffreda et al[15] in which they examined 60 patients with CVA. They found that 55% had binocular vision disorders, and convergence insufficiency was the most common binocular vision problem (37%). Fifty-seven percent had eye movement problems (saccadic and pursuit deficits and nystagmus), and 13% had accommodative disorders.

Visual System Model: Functional Based

As explained in earlier chapters of this book, a comprehensive understanding of vision includes visual acuity, refraction, eye health, visual efficiency, and visual processing. To help understand functional performance of patients with brain injury, clinicians and researchers have found it useful to view the visual system from an additional perspective or model. This model consists of two modes of visual processing: a central or focal process and a peripheral or ambient process.[23] The two modes of processing involve separate neurological pathways that simultaneously process visual input. Together, the two systems provide integration of visual input.

The focal mode is made up of the foveal, parafoveal, and primary visual cortex inputs. The focal mode contributes to the "what" of vision (object recognition and identification). The focal mode is attention oriented and centers on detail in small areas of space. The focal mode can be measured by more traditional tests such as visual acuity and color perception.

The ambient mode (more midbrain in location) is concerned with the "where," or the location of objects. Information about movement and position of objects is transmitted to the posterior parietal cortex, which provides a reference of where objects are located in space. The ambient mode is important in posture, motion, and spatial orientation. It is more peripheral and is involved in object localization and mobility. It receives input from the other sensory systems, including tactile, kinesthesia, and proprioception. It is difficult to assess the ambient function other than through observation about how the patient moves.[24]

To understand these two different visual processes, try the following demonstration: stand up, look straight ahead, and hold each index finger as close to each eye as possible to effectively block out central vision when looking straight ahead. You should still be able to see peripherally. For example, if you hold your finger in front of your eye and look directly at a person, you cannot see the person; however, you are still able to see the room around the person. Now walk around the room, keeping your fingers in front of your eyes. Move your fingers from your eyes and make each hand into a loose fist so as to form a small "telescope" with each hand. Hold each hand up to each eye, so that you can see straight ahead but very little peripherally. Now walk around the room. Which way is easier to move, with your fingers blocking central vision or blocking peripheral vision? Why?

Most people find it much easier to move when central vision is blocked and when peripheral vision is not affected. This is because the ambient system, which is more closely related to peripheral processing, is integrated with movement and balance systems. Therefore, if a person has an injury or damage to the focal system (such as loss of visual acuity due to cataracts, retina, macular degeneration), he or she may have problems reading or watching TV, but movement is often not affected unless there are other motor problems. If a person has injury or damage to the ambient system (ie, field loss, poor ocular motor control, etc), then movement through space may be hindered.

The ability to match information between the visual and motor processes is essential for the coordination of motor function. For example, a problem in either the focal or ambient systems described above will have a negative effect on the motor system. There is a constant interchange between focal and ambient function of vision throughout life. This interchange is often affected when there is brain injury. It is thought that this disruption may occur at the level of the midbrain. Padula[24,25] termed the condition *post-traumatic vision syndrome* (PTVS). Symptoms include asthenopia (eyestrain), diplopia (double vision), complaints that objects appear to move, poor tracking abilities, staring behavior, and visual memory problems. The syndrome is characterized by accommodative dysfunction, balance and posture difficulties, convergence insufficiency, exophoria, lowered blink rate, and spatial disorientation.

Types of Brain Injuries

The anatomy and physiology of the skull, the vascular network for the brain, as well as the dynamics of head trauma all contribute significantly to the effects of insult to the visual system.[3] This neurological insult affects the patient's neurological integrity and ability to process visually related or visually guided information.

To understand the types of visual dysfunctions that may be present, one needs to have a basic understanding of the brain and the effect of various types of injury on the visual system. Not all injuries result in the same type of deficit. For example, CVA patients often have more of a focal injury, whereas patients acquiring a TBI from a motor vehicle accident often exhibit diffuse injury resulting in multiple deficits. Focal damage is the result of direct injury to a structure that can be localized by observation, computed tomography (CT) scan, or magnetic resonance imaging (MRI). Diffuse damage is not always associated with specific objective abnormalities (on CT or MRI). Instead, it is presumed to occur as axons are stretched or sheared. Diffuse or focal damage can result in sensory, motor, cognitive, or other disorders.

Direct optic nerve dysfunction is highly correlated to injury site. Supraorbital and frontal head injuries are most likely to cause optic nerve dysfunction. This type of injury could result in partial or complete loss of vision. Optic nerve dysfunction is also often seen with other types of neurological diseases, such as multiple sclerosis.[26-30]

Concussion resulting in diffuse axonal injury can cause sensory motor impairments. If the injury is localized more in the left hemisphere, language deficits often result, whereas right hemisphere insult often causes more visual spatial difficulties. Injury to the frontal lobe may affect intellectual thinking, planning, and motor planning. The left hemisphere is often involved in analytical, sequential, time-oriented, organizational processing, and processing of letters and words. The right hemisphere is involved in nonverbal behavior such as visual spatial tasks and nonlinguistic functions (depth, color, and shape discrimination).

CVA results in deficits of varying severity depending on the location and extent of injury. A transient ischemic attack may be a presentation of an impending stroke. Strokes that occur in the areas supplied by the middle cerebral artery often result in hemiparesis. Eye movement control, memory, and consciousness will be affected if the anterior cerebral artery supply is involved. These vessels serve the frontal lobes, the upper portion of the chiasm, and the intracranial portions of the optic nerve.[31] Part of the lateral geniculate nucleus, optic tracts and radiation, portions of the midbrain, and the parietal and occipital lobes are supplied by the posterior cerebral arteries. Infarcts of the posterior cerebral arteries result in color anomia and visual field deficits (homonymous hemianopia with macular sparing). Sections of the temporal lobes, the cerebellum, significant portions of the brainstem (subthalamic nucleus, midbrain, pons, and medulla), and the optic radiation are supplied by the vertebrobasilar system. Obstruction of this system will lead to dysfunction of the eye muscles, balance, and vision.[32]

Ocular Health

Disruption of the visual system results from injury to the ocular structures (including the cornea, iris, lens, sclera, choroid, and retina), ocular orbits, ocular muscles (medial rectus, lateral rectus, superior rectus, inferior rectus, superior oblique, and inferior oblique), optic nerves, chiasm, tracts, radiation, and primary and associated visual cortical areas. The residual effects range from minimal, such as a mild abrasion, to a more severe vision-threatening injury. Loss of acuity and change in refraction or visual field may occur, resulting in decreased acuity, ocular discomfort, visual confusion, double vision, blurriness, light sensitivity, and decreased visual awareness. Sometimes the injuries may improve spontaneously with time, but medical treatment is often necessary immediately.

It is not uncommon to encounter an elderly patient with visual conditions such as glaucoma, macular degeneration, and/or cataract present before brain injury. Even though these types of visual conditions may or may not have been secondary to the injury, visual treatment is necessary. As an example, a 78-year-old patient after CVA was referred by his occupational therapist for a vision evaluation because of suspected "visual spatial and eye-hand coordination difficulties." The referral for functional reasons resulted in a visual evaluation, at which time the diagnosis of cataracts was made and surgery was recommended. After cataract extraction, the patient was much more accurate with eye-hand tasks because his eyesight was much improved. The improvement in vision affected his entire rehabilitation program.

Another common condition is "dry eyes." This condition may be due to poor blinking or incomplete lid closure when sleeping, or it may be a side effect of other medications. Artificial tears, ointment, and other treatment methods may be prescribed by the eye doctor.

Visual Symptoms

A number of visual symptoms and observations are noted with patients with diagnosed visual dysfunctions. Symptoms include double vision, difficulty seeing, ocular discomfort, an inability to follow or track an object, bumping into objects, and difficulty judging size or space. Table 9-1 summarizes patient symptoms, professional observations, and possible areas of visual dysfunction.[33]

The occupational therapist is often called upon to provide the vision screening for a patient with brain injury. This patient observation and the symptom checklist provide very valuable information regarding the patient's visual status. Refer to Chapter Six for the vision screening protocol.

Table 9-1

Patient Symptoms, Professional Observations, and Possible Area of Visual Dysfunction

Binocular Problems

(Pointing system)
Closing one eye

Double vision
Muscle palsy
Headaches
Pain
Reading problems

Print blurry
Ocular discomfort

Accommodation Problems

(Focusing system)
Focusing problems

Headaches
Pain
Double vision
Squinting
Closing one eye

Reading problems
Ocular discomfort

Motilities

(Tracking system)
Inability to follow objects smoothly
Reading problems
Skipping words
Re-reading words
Reversals
Nystagmus involuntary movement or rotation of the eyes

Strabismus

(Eyeturn)
Closing of one eye
Double vision
Head tilts or turns
Sudden onset of eye turn

Muscle palsy
Difficult judging depth and 3-D view

Visual-Perceptual

Problem judging size
Problem judging distances
Coordination problems
Left-right confusion

Visual Field Defects

Bumping into chairs, objects, etc
Difficulty seeing at night
Tunnel vision
Holding onto walls, other people, etc

Reprinted from Cohen AH, Soden R. An optometric approach to the rehabilitation of the stroke patient. *J Am Optom Assoc.* 1981;52(9):795-800. © 1981 by the American Optometric Association. Reprinted with permission.

Visual Disorders

As stated earlier the most common visual problems associated with brain injury include nonstrabismic binocular dysfunction such as convergence insufficiency, accommodative dysfunction, eye movement deficits, visual field loss, and visual information processing disorders.[3,14-18,34-62] Other common problems include visual acuity loss, and double vision. Table 9-2 is adapted from Zoltan.[45] It summarizes the more common types of visual deficits found with patients with brain injury.

Binocular Disorders

Acquired strabismus or nonstrabismic binocular vision problems often occur after trauma and result in double vision, blurriness, or visual confusion. The strabismus is often noncomitant (ie, variable depending on the direction of gaze). Paresis of cranial nerves III, IV, and/or VI are often associated with this type of strabismus. A patient with an acquired strabismus may close one eye, request a patch, or develop an awkward head turn to reduce symptoms. Common nonstrabismic binocular vision problems include convergence insufficiency, decrease in fusional amplitudes, and suppression. Patients with these problems often fatigue quickly with sustained visual tasks.

Table 9-2

Types of Visual Deficits

Deficit	Underlying Mechanism	Clinical Manifestation/ Resulting Deficit
Blurred or decreased visual acuity	Ocular injury (cornea, lens, retina), optic nerve (II), and/or pathway injury, III nerve, midbrain, refractive error, amblyopia	Vision blurred either full- or part-time in one or both eyes, may have fatigue with sustained visual tasks
Strabismus or binocular dysfunction (convergence/ divergence)	Decreased ocular motor control (eg, III, IV, or VI nerve paresis or dysfunction), midbrain injury affecting medial longitudinal fasiculus and/or ocular motor nuclei	Patient may see double part- or full-time, may close or cover an eye, may learn to suppress an eye, may have decreased or inaccurate depth perception, difficulty with localizing objects in space, confusion with sustained visual activities
Nystagmus	Brainstem damage (especially vestibular), cerebellar damage	Abnormal oscillations of the eyes, resulting in blurred vision, nausea, visual confusion
Decreased ocular motor skills: 1. Ocular pursuits	Lesion in either hemisphere with or without brainstem damage	Difficulty tracking in any or all of the planes
2. Saccadic eye movements	Lesion in frontal cortex (area 8) or parietal lobe	Difficulty or inability in quick localization, difficulty with reading

Adapted from Zoltan B. *Vision, Perception, and Cognition: A Manual for the Evaluation and Treatment of the Neurologically Impaired Adult.* 3rd ed. Thorofare, NJ: SLACK Incorporated; 1996.

Accommodation Disorders

Accommodative disorders frequently occur after trauma. The most common condition is accommodative insufficiency. Patients complain of visual fatigue with sustained near work, of difficulty changing focus from one distance to another, and sometimes of variability in clearness of vision. Even patients with mild TBI or whiplash injuries may show accommodative disorders.

Eye Movement Deficits

Patients with brain injury may show smooth pursuits and saccadic fixation abnormalities. These patients have difficulty tracking or following an object or may have problems fixating or locating objects. Deficits in scanning result in an inefficient gathering of visual information. Scanning deficits can impact on visual perceptual skills including visual closure, figure ground, and visual memory.

Nystagmus is sometimes present, especially with patients who have suffered brainstem or cerebellar damage. Patients with acquired nystagmus are quite uncomfortable and often experience nausea.

Visual Field Loss

Visual field loss and neglect may be present secondary to a brain injury, especially after CVA. Functional observations of patients with field loss include:

- Problems in mobility in a certain field (patient keeps bumping into things on the side of loss)
- Inattention to an area in space (patient not aware of objects or people; eg, patient may only eat part of food on plate)
- Startle response (surprised when object appears, as patient was unaware of object in loss field)
- Difficulty reading (cannot accurately find end of column)

Vestibular/Balance/Movement Problems

If a patient presents with balance, dizziness, and/or movement problems, rehabilitation needs to be carefully coordinated with all therapists and physicians. Some patients may be suffering from vestibular, cerebellar, and/or other neurologic disorders, and the patient may need to depend on visual input to compensate and stabilize the system. In such cases, the individual's visual skills need to be at maximum performance levels. If vision problems are present in addition to vestibular/balance/movement problems, the patient may be even more symptomatic.

Visual Perceptual Deficits

Visual perceptual problems occur when there has been injury in the cortical or midbrain areas. It is inappropriate to diagnose a visual perceptual dysfunction until a full visual evaluation is completed, as ocular health and visual efficiency problems can affect a person's visual input and thereby interfere with the ability to process and respond to the visual information.

Visual perceptual deficits can include body scheme disorders and disorders of higher level visual perceptual skills, such as discrimination, spatial relations, and so on.[2] These deficits usually involve parietal and/or occipital lobe lesions. Table 9-3 summarizes the more common visual perceptual deficits found with patients with brain injury.

Effect of Visual Function on Rehabilitation

Vision, which is considered to be the primary sense for gathering information, is often overlooked or ignored in the rehabilitation program. During the acute phase of medical treatment, management of life-threatening conditions and physical injuries is certainly the priority. If there is damage to ocular structures or to the ocular motor system, an ophthalmologist or neuro-ophthalmologist will often be called to provide diagnostic and therapeutic care. This is appropriate, as surgical or medical treatment may be necessary to minimize loss of sight.

However, once the patient is medically stable, the functional aspects of vision are routinely overlooked. Hundreds and thousands of dollars may be spent in rehabilitation without addressing the visual system. Common examples include the following:

- Patients with a field loss may be given the task of learning to feed themselves without first being taught how to scan or locate objects in the affected field.
- Patients may be taught to read or to use the computer even though they lack appropriate glasses to "see" the task.
- Patients with constant double vision are patched full-time and then are asked to walk. This could have a negative effect on balance.
- Patients who have vestibular dysfunctions causing dizziness, vertigo, or balance problems may still wear their "invisible, no-line bifocals" that can often exaggerate or aggravate the dizziness and balance condition.

Table 9-3

Visual Perceptual Deficits

Deficit	Clinical Manifestation
Agnosia	Inability to recognize an object by sight despite adequate cognition, language skills, and visual acuity/field
Prosopagnosia	Inability to recognize a familiar face
Object agnosia	Inability to recognize objects by visual inspection alone
Achromatopsia agnosia	Inability to discriminate between different colors
Simultanagnosia	Inability to perceive entire picture or to integrate its parts
Alexia	Inability to recognize or comprehend written or printed words
Apraxia (optic)	Inability to execute purposeful movement
Ataxia (optic)	Inability to visually guide limbs (mislocalization when reaching or pointing for objects)
Constructional apraxia	Inability to copy or build a simple design
Depth perception	Inability to judge depths and distances
Figure ground	Inability to distinguish foreground from background
Form perception/constancy	Inability to judge variations in form
Spatial relations	Inability to perceive the position of two or more objects in relation to self and to each other
Unilateral spatial neglect	Inability to attend to or respond to meaningful sensory stimuli presented in the affected hemisphere

---

Many patients who have been diagnosed with mild brain injuries are often not aware of their visual problems, nor are they visually evaluated until many years post-injury.

Few rehabilitation facilities currently use rehabilitative optometric services on a regular basis. With the high prevalence of visual system dysfunctions, optometric rehabilitative assessment and management is essential although this does not replace the need for ophthalmology and neuro-ophthalmology intervention.

Summary

A primary objective of this chapter is to demonstrate the need for a comprehensive vision evaluation for a patient as soon as possible after brain injury. There are also many visual compensation strategies and adaptive techniques that may significantly help patients in their recovery. Prompt attention to the visual system in patients with ABI will lead to early identification and treatment of vision problems that can potentially interfere with rehabilitation. There are also many compensatory and adaptive techniques that can be implemented once the nature of the vision problem is identified. The next chapter will review vision rehabilitation for ABI.

References

1. Lehmkuhl DL. *Brain Injury Glossary*. Houston, TX: HDI Publishers; 1993.
2. Rosenthal M, Griffith ER, Bond MR, Miller JD. *Rehabilitation of the Adult and Child With Traumatic Brain Injury*. Philadelphia, PA: FA Davis Co; 1990.
3. Cohen AH, Rein LD. The effect of head trauma on the visual system: the doctor of optometry as a member of the rehabilitation team. *J Am Optom Assoc*. 1992;63:530-536.
4. Thurman DJ, Sniezek JE, Johnson D, et al. *Guidelines for Surveillance of Central Nervous System Injury*. Atlanta, GA: US Department of Health and Human Services, Public Health Service, Centers for Disease Control and Prevention, National Center for Injury Prevention and Control; 1995.

5. Kraus JF, MacArthur DL. Epidemiologic aspects of brain injury. *Neurol Clin.* 1996;14(2):435-450.

6. Sosin DM, Sniezek JE, Thurman DJ. Incidence of mild and moderate brain injury in the United States, 1991. *Brain Inj.* 1996;10(1):47-54.

7. National Institutes of Health. *NIH Consensus Statement on Rehabilitation of Persons With Traumatic Brain Injury.* Bethesda, MD: Author; 1998.

8. Greenspan AI, Wrigley JM, Kresnow M, et al. Factors influencing failure to return to work due to traumatic brain injury. *Brain Inj.* 1996;10(3):207-218.

9. Ip RY, Dornan J, Schentag C. Traumatic brain injury: factors predicting return to work or school. *Brain Inj.* 1995;9(5):517-532.

10. Alexander MP. Mild traumatic brain injury: pathophysiology, natural history, and clinical management. *Neurology.* 1995;45:1253-1260.

11. Whyte J, Hart T, Laborde A, et al. Rehabilitation of the patient with traumatic brain injury. In: DeLisa J, Gans BM, Bockenek WL, et al, eds. *Rehabilitation Medicine: Principles and Practice.* 3rd ed. Philadelphia, PA: Lippincott-Raven; 1998:1191-1239.

12. Kraus JF, MacArthur DL, Silverman TA. Epidemiology of mild brain injury. *Semin Neurol.* 1994;14:1-7.

13. Hellerstein LF, Freed S, Maples WC. Vision profile of patients with mild brain injury. *J Am Optom Assoc.* 1995;66:634-639.

14. Suchoff IB, Kapoor N, Waxman R, Ference W. The occurrence of ocular and visual dysfunction in an acquired brain injury patient sample. *Optometry.* 1999;70:301-309.

15. Ciuffreda KJ, Kapoor N, Rutner D, et al. Occurrence of oculomotor dysfunctions in acquired brain injury: a retrospective analysis. *J Am Optom Assn.* 2007;78:155-161.

16. Goodrich L, Kirby J, Cockerham G, Ingalla SP, Lew HL. Visual function in patients of a polytrauma rehabilitation center: a descriptive study. *J Rehabil Res Dev.* 2007;44:929-936.

17. Brahm KD, Wilgenburg HM, Kirby J, Ingalla S, Chang CY, Goodrich GK. Visual impairment and dysfunction in servicemembers with TBI. *Opt Vis Sci.* 2009;86:817-825.

18. Stelmack JA, Frith T, Van Koevering D, Stelmack TR. Visual function in patients followed at a Veterans Affairs polytrauma network site: an electronic medical record review. *Optometry.* 2009;80:419-424.

19. Warlow CP. Epidemiology of stroke. *Lancet.* 1998;352(Suppl 3):1-4.

20. Wolf PA, D'Agostino RB, Belanger AJ, Kannel WB. Probability of stroke: a risk profile from the Framingham Study. *Stroke.* 1991;22:312-318.

21. American Heart Association. *2001 Heart and Stroke Statistical Update.* Dallas, TX: Author; 2001.

22. Kuller LH. Epidemiology of stroke. *Adv Neurol.* 1978;19:281-311.

23. Trevarthen C, Sperry RW. Perceptual unity of the ambient visual field in human commissurotomy patients. *Brain.* 1973;96:547-570.

24. Padula WV. *A Behavioral Vision Approach for Persons With Physical Disabilities.* Santa Ana, CA: Optometric Extension Program; 1988.

25. Padula WV. Neuro-optometric rehabilitation for persons with a TBI or CVA. *J Optom Vis Devel.* 1992;23:4-8.

26. Barron C. Low vision rehabilitation of multiple sclerosis: a case report. *J Am Optom Assoc.* 1993;64:38-44.

27. Gray L, Winkelman AC. Multiple sclerosis: recent developments. *Ocul Dis Update 2.* 1991:81-95.

28. Harkins T. Treating multiple sclerosis. *Clin Eye Vis Care.* 1994;6(3):133-136.

29. Sherman J, Morschauser D. A clinical update on multiple sclerosis. *Rev Opt.* 1994;131:55-63.

30. Wall M. Multiple sclerosis. In: Albert DM, ed. *Principles and Practice of Ophthalmology.* Philadelphia, PA: WB Saunders; 1994:2682-2688.

31. Wolff E, ed. *Anatomy of the Eye and Orbit.* Philadelphia, PA: WB Saunders; 1976.

32. Zost MG. Diagnosis and management of visual dysfunction in cerebral injury. In: Maino D, ed. *Diagnosis and Management of Special Populations.* St. Louis, MO: CV Mosby; 1995.

33. Cohen AH, Soden R. An optometric approach to the rehabilitation of the stroke patient. *J Am Optom Assoc.* 1981;52:795-800.

34. Carroll RP, Saeber JH. Acute loss of fusional convergence following head trauma. *Am Orthop J.* 1974;24:57-59.

35. Fowler MS, Richardson AJ, Stein JF. Orthoptic investigation of neurological patients undergoing rehabilitation. *Br Orthopt J.* 1991;48:8.

36. Harrison RJ. Loss of fusional vergence with partial loss of accommodative convergence and accommodation following head injury. *Binoc Vis.* 1987;2:93-100.

37. Horwich H, Gables C. The ocular effects of whiplash injury. *Transactions of the Section on Ophthalmology: American Medical Association.* 1961:86-90.

38. Krasnow DJ. Fusional convergence loss following head trauma: a case report. *Optom Mon.* 1982;73:18-19.

39. Kelley JS, Hoover RE, George T. Whiplash maculopathy. *Arch Ophthalmol.* 1978;96:834-835.

40. Mazow ML, Tang R. Strabismus associated with head and facial trauma. *Am Orthop J.* 1982;32:31-35.

41. Pratt-Johnson JA. Central disruption of fusional amplitude. *Br J Ophthalmol.* 1973;57:347-350.

42. Padula WV, Shapiro JB, Jasin P. Head injury causing post trauma vision syndrome. *N Engl J Optom.* 1988;Dec:16-21.

43. Roberts SP. Visual disorders of higher cortical function. *J Am Optom Assoc.* 1992;63:723-732.
44. Roca PD. Ocular manifestations of whiplash injuries. *Ann Ophthalmol.* 1972;4:63-73.
45. Zoltan B. *Vision, Perception and Cognition: A Manual for the Evaluation and Treatment of the Neurologically Impaired Adult.* 3rd ed. Thorofare, NJ: SLACK Incorporated; 1996.
46. Roy RR. The role of binocular stress in the post-whiplash syndrome. *Am J Optom Arch Am Acad Optom.* 1961;11:625-635.
47. Seabrook C. Surviving a stroke—25% decline in death signals a big success story? *The Atlanta Journal.* 1985;103:22A.
48. Stanworth A. Defects of ocular movement and fusion after head injury. *Br J Ophthalmol.* 1974;58:266-271.
49. Swanson M. Neuro-rehabilitation. *Eye Quest Magazine.* 1995;Jan-Feb:50-55.
50. Thomann KH, Dul MW. The optometric assessment of neurologic function. *J Am Optom Assoc.* 1993;64:421-430.
51. Tierney DW. Visual dysfunction in closed head injury. *J Am Optom Assoc.* 1988;59:8.
52. Uzzell BP, Dolinskas CA, Langfitt TW. Visual field defects in relation to head injury severity. *Arch Neurol.* 1988;45:420-424.
53. Wiesinger H, Guerry D. Ocular aspects of whiplash injury. *Virg Med Mon.* 1962;89:165-168.
54. Vogel MS. An overview of head trauma for the primary care practitioner, part I: etiology, diagnosis, and consequences of head trauma. *J Am Optom Assoc.* 1992;63:537-541.
55. Vogel MS. An overview of head trauma for the primary care practitioner, part II: ocular damage associated with head trauma. *J Am Optom Assoc.* 1992;63:542-546.
56. Aksinoff EB, Falk NS. The differential diagnosis of perceptual deficits in traumatic brain injury patients. *J Am Optom Assoc.* 1992;63:554-558.
57. Hellerstein LF, Freed S, Maples WC. Vision profile of patients with mild brain injury. *J Am Optom Assoc.* 1995;66:634-639.
58. Hellerstein LF, Kadet TS. Visual profile of patients presenting with brain trauma. *J Opt Vis Devel.* 1999;30:51-54.
59. Freed S, Hellerstein LF. Visual electrodiagnostic findings in mild traumatic brain injury. *Brain Inj.* 1997;11(1):25-36.
60. Suchoff IB, Kapoor N, Waxman R, et al. The occurrence of ocular and visual dysfunctions in an acquired brain injury sample. *J Am Optom Assoc.* 1999;70:301-308.
61. Suchoff IB, Gianutsos R, Ciuffreda KJ, Groffman S. Vision impairment related to acquired brain injury. In: Silverstone B, Lang MA, Rosenthal BP, Faye EE, eds. *Vision Impairment and Vision Rehabilitation.* Vol 1. New York, NY: Oxford University Press; 2000:517-540.
62. Langerhorst CT, Safran ASB. Progressive shrinkage of the visual field during automated perimetry following traumatic brain injury. *Neuro-ophthalmology.* 1998;20:177-185.

Chapter Ten

Visual Rehabilitation for Patients With Brain Injury

Lynn Fishman Hellerstein, OD, FCOVD, FAAO;
Mitchell Scheiman, OD, FCOVD, FAAO; Beth I. Fishman, OTR, COVT;
and Stephen G. Whittaker, OTR, PhD, CLVT

Overview

When brain injury occurs, a comprehensive rehabilitation program that provides for evaluation, training, and interaction in all routine activities of daily living is often recommended.[1] All deficit areas need to be addressed by retraining an existing process or teaching a new one if the existing process is untrainable. The rehabilitation team is generally composed of physicians (including general physicians, internists, physiatrists, neurologists, neurosurgeons, ophthalmologists, and optometrists), psychologists, neuropsychologists, and therapists (physical, occupational, speech, and cognitive).

In order to make the complex visual decisions necessary for activities of daily living, such as reading, math, driving, and vocations, integration of basic sensory systems is critical. For example, what appears to be a deficit in a visual cognitive skill, such as figure ground (ie, finding an article of clothing in a drawer), may actually be caused by refractive, binocular, accommodative, ocular motility, or pattern recognition problems. Therefore, to help patients regain complex functions, treatment must be started at the basic processing level and proceed through a hierarchy of skills. Throughout this book, we have emphasized that ocular health, refractive, visual acuity, and visual efficiency skills should be addressed before visual information processing problems. Direct treatment of the higher level skill (figure ground) in the example above would not be effective unless the underlying deficits are addressed first.

Determining the cause of the visual deficit requires an understanding of the brain injury effect on the entire visual process from input to output. Some patients require treatment based on a developmental model and might also include sensory integration treatment. Other patients, however, have such severe deficits that function cannot be regained, and strategies to teach the patient to compensate for the impairment are appropriate. All patients who have suffered a brain injury should have a complete vision evaluation by an optometrist who has extensive experience in vision rehabilitation and functional vision care.[2,3] Treatment strategies can then be established.

Optometric Treatment Methods

The goals of optometric intervention are to improve visual acuity, eliminate diplopia, and improve visual awareness and visual cognitive function[4] so that visually related performances are enhanced, allowing the patient to maintain the highest quality of life. Techniques used in optometric rehabilitation include: lenses, prisms, absorptive filters, selective occlusion for specific tasks and distances, low vision aids, and vision therapy (see Chapter Seven).

Ocular Health

Appropriate medications and surgery should be a priority if necessary. Artificial tear regimen and/or taping lids closed for dry eyes may be necessary and sight saving. The therapist has little responsibility in the ocular health areas, and the optometrist or ophthalmologist should be consulted for treatment of patients with ocular health issues. However, it is quite useful for the therapist to be knowledgeable about the type of ocular health problem present and its impact on function.

Lenses

One of the most effective tools that the optometrist uses in practice are lenses.[5] Lenses can be used to improve clarity and sight, reduce or eliminate double vision, and reduce visual discomfort and/or stress, and they affect body posture and weight shifting. A good rule of thumb is that almost all people over the age of 40 years old will need glasses for either distance, near, or full-time wear. You should be suspicious if you are working with a patient over 40 years old who is not wearing glasses for any task. The following are some of the common reasons why patients may need new glasses.

- A patient arrives in the hospital without his or her glasses.
- His or her glasses were broken or lost as a result of the injury.
- His or her glasses are many years old and are an outdated prescription.
- The brain injury has caused a change in prescription and current glasses are not correct.
- The patient cannot utilize the glasses properly because of injury. For example, the brain injury resulted in restriction of movement of eyes in downward gaze, and so the patient cannot move his or her eyes into the part of the bifocal lens that allows for vision at near.

If you wear prescription glasses or contact lenses currently, try spending a day functioning without your proper prescription. It may cause fatigue or nausea, or it may make you less efficient or even nonfunctional! Imagine what it would be like if you have other motor and cognitive impairments in addition to the visual problems.

The best lens for "seeing" is not always the best lens for all tasks. For example, people may see clearly to drive with a certain prescription glass, but they may not be able to read with that prescription. Some patients see clearly at near, but read much more comfortably and efficiently with a special reading lens. Have you ever received a new pair of glasses that allowed you to see clearly yet make you feel uncomfortable when you walked?

Eyeglass prescriptions may need to be modified throughout the rehabilitation program.

Prism

Prism may be prescribed for temporary or permanent use. Fresnel prism, described in Chapter Seven, is a relatively inexpensive, temporary type of prism that can immediately be placed on a current prescription lens. Fresnel prism can also be removed very easily, making it very useful for temporary situations. A disadvantage of Fresnel prisms is that they may distort visual acuity. Prism that is ground into a glasses prescription is a more permanent type of prism prescription.

Prism is used for three main purposes:

1. To neutralize or compensate for patients with acquired strabismus or significant heterophoria (compensatory)
2. To affect spatial awareness and midline awareness (yoked)
3. To expand visual field

COMPENSATORY PRISM

Neutralizing or compensatory prism may be utilized for patients with acquired strabismus or significant heterophoria. Compensatory prism is sometimes difficult to prescribe because the patient's visual condition may be intermittent, variable, or noncomitant. Fresnel prism may be used initially. However, if compensating prism is needed over a longer period of time, the prism is often incorporated into the lens of a pair of glasses. If the compensating prism eliminates the strabismus condition, it will often alleviate double vision. In some cases, a patient may have an abnormal head tilt or turn due to strabismus. If the compensating prism is effective, the head turn or tilt may also be reduced.

When prescribing compensatory prism, we generally describe the prism as either base-in, base-out, base-up or base-down. This refers to the location of the base of the prism relative to the patient's eye (refer to Chapter Seven for more details).

For exophoria, we prescribe base-in prism for both eyes while base-out prism is used for esophoria. For vertical deviations, base-down is used in front of one eye and base-up in front of the other.

PRISM TO AFFECT SPATIAL AWARENESS: YOKED PRISM

Yoked prism differs from compensatory prism because the base of the prism will always be on the same side of each eye (see Chapter Seven). Yoked prism is often utilized to alter a patient's spatial awareness, to modify a patient's midline perception, or to change weight shifting.[6-8] The yoked prism may be temporary and used for certain activities during the rehabilitation process, or it may be permanent for full-time wear. Yoked prism may also be beneficial with field loss patients.

PRISM TO EXPAND VISUAL FIELD

One of the most significant vision problems associated with traumatic brain injury and cerebrovascular accident is visual field loss. One of the treatment modalities available to help a patient compensate for this loss is prism. In recent years studies[9,10] have demonstrated that a prism field expansion system called the Peli Visual Field Expansion Device for Hemianopia is an effective treatment for patients with hemianopia (see Chapter Seven). This prism can expand the visual field by as much as 30 to 40 degrees and allows the patient to be aware of potential obstacles in the periphery.

Filters and Lighting

Absorptive filters or "tints" are often utilized in patients with brain injury. Light sensitivity is a common complaint after injury. Different colors, such as yellow, amber, gray, brown, and green, and other shades of tints are used to decrease light sensitivity symptoms. Pink tints are often helpful for patients working on computers or under fluorescent lights. Anti-reflection coatings reduce glare, especially at night. Some patients, especially elderly patients with age-related decrease in vision, need more light. Better lighting is recommended in addition to yellow tints.

Occlusion

Patients suffering a neurological insult often complain of double vision. Strabismus, including paresis, muscle restrictions, and globe injury are among the leading causes. Patients may squint, cover one eye, or assume an awkward head position to avoid double vision. Physicians or therapists may try to remedy the situation by having the patient wear a patch over one eye. "Which eye should be covered?", "How often should the patient wear the patch?", and "What type of patch should be used?" are common questions that rehabilitation personnel ask. A patient's visual status, in addition to his or her demands in activities of daily living, need to be considered when occlusion is recommended. Therefore, merely telling a patient to patch an eye is an inappropriate recommendation. Optometric consultation is critical when occlusion is being considered.

TOTAL OCCLUSION

If possible, total occlusion (patching) should be avoided.[11] Total occlusion should be utilized only when double vision is constant and no other treatment strategy (lenses, prisms, partial occlusion) is successful. If total occlusion is deemed to be the treatment of choice, the optometrist may recommend alternate occlusion (occluding left eye one day or part of a day and then changing to the right eye). If the vision is exceptionally poor in one eye, the optometrist may recommend occlusion of the poorer eye so that the patient can visually function, or occlusion of the better seeing eye may be recommended so that the patient has a chance to improve visual functioning of the poorer eye.

Figure 10-1a illustrates total occlusion of a patient's left eye. Observe the significant change in head posture when the occluder is changed to the right eye in Figure 10-1b.

Several different methods of occlusion are listed below.

- The black patch with an elastic string, as seen in Figure 10-2a, is an inexpensive, easy method. The main disadvantage is the cosmesis of the patch.

- Clip-on patches as pictured in Figure 10-2b may be utilized. Clip-on patches are also easy and inexpensive but are susceptible to becoming dislodged.

- Figure 10-2c shows tape over the lens of the patient's glasses. Tape is effective and inexpensive, however, it is difficult to clean off a lens, especially when it is necessary to alternate occlusion.

- A Bangerter occlusion foil (see Appendix A) is pictured in 10-2d. This is a very thin plastic-like material that can be ordered in a variety of gradations. These different gradations can create minimal, moderate, or significant decrease (including no light perception) in contrast and acuity. The Bangerter foils can be cut for any size lens and can be easily removed or changed.

PARTIAL OCCLUSION

If a patient has intermittent double vision, full-time occlusion is not recommended. Partial occlusion, like total occlusion, is used only when necessary and allows the patient to be binocular at least part of the day. The types of occluders are the same as described above with one difference. The tape or Bangerter occluder may be cut in such a way as to block only part of the field of vision as pictured in Figure 10-3. This type of occluder allows a patient to still use each eye, but will eliminate double vision in certain fields of gaze. This technique is especially useful to noncomitant strabismics who may have double vision in just certain gazes.

Low Vision Aids

Brain injury can actually damage optical and neural pathways affecting visual acuity at distance and near. In addition, the premorbid state of the patient may include pathology that could also cause decreased visual acuity. There are numerous types of lenses, optical devices (magnifiers, telescopes), computers, and lighting that may be useful to a patient with low vision.[12] Some of these low vision techniques are discussed in Chapters Thirteen and Fourteen.

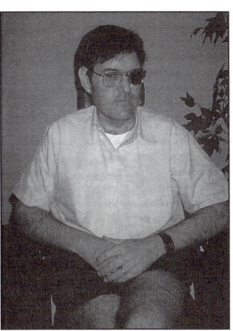

Figure 10-1a. Total occlusion of a patient's left eye.

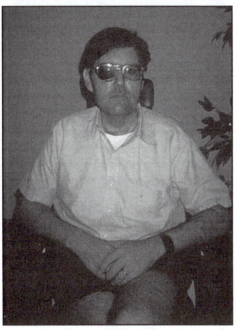

Figure 10-1b. Observe the significant change in head posture when the occluder is changed to the right eye.

Figure 10-2a. Black patch with an elastic string.

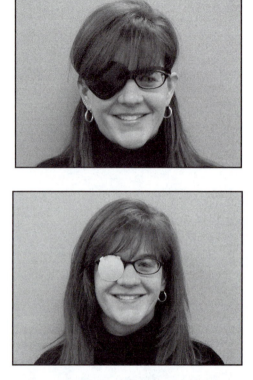

Figure 10-2b. Clip-on patches.

Figure 10-2c. Tape over the lens of the patient's glasses.

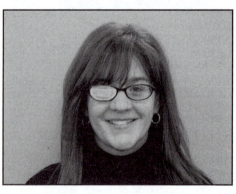

Figure 10-2d. Bangerter occlusion foil.

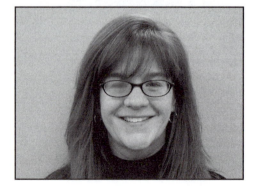

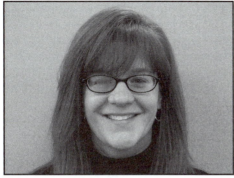

Figure 10-3. The Bangerter occluder may be cut in such a way as to block only part of the field of vision.

Vision Therapy

Vision therapy is an integral part of the rehabilitation treatment for many brain injury patients.[2,13-35] When should vision therapy be started? It is quite ironic that many physicians suggest that patients wait to have a vision evaluation for 6 to 12 months post-trauma because "the vision may change over time." This is comparable to telling a patient who has suffered a paralysis of one side not to use a wheelchair or exercise for at least 6 months because motor function may return. Vision may change, however, it is of questionable value to rehabilitate in other areas when patients have significant vision dysfunction as indicated by the following examples. If double vision is present, patients have more difficulty with balance and movement. If a patient has reduced visual acuity or inappropriate glasses, the use of computers for rehabilitation may be limited. It is frustrating for both the patient with visual field loss and the therapist to perform daily living activities if appropriate scanning and visual compensations are not initiated first. These examples demonstrate that patients should be evaluated very early in the rehabilitation process. This does not mean vision therapy will be initiated immediately, but appropriate lenses, prisms, occlusion, and consultation may be helpful.

If the optometrist prescribes vision therapy, direct supervision and guidance by the optometrist is essential. The occupational therapist may perform daily therapy techniques prescribed by the optometrist, and most importantly, can help the patient generalize visual skills into daily living activities as well as assist in adaptations. Techniques, especially those involving binocularity, should only be attempted by a therapist under direct supervision of an optometrist. The therapy procedures included in this chapter are those that could be provided by the occupational therapist. The more advanced vision therapy techniques requiring direct optometric supervision are not discussed in this book.

When treating a patient with acquired brain injury using vision therapy, the following guidelines are important:

- Obtain visual attention before initiating the therapy procedure.
- All techniques should provide feedback to the patient.
- Work at the level of the patient's current performance.
- Progressively increase the demand of the technique.
- Integrate the visual skill into activities of daily living.

OVERVIEW OF VISION THERAPY FOR BRAIN-INJURED PATIENTS

Vision therapy procedures are organized in a sequence starting from gross motor movements, which are the foundation from which visual skills develop. Gross motor movements, which often include vestibular and balance techniques, begin as reflexive and spontaneous movements and then become more organized with an attempt to use both sides of the body. If the patient has significant tactile and proprioceptive issues as well, techniques in those areas should also be included. The therapy techniques provide a basis for body schema and laterality.

Fine motor and eye movement skills therapy are initially practiced independently and are then integrated with movement. Appropriate eye movement therapy includes emphasis on visual attention, saccadic fixations, and scanning, in addition to smooth, efficient pursuit movements. Without these basic skills, higher level visual perceptual functioning is compromised. Visual perceptual skills often improve as foundation skills improve, even without specific perceptual activities. As foundation skills are integrated, higher level perceptual activities, if necessary, may be included with the goal of improving visual manipulation and visualization abilities. These skills are required in academic areas such as reading, writing, and math and for many vocations. Depending on the neurologic injury and recovery, adaptations or compensatory skills may also be necessary in addition to remedial techniques discussed above.

The sequence of therapy techniques is based on clinical judgment but needs to begin at the level at which the patient can succeed. The key to success is to work at the level of the patient's current performance and gradually increase the demands of the tasks.

VISION REHABILITATION TECHNIQUES FOR PATIENTS WITH BALANCE/MOVEMENT DISORDERS

When a patient presents with a balance and movement disorder, there is often a problem with integration of the visual, vestibular, and somatosensory systems.[36] Somatosensory and vestibular interaction, rather than the visual system, should control balance in the adult. However, with a patient who has suffered a cerebrovascular accident or traumatic brain injury that results in decreased proprioceptive and tactile cues, the visual system is often the predominant system for balance. These patients need an integrative therapy program that includes vision, physical, and occupational therapy. Too often, vision is not appropriately addressed during vestibular rehabilitation programs. Vision therapy treatment can enhance vestibular therapy since vestibular therapy can enhance vision therapy.

The goals of vestibular therapy are to[37]:

- Develop proprioceptive and visual mechanisms to compensate for a disturbance in labyrinthine function.
- Improve muscle coordination.
- Practice balancing under everyday conditions with special attention to developing the use of the eyes, muscles, and joints.
- Train movement of the eyes independent of the head.
- Loosen the muscles of the neck and shoulder to overcome the protective muscular spasm and tendency to move "in one piece."
- Practice head movements that cause dizziness and thus gradually overcome the disability.
- Become accustomed to moving about naturally in daylight and in the dark.
- Encourage the restoration of self-confidence and easy spontaneous movement.

Physical and occupational therapy usually involves techniques for the vestibular system (balance/equilibrium and toleration of movement in different planes) and muscle control/coordination. The vision therapy emphasizes visual skill efficiency. Lenses and prisms are continually evaluated throughout the vision therapy program. Eye movement skills are then integrated with motor skills.

The program should progress from matching all three sensory inputs, decreasing the amount of input from any or all three systems and, finally, using techniques that have conflicts within the three systems.

Tactile, proprioceptive, and vestibular issues need to be addressed early in treatment. A sensory integration approach including brushing and massage techniques may be beneficial. If the vestibular dysfunction is severe, the patient may need to start treatment in the supine position with no movement initially (patient receives tactile and proprioceptive clues from the floor). Start with eye movement movements only, discussed later in this chapter, or head movements only.[38,39] As the patient can tolerate, progress to eye and head movement. Gradually, move the patient to a supported sitting position, then standing. Use proprioceptive activities, such as wall push-ups, crawling, and holding onto or pushing in the chair with hands, to help toleration of movement. Allow the patient to suck on peppermint or to take ginger to decrease nausea. Once the patient can integrate eye movements with body movements, therapy can continue in visual motor, bilateral integration, fine motor, and motor planning areas, if necessary.

EYE MOVEMENT TECHNIQUES
Chapter Seven describes sample vision therapy techniques for pursuits and saccades. For many patients with brain injury, however, these techniques may be too high level.[40] Therefore, the techniques described below should be initiated first.

Eye Calisthenics
Objective. Large ocular calisthenics are used to restore muscle action or to prevent secondary contractures or adhesions of paretic muscles.

Equipment Needed. No equipment necessary. Have the patient remove his or her glasses.

Description and Setup. Have the patient look as far to the right as possible and to hold in that position for several seconds. Then have the patient look to the left, again holding for several seconds. Continue with looking up, down, and in oblique locations. Try to have the patient "stretch" as far as possible. It may be uncomfortable at first, but it often improves with time and practice. The patient should do these procedures at least twice a day for several minutes each time.

Pursuit Procedure
Objective. The goal of this activity is for the patient to move his or her eyes smoothly, accurately, and without discomfort or restriction in all fields of gaze. Pursuits procedures should be started very early in treatment program.

Equipment Needed. Small hand-held object or finger puppet. The patient may need to use glasses for near.

Description and Setup. Pursuit procedures may be given with the patient lying, seated, or standing, whichever posture is the most comfortable initially. The patient should keep his or her head still, as these are eye movements, not "head" movements. Hold the puppet directly in front of the patient's nose, approximately 14 to 16 inches from the patient's face. The therapist should slowly move the puppet in all directions, starting with horizontal movements, vertical movements, then diagonal movements. The pursuits pattern should resemble a star. Now move the object in a circular fashion. In the event of restriction of ocular movement, ocular discomfort, or nausea, the optometrist should be consulted immediately.

Saccadic Fixations
Objective. The objective of a saccadic fixation procedure is to improve the accuracy of saccades as well as to improve visual attention.

Equipment Needed. Two different colored pens or two different objects such as hand-held puppets.

Description and Setup. Hold the pens or objects approximately 14 to 16 inches from the patient's face. Call out the color of one of the pens or the name of one of the objects. Have the patient look at the pen or object you called until you call out the second color or object. The patient should then look to the second pen or object. Continue calling each pen or object while you periodically change the location of one of them so the patient fixates in all fields of gaze. The patient should maintain fixation on the object requested by the therapist and should not be distracted, anticipate, or take several jumps to locate the object.

Spotting Techniques

Spotting is a technique used by dancers or ice skaters. When a dancer moves or spins rapidly, he or she is taught to spot and fixate on an object to help stabilize and stop the feeling of motion. This same technique is used for people who have motion sickness, which is often a result of vestibular dysfunction. A person in a car may suffer from motion sickness when riding in the back seat, but may not show symptoms when riding in the front seat. Sitting in the front seat allows a person to visually fixate in the straight ahead field, rather than see constant motion peripherally as when riding in the back seat of a car. Therefore, even though a person may have a vestibular dysfunction, the use of visual spotting or fixation can relieve symptoms and improve balance control.

Objective. The objective of spotting techniques is to teach the patient how to visually fixate and maintain fixation on an object.

Equipment Needed. None.

Description and Setup. Have the patient look at an object in straight ahead gaze and maintain fixation on a target. Do not merely ask a patient to just look at a wall or door. Rather, have the patient look specifically at a spot or object on the wall or at the light switch. Encourage the patient to use spotting when moving, especially when the patient is dizzy or disoriented.

Scanning Techniques

Objective. The objective of the scanning technique is to teach a person how to be aware of his or her full field of vision. This is most important with the patient with field loss.

Equipment Needed. Four colored stickers or pictures.

Description and Setup. Place colored stickers or pictures on each corner of a door jam. Before a person moves through the door jam, he or she needs to scan and look for all four stickers. This technique should be used consistently when moving through space or for dressing or eating. The pictures can be put on four corners of the food tray and the patient must look for all four pictures before eating. This gives the patient information about what is on the food tray and helps to decrease spilling and misgrabbing for food. Figure 10-4 demonstrates the four corner setup on a food tray.

Binocular Techniques

Procedures may include specific lenses, prisms, occlusion, and vision therapy. A patient should have an immediate vision consultation with an optometrist or ophthalmologist if double vision is suspected. Vision therapy for binocular disorders is prescribed by the optometrist. Therapy techniques may be prescribed for the occupational therapist to implement with the patient on a daily basis, however, the prescription and management of vision therapy is under direct

Figure 10-4. The four corner setup on a food tray.

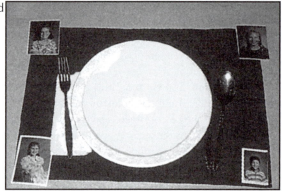

optometric supervision. At times, strabismus surgery may be necessary for a patient who still demonstrates a large angle strabismus 6 months to 1 year post-injury.

ACCOMMODATION TECHNIQUES

Treatment recommendations are similar to those for binocular disorders, except surgery is not necessary.

VISUAL MOTOR TECHNIQUES

Numerous visual motor activities can be found in occupational therapy literature. Techniques may include ball roll, catch, and ball hitting.

BILATERAL INTEGRATION TECHNIQUES

Activities can be found in *Brain Gym*[41] and include cross marches, bilateral circles and lines, and lazy eights.

FINE MOTOR TECHNIQUES

Numerous techniques can be found in the *Fine Motor Dysfunction* manual.[42] Other recommendations include working with Silly Putty (Crayola, Easton, PA), games like Finger Thinking or Tricky Fingers (Edushape, Deer Park, NY), and utilizing pencil grips.

MOTOR PLANNING TECHNIQUES

Sequencing games such as Simon Says, clapping patterns, rope jumping, and scavenger hunts may be beneficial.

VISUAL PERCEPTUAL TECHNIQUES

The higher level perceptual skills are addressed by the optometrist and the occupational therapist, in conjunction with other members of the rehabilitation team. The importance of starting with treatment at the foundation levels (tactile, proprioceptive, motor movements, and eye movement skills) before visual perceptual techniques cannot be overemphasized. Educating the patient about the deficit is an important first step to help the patient learn to use compensatory techniques.

Chapter Seven contains a number of vision therapy techniques for the treatment of visual perceptual dysfunctions. Additional procedures can be found in many references.[43-49] There are many activities and games that can be found in toy or teacher supply stores that are used to work on visual perceptual skills. They are listed in Table 10-1. Even though the techniques may be designed for a child, the techniques can be adapted to the level of a patient of any age and then modified as the patient improves. Table 10-2 summarizes compensatory techniques for patients with visual perceptual deficits.

Vision Field Loss Rehabilitation

Can Visual Field Loss Be Remediated?

In a series of reports, Sabel and colleagues described partial recovery of homonymous visual field defects by intensive computer-based rehabilitation therapy.[50-52] In this approach, patients use a software program at home for an hour a day, 6 days a week, for 6 months. A chin support is used for head stability and a monitor is placed 30 cm away. Stimuli are white lights shown against a dark background. The patient has to press a button every time he or she sees the white target appear. Protocols are tailored for each patient to present most stimuli near the border of the field defect to maximize potential therapeutic benefit. Sabel subsequently founded a company (NovaVision) that offers this visual rehabilitation therapy. The idea behind visual restoration therapy is that after stroke or traumatic brain injury, a region of salvageable vision exists between

---

Table 10-1

Visual Perceptual Activities and Games

Area of Emphasis	Activity
Visual discrimination	Games that emphasize pattern recognition, such as parquetry blocks, matching, sorting, Perfection game (Milton Bradley, East Longmeadow, MA)
Visual form constancy	Geoboards, tangrams, parquetry blocks, dot-to-dot
Visual closure	Word search, dot-to-dot, Hangman
Visual figure ground	Hidden picture, Where's Waldo?
Visual memory	Checkers, chess, Tic Tac Toe
Visual spatial perception	Obstacle course, road map
Visualization strategies	Puzzles, tangrams

Table 10-2

Compensatory Strategies for Patients With Visual Perceptual Deficits

Type of Deficit	Compensatory Techniques
Agnosia	Augment visual with tactile/auditory stimuli when possible
Alexia	Utilize pictures and multisensory stimuli
Apraxia	Ocular motor techniques; augment with verbal and tactile stimuli
Ataxia	Provide additional proprioceptive and kinesthetic input and cuing
Depth perception	Emphasize safety issues; use tactile and kinesthetic reinforcement for tasks such as walking down stairs; use landmarks for location; reduce impulsivity with movement
Figure ground	Reduce clutter in visual environment; use high-contrast markers or tape to identify figure; teach patient to be very systematic when examining a small area
Form perception/constancy	Augment visual with tactile, kinesthetic stimuli
Spatial relations	Use landmarks for location; have patient orient him- or herself in space and then proceed from object to object
Unilateral spatial neglect	Important communication should take place in the field of awareness; advise safety issues; augment with verbal and tactile cues

---

areas of the visual field served by normal and damaged brain tissue. Visual stimulation in this zone with more than 1000 trials a day is postulated to resuscitate its functional potential. After treatment, homonymous field defects have been reported to show a mean gain of about 5 degrees.

However, there are a number of major problems with the data reported by Sabel et al[53,54]:

- Even if the treatment truly leads to a mean gain of 5 degrees, the question is whether such a gain is clinically meaningful. Most clinicians would suggest that an increase in visual fields of 5 degrees is not meaningful.

- The studies were conducted by individuals with a commercial interest in the software company.

- The same software program used for visual restoration therapy was also used to show improvement in the visual fields. Obviously, the data would be more compelling if visual field improvement could be demonstrated with any standard clinical visual field instrument. When patients with visual field loss were tested before and after visual restoration therapy with a standard visual field instrument, no benefit of treatment could be detected.[55]

- The authors did not control for eye movements. Therefore, the visual field recovery can simply be attributed to teaching the patient to make small eye movements. In a study designed to control for eye movements, 17 patients with stable homonymous field defects were treated according to the visual restoration therapy protocol.[55] Independent visual field testing was done before and after treatment to assess the outcome. A crucial innovation was that perimetry was performed using a scanning laser ophthalmoscope, which allows the examiner to control fixation. The study found no significant improvement in visual field defects, although most patients had the subjective impression that they had benefited from visual restoration therapy. This discrepancy underscores a limitation of outcome satisfaction surveys: patients can be swayed by placebo effects.

It remains true, therefore, that no therapeutic intervention can effectively correct the underlying visual field deficit.[55] Thus, remediation and compensation must be used in visual rehabilitation for visual field loss. We can help patients by teaching them compensatory techniques to function more effectively in activities of daily life in spite of the field loss. Gianutsos and Suchoff stress that intervention must emphasize compensation, rather than restoration.[56] They conceptualize visual field defect cases on a continuum. At one end, there are those patients who are quite aware of the hemianopia, while at the other end are those individuals who are totally unaware of the deficit.[56] The goal of visual rehabilitation, therefore, is to move the patient from one end of the continuum (lack of awareness) to as close to awareness as possible.

To develop effective treatment, sensory deficits must be differentiated from perceptual, attention, linguistic, and other cognitive deficits.[57] Brain injury affects a variety of cognitive and linguistic functions that might affect visual function such as letter identification and reading. People may have difficulty reading because of damage to linguistic processing areas. They may not respond to objects in the periphery because of impaired visual attention or unilateral inattention and neglect.[58,59] Since unilateral field loss is often associated with unilateral inattention, the treatments often address unilateral attention as well as unilateral field loss.

Unilateral field loss usually does not cut the field down the middle but rather leaves central vision intact, called central sparing. Functionally, an individual with a unilateral field loss "with central sparing" will see most of a person's face at about 1 meter (3 feet) but see nothing to one side or the other of the face. People with field cuts and central sparing usually have normal acuity and only minor problems with reading. These individuals will read a single line of text normally but might lose their place when reading, or may have difficulty scanning a page for information. In some cases, people with unilateral field loss have a unilateral field loss that also bisects the central field. These individuals will report that one-half of the examiner's face can be seen during field testing. People with "split central fields" will only see half of a letter or words they are trying to identify as well. The resultant loss of basic shape, letter, and face recognition may be confused with higher order perceptual deficits. People with a right unilateral field loss with a split central field will have severe problems with reading even though other linguistic functions are intact.[57]

Functionally, people with unilateral field loss will present with a disabled visual scanning and peripheral warning system, often with the functional effects compounded by an overlay of unilateral visual inattention. In addition a person with unilateral field loss may present with "wayfinding deficits," and often cannot even retrace his or her steps. A person may have basic problems with wayfinding primarily due to a unilateral field loss rather than cognitive deficit. For example, if a client with a left field loss walks down a hall for the first time he or she will see one side of the hall to his or her right. When he or she turns around to retrace his or her steps, the formerly right side of the hall will now be to his or her blind, left visual field. The side of the hall that is now in his or her intact right field would never have been seen before. In effect, the client has never seen the route he or she is retracing. This problem is exacerbated for people who have split central fields and/or unilateral inattention.[57]

The following is a sequential list of treatment for visual field loss rehabilitation:

- Awareness training
- Prism field expansion
- Eye movement therapy
- Scanning training
- Wide field eye movement therapy
- Adaptations

Awareness Training
COMPUTER SOFTWARE

The goal of awareness training[56] is to bring about an intellectual appreciation of the visual loss. Gianutsos has developed computer software that can be used for awareness training. One program is called REACT[60] and is a useful first task. In this procedure targets appear randomly in the four quadrants (up and to the right, up and to the left, down and to the right, down and to the left). The patient must press the appropriate key as the target appears. The main part of the therapy, however, occurs after completion of the task. The patient is given many opportunities to perform and attempt to compensate for the loss. The therapist attempts to teach the patient how to tabulate the results (eg, counting how many trials took longer than 0.5 seconds on the left and right sides, respectively). This tabulation draws attention to the problem, and, for some, it is also a challenging visual search exercise. Other techniques such as SOSH,[61] SEARCH,[62] and FASTREAD[63] can be used.

Gianutsos and Suchoff stress that throughout this practice, the therapist should elicit evaluative statements from the patient, fading the level of prompting. For instance, "Where did you have the most difficulty?" or "Did you notice that you had difficulty on one side?" An intermediate level prompt might be, "Where would I be telling you to look, if I were to do so?" A minimal prompt might be, "What do you think I am thinking?"[56]

NON-COMPUTER TECHNIQUES
Awareness Training With a Laser Pointer

The therapist has the patient sit facing a wall 2 meters away. The patient is instructed to fixate a small target—a drawing on a sticky note will do. The patient also holds a laser pointer of a different color. The patient is instructed to "tag" the therapist's laser spot when he or she sees it, without moving his or her eyes from the fixation target. Starting in the blind area of the visual field, the therapist moves the laser spot to the edge of the blind area, and marks with a small sticky note the place on the wall where the patient first responded to the light. The therapist then moves the laser spot along a different trajectory to another point on the suspected edge of the blind area (eg, just above or below the previously placed sticky note) until it is first detected and places another sticky note. The therapist then keeps moving the laser spot to different points on the edge of the blind area until the edge of the blind area is defined vertically and horizontally by a string of sticky notes. Once this testing is completed, a person with a complete left homonymous quadrantopsia will have a string of sticky notes along the vertical midline, around the central visual area (if central sparing), and along the person's horizon to the left forming an area that resembles a quarter of a pie. Once the blind area is defined by sticky notes, then the patient is instructed to look over and observe the extent of the blind area.

This process can then be repeated with the patient looking from the center fixation target to the peripheral laser spot as soon as it is detected. This helps patients understand the extent of the blind area, which they often find surprising.

Patients can purchase a laser pointer and perform this at home with a helper. Often patients are anxious for a prognosis; this procedure allows them to monitor progressive changes in visual fields at home.

Detecting Sticky Notes on Both Sides

Sticky notes can also be used for an awareness training procedure. Before the therapy session, the therapist places 20 sticky notes on the right and left walls of a hallway. The sticky notes are numbered (in the back) from 1 to 20. The 10 even-numbered sticky notes are placed on the right side of the hallway wall while the 10 odd-numbered sticky notes are placed on the left side of the wall. The patient is asked to walk down the hallway and find all of the sticky notes. The typical patient with visual field loss and left visual inattention will only find 10 of the 20 sticky notes on the right wall. The therapist would have the patient repeat the procedure trying to be more aware of the left side.

Coupons, Photographs, and Playing Cards

Coupons, family photographs, and playing cards can be used in a similar fashion. The playing cards can be scattered in a particular pattern (red on right, black on left, kings on one side, queens on the other) and the only way the patient can successful complete the task is to be aware of both sides of the visual field.

Throughout this awareness training, the therapist would stress the questions suggested by Gianutsos and Suchoff[56]: "Where did you have the most difficulty?", "Did you notice that you had difficulty on one side?", "Where would I be telling you to look, if I were to do so?", "What do you think I am thinking?

Prism Field Expansion

The prism field expansion system called the Peli Visual Field Expansion Device for Hemianopia, described earlier, is an effective treatment for patients with hemianopia.[9,10] This prism can expand the visual field by as much as 30 to 40 degrees and allows the patient to be aware of potential obstacles in the periphery. However, it has not been evaluated with visual neglect. Thus, awareness training must occur first and if the patient develops an awareness of his or her visual field loss, prism expansion can be considered. This technique requires gradual introduction, first with the upper prism and then with the lower prism. When each prism is first introduced, the above field awareness training procedures are recommended to enable the patient to learn to recognize the ghost image of an object that is just outside of the field of view.

Eye Movement Techniques for Patients With Visual Field Loss

The eye movement techniques described in this chapter and in Chapter Seven are utilized with patients with visual field loss. Begin with all stimuli placed on the side that has normal vision. Thus, with a left hemianopia, all stimuli are placed on the right side at first. Once the patient can master all of the saccadic and pursuit techniques described in Chapter Seven, stimuli can be scattered across both sides of the visual field. After completion of this aspect of the therapy, wide field eye movement techniques should be used.

Scanning Training and Wide Field Eye Movement Techniques

The method that seems to produces the largest and functionally greatest increase in peripheral awareness is called compensatory visual scanning. In this technique, the therapist teaches the client to look with quick saccades in the direction of the blind hemifield.[64] Compensatory visual scanning does not actually increase the size of the intact field.

To compensate for a unilateral field loss the client must change habitual eye movement patterns. Normally we look at an object and depend on our peripheral vision to see on either side. Compensatory visual scanning involves frequently and consistently looking in the direction of the blind hemifield much like a driver uses rearview and sideview mirrors when driving to get a sense of what is going on around the car and beyond the range of peripheral vision. As with any therapeutic intervention, the client must be educated about the deficit and provided with an explanation for the compensatory strategy. Understanding and verbalizing the problem or demonstrating improved performance during instructional protocols is not sufficient. The client must demonstrate compensatory scanning as an ingrained habit during real-life activities when attention is on the activity not the eye movement.

If a patient does not quickly respond to the following treatments, visual neglect may be an issue. Visual neglect is sometimes referred to as visual inattention. Visual neglect, however, involves a variety of spatial, perceptual, and cognitive problems including peripheral inattention. More common in our experience is left visual neglect associated with right hemisphere damage. Bilateral neglect is associated with bilateral damage, dementia, and diffuse cortical damage due to, for example, dementia and encephalopathies. Right field neglect is rare and usually transient.[58] With visual neglect, the patient may need external prompting. Eventually, we want the patient to self-direct; for example, the patient knows to scan and look in the area of loss without external prompting.

Scanning With Expected Then Unexpected Objects
We suggest a three-step sequence for teaching this skill.

Step One
The first stage in treatment is to engage the client in various search tasks, looking for specified objects in a room, looking for cooking or self-care items, simple puzzles, dominos, and completing cancellation and drawing tasks. Examples of these treatment strategies have been well described in the occupational therapy literature.[59,65] This step is quickly mastered by people with intact visual attention, less easily recovered with clients who have attention deficits. When grading the activities, easier tasks should be familiar and meaningful activities such as brushing teeth. Using tasks with expected objects (the brush, toothpaste, and glass) will encourage the client to continue looking until all the components in the visual task are found.

To remediate inattention deficit, first one might force fixation to the side where there is inattention by occluding one-half of each lens on the intact side with translucent tape (Figure 10-5). This forces the client to look past the midline in the direction of the visual field loss, if the head is straight ahead. Nonvisual cues such as making noise and tapping the patient's left shoulder might be added to direct attention to the affected side as well. Often patients with visual neglect have attention deficits as well. Attention to the left can be increased by decreasing stimulation on the person's unaffected right side and increasing stimulation on the person's affected left side. This could be done, for example, by having the person sit with his or her right side next to a wall, and then have the therapist and other activities in the clinic on the person's left side. Stimulation on the affected left side might also be increased by tapping the shoulder, using mild electrical stimulation, positioning items of interest during activities (eg, toothpaste and toothbrush) on the left side, and positioning food items during eating on the left.

Next directly instruct the patient to adopt a strategy for scanning to the affected side like a "lighthouse,"[66] and have the patient use visual imagery to scan to the affected side as well as describe the strategy. It often helps to have the patient with visual neglect have a target to define how far to the affected side he or she must scan. A classic strategy is to place a brightly colored line and

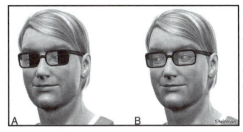

Figure 10-5. Two techniques to facilitate adaptive scanning into an affected hemifield. (A) Partial lens occlusion forces the he to look into the affected hemifield. (B) The Sarah Appel technique uses colored translucent filters to cue the client when he or she is looking in the correct direction. (Reprinted with permission from Scheiman M, Scheiman M, Whittaker SG. *Low Vision Rehabilitation: A Practical Guide for Occupational Therapists*. Thorofare, NJ: SLACK Incorporated; 2007.)

tactual marker down the edge of the page or field being scanned and telling the client to keep looking until the line is seen; this reference stimulus is sometimes called an anchor. We find using naturally occurring stimuli are more generalizable. For example, a person with left visual neglect can use his or her left shoulder as an anchor. A person with left neglect trying to read can be instructed to move the left finger down the left margin of the page and use the right finger to point to the words being read. When scanning to the next line, the patient is instructed to "touch fingers." Once the client can consistently scan for objects even with less familiar tasks, the searching and scanning function has been restored for expected objects that are necessary for completion of a task.

Step Two
Step Two involves having the client scan a room where unexpected objects might be found, trying to find hazards in a kitchen, or picking up objects on the floor, for example.

Step Three
Step Three, Behavior Modification Methods, re-establishes the warning function of the peripheral retina. This step presents a greater challenge because responding to approaching objects from the affected side usually requires performance during divided attention, which is often impaired with brain injury or in older individuals. One approach we have successfully used involves behavior modification of scanning eye movements. The goal is to establish the habit of frequently and quickly looking in the direction of the field defect. Computer programs and equipment[56] have been developed that allow the client to be set up to perform this task independently, but there is question as to how well the habits generalize into real-life situations.

Laser tag transitions the client to more real-life situations. The therapist and client each hold a laser pointer. The therapist presents the laser spot on a surface such as an uncluttered wall. The client responds by pointing to the light and tagging the spot with his or her laser pointer. At first the light is flashed at two predictable points in the right and left fields. The task is graded to become more challenging and realistic by moving from predictable positions in an uncluttered area to unpredictable locations in a cluttered area. To further increase difficulty, the laser spot targets can be presented at different distances. Finally, the task is performed when the client's attention is divided such as in a visually busy environment with people walking around. During this task, the therapist gradually decreases the frequency of presentations and varies the interval between laser spot presentations as well, pausing up to a minute or two between presentations. At this point, the client should be walking with frequent automatic glances into the affected hemifield, so that when the light eventually appears he or she detects it within 2 seconds. This instructional sequence should result in the client frequently and habitually looking in the direction of the field deficit. Generalization requires frequent instruction outside of the clinical context and in the context of naturally occurring activities. It is important to have a caregiver or family member involved in training.

Holding fixation in the direction of the deficit is another strategy that provides early warning in the direction of the field loss. In this procedure the client must look over and maintain fixation in the direction of the field deficit, use peripheral vision in the intact field to look straight ahead, and to see into the unaffected hemifield. The client could be encouraged to play two-on-one ball games such as soccer or basketball, practice walking in crowds, practice crossing intersections, and when walking down the street, a partner might intermittently and unexpectedly veer into the client and playfully bump shoulders if not detected. Success is achieved if the client automatically maintains most of the fixation between straight ahead and the affected side so as to detect an approaching target within a second or two.

If the patient does not progress through either Step One or Step Two, then the patient likely has a moderate to severe visual inattention or neglect. Two procedures now have been shown effective for treating visual left neglect. Prism adaptation therapy involves placing 20 to 40 diopter yoked prisms on the patient with the base of the prism toward the left side. This will shift the apparent location of the visual scene to the right so that the patient will tend to mislocalize to the right of an object. Then the patient adapts by training until he or she no longer mislocalizes. Finally, the prisms are removed. This is repeated daily for several days. It is important that the visual localization tasks used during training DO NOT involve continuous visual feedback. For example, one task requires a patient to reach forward and knock down a domino that the therapist taps. To eliminate continuous visual feedback, the arm is masked by, for example, reaching through a box with both ends open. Other tasks involve throwing objects, again with the throwing arm covered from view. You know the prism adaptation has been effective if after the prism has been removed there is a mislocalization to the opposite direction. Prism adaptation has been shown by several studies to ameliorate a visual neglect in the short term and have more prolonged effects with repeated, daily, application.[67-71]

WIDE FIELD EYE MOVEMENT TECHNIQUES

These methods would be useful in Step One and in transitioning to Step Two in the wide field technique described above.

The Wayne Saccadic Fixator

The Wayne Saccadic Fixator (Wayne Engineering, Skokie, IL) is a wall-mounted instrument (Figure 10-6) with a touch-sensitive membrane panel containing 33 LED lights arranged in three concentric circles with one light at the center. The user responds to the appearance of a light by pressing the membrane button surrounding it. The built-in computer provides a large variety of activities. Both random and fixed light presentation patterns are available. All activities can be time limited. The number of lights used in an activity is adjustable (all lights, outer circle only, four quadrant lights, etc). The unit can store 203 activity programs, of which 172 are preprogrammed with activities for developing rapid saccadic fixations, eye-hand coordination, accuracy, speed, sequencing, directionality, pattern recognition, visual memory, anticipation, reaction time, peripheral awareness, and more.

One of the key features of the Wayne Saccadic Fixator is an attachment called Visual Stick-ups, which integrate all Wayne Saccadic Fixator activities into real space. Stick-ups provide realistic use of available space to enhance training. Each Stick-up is a small box with a photosensitive light that acts as an extension of one of the lights/switches on the Fixator. Stick-ups can be mounted on any surface and spaced up to 8 feet apart in any order. A gun-like device is used by the patient to "shoot out" the light box that is illuminated. Thus, the patient is free to move and is not required to be right in front of the instrument.

Once the patient has made progress with the wall-mounted Wayne Saccadic Fixator, the task can be made more relevant to everyday activities using the Visual Stick-ups. The patient can stand 10 to 20 feet from the wall and while standing still has to use the entire field to locate the lights as they randomly become illuminated. This is accomplished by scanning the field using both head and body movement. The next level of difficulty would be to have the patient walking forward and

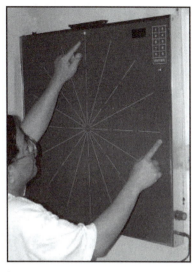

Figure 10-6. The Wayne Saccadic Fixator is a wall-mounted instrument with a touch-sensitive membrane panel. (Reprinted with permission from Wayne Engineering.)

backward while performing the task. Finally, obstacles can be place in the patient's way as he or she tries to locate and extinguish the illuminated Stick-ups.

Wide Field Chalkboard Saccadic

Gianutsos and Suchoff suggest the following therapy technique.[56] Place 15 to 20 numbers, letters, or other targets randomly on the side of a full-size chalkboard corresponding to the patient's field defect. The patient is centrally positioned in front of and at least 10 feet from the board and locates targets with a flashlight that are called out by another person. As the patient gains mastery of this task, the board is erased and new targets are written, still mainly in the affected hemifield but with some on the unaffected side. The patient is first instructed to scan the board in a circular manner and then to "pay more attention" to the affected side during the task. Gradually, the targets are evenly distributed between the two sides. Sticky notes could be used for this procure instead of a chalkboard.

Wide Field Near Saccadic Activities

Similar activities can be accomplished at near with targets linearly arranged and the patients locating specified numbers or letters with a pencil in the same manner (ie, with targets first being contained on the side of the compromised field and gradually distributing them so that an equal number appear in both fields).[56]

Adaptations

READING ADAPTATIONS FOR PATIENTS WITH VISUAL FIELD LOSS

Patients with visual field loss complain of frequent loss of place when reading. The following adaptations may be useful.

- Use an L-shaped marker with Velcro so that the patient can "find and feel where the boundaries are" (Figure 10-7).
- Turn the book 45 to 90 degrees. This moves the print into a field of awareness. If the patient has a right hemianopsia, he or she has difficulty following a line of print. By turning the book so that the print reads up and down, he or she may now be able to follow the line better since the next words to be read are now in his or her visual field (Figure 10-8).

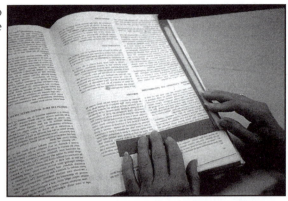

Figure 10-7. L-shaped marker with Velcro so that the patient can "find and feel where the boundaries are" when reading.

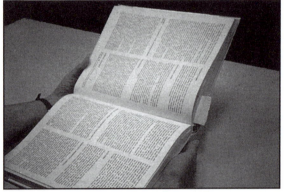

Figure 10-8. By turning the book so that the print reads up and down, the patient may now be able to follow the line better because the next words to be read are now in his or her visual field.

ADAPTATIONS FOR DRIVING

Patients with hemianopsia cannot drive legally and safely. It is possible for people with less than a homonymous quadrantanopia to drive legally. The field requirement for driving varies from state to state but often is 120 degrees on the visual horizon. In other words, if a patient is fixating a point on a wall while sitting 1 meter away (3 feet), the person can see flashes of light along a 2.5 meter straight horizontal line through the fixation point without any interruption. Only an ophthalmologist or optometrist can certify a patient meets the visual requirements for driving. A special field wide field binocular test is appropriate for driving; standard field tests are not adequate. The patient needs, therefore, to specifically request a vision evaluation for driving. Patients with a quadrant loss or less may be remediated only if other cognitive and motor skills are appropriate.[72] Care must be taken to rule out even mild visual neglect. The vision therapy techniques for driving would include the following (all of the techniques have been previously described in this chapter or Chapter Seven).

- Eye movement therapy techniques
- Spot stationary objects while patient is stationary
- Locate and follow moving objects while patient is stationary
- Learn to locate and track stationary objects while patient is moving
- Track moving objects while patient is moving and using scanning skills to gather visual information
- Include eye-hand-foot activities

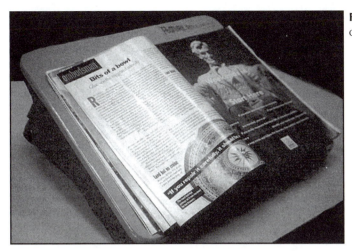

Figure 10-9. Slanted lapboards can be used for near activities.

- Practice with stress (ie, different light conditions, talk to the patient, turn on music)
- Develop visual memory skills (speed/span of recognition)
- Plan routes verbally/visually; visualize

ADAPTATIONS/COMPENSATIONS FOR PATIENTS WITH VISUAL DYSFUNCTION

The following suggestions are useful when working with patients with visual dysfunction.

- Working distance: The distance from the patient to the object is critical whether it be for near activities or distance. Especially with patients wearing bifocals or trifocals, the lenses are very distance specific. Normal working distance at near is the measurement from the elbow to the second knuckle, approximately 16 inches. If an object is outside of the normal working distance for which the glasses have been prescribed, the patient may not be able to accurately see the object.
- Posture: The patient needs to comfortable and supported. Slanted lapboards can be used for near activities (Figure 10-9).
- Lighting: Most elderly patients need more light to see. However, it is not uncommon that brain injury patients are light sensitive and request less light. Use a light that can be adjusted.
- Contrast: Elderly patients and patients with vision loss may function better if there is better contrast. For example, at the dinner table, do not use white placemats and white plates on a white tablecloth. Use different colors for better contrast.
- Reduce demands: If the task is too difficult for the patient, reduce the demands. For example, if a patient cannot fixate and walk at the same time, work on visual fixations while sitting or lying before integrating visual fixation with walking.
- Pencil grips: If a patient has difficulty gripping an object, a variety of pencil and utensil grips are available from occupational therapy supply catalogs.
- Enlarge print, enhance print quality: Large-print books and talking books are available through local libraries for the visually impaired. Use a copy machine to enlarge print if necessary.
- Reinforce with multisensory: If a patient cannot understand the task by just telling him or her, make sure multisensory stimuli is used (ie, show it, tell it, experience it, feel it).
- Markers: If patient loses his or her place when reading, use markers to help the patient stay on line.

Case Histories

Five different types of case histories are presented below. These patients have different types of brain injuries and visual dysfunctions. Vision evaluation and treatment recommendations differ depending on the patient diagnosis, severity of injury, and patient goals. Some patients are in hospital or rehabilitation settings and others are not in formal programs and live at home.

Case One

Jeannie, a 32-year-old female, received a mild traumatic brain injury, whiplash, and cervical strain secondary to a fall. She was referred for an optometric evaluation 2½ years post-injury by her neurologist. Jeannie complained of frequent frontal headaches, double vision, blurred vision, motor function decrease, poor balance, and attention/concentration and organizational deficits. She experienced difficulties with grocery shopping, cooking, and writing. She was unable to drive. Jeannie had received occupational, physical, and speech therapy immediately after her injury but was no longer receiving treatment. She was living at her home with her family.

Her general medical health was unremarkable with no known allergies. She was taking Depakote (divalproex sodium) and ibuprofen. There was no history of previous eye or head trauma, and social history was unremarkable. Jeannie had been evaluated by several ophthalmologists prior to my evaluation. She received no vision treatment other than the recommendation to buy a pair of reading glasses at the drug store.

VISUAL ACUITY, REFRACTION, EYE HEALTH

The external and external ocular evaluation was unremarkable. Pupils were equal, round, and responded to light. Visual acuity was:

	Distance	Near
Right eye	20/20	20/30
Left eye	20/25	20/60

Refraction revealed a low amount of hyperopia (farsightedness).

VISUAL EFFICIENCY TESTING

A high amount of exophoria that decompensated to an exotropia at near was measured. Near point of convergence was receded with a break at 10 inches and a recovery at 14 inches. Accommodation was found to be quite poor. Pursuits were full and unrestricted, but they were not smooth or accurate. Jeannie could not dissociate eye from head movement. She demonstrated tearing and discomfort during pursuit and saccade testing.

VISUAL FIELD EVALUATION

A generalized constriction on all isopters was shown in addition to a homonymous, incongruous lower right quadrantanopia (Figures 10-10a and 10-10b).

VISUAL INFORMATION PROCESSING

Jeannie could respond to the visual perceptual tests if given extra time and many rest breaks. Extreme fatigue, blurriness, and ocular discomfort were present. Figure ground and visual motor integration testing, in particular, presented difficulty for Jeannie.

ASSESSMENT AND DIAGNOSIS

1. Mild traumatic brain injury by history (diagnosed by her neurologist)
2. Hyperopia
3. Intermittent exotropia at near
4. Accommodative dysfunction

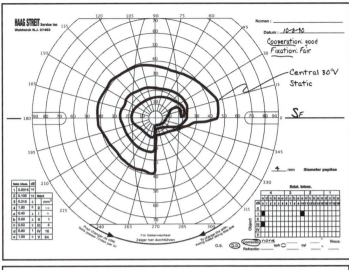

Figure 10-10a. A generalized constriction on all isopters in addition to a homonymous, incongruous lower right quadrantanopia.

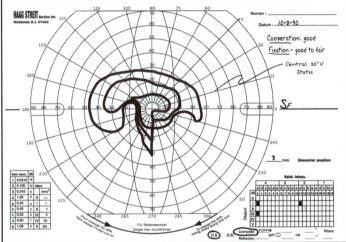

Figure 10-10b. A generalized constriction on all isopters in addition to a homonymous, incongruous lower right quadrantanopia.

5. Binocular dysfunction
6. Ocular motor dysfunction
7. Homonymous, incongruous, lower right quadrantanopia
8. Visual perceptual deficits

Treatment Plan

Two pairs of glasses were prescribed. One was for distance and a different prescription for near was prescribed that included base-in prism in addition to a plus lens. A program of vision therapy was initiated. The patient was seen in vision therapy once a week for 45 minutes and home vision therapy activities were given. Throughout the vision therapy, distance and near glasses were re-evaluated and changed periodically. After 8 months of vision therapy, subjective symptomology revealed less blurry vision, no diplopia, and a decrease in headache frequency and severity. Jeannie could now read, write, cook, and drive. Visual efficiency and visual perceptual evaluation showed significant improvement. Visual fields also improved, showing no overall constriction, although a lower right incongruous quadrantanopia was still found (Figures 10-11a and 10-11b).

Figure 10-11a. Visual fields are improved, showing no overall constriction, although a lower right incongruous quadrantanopia was still found.

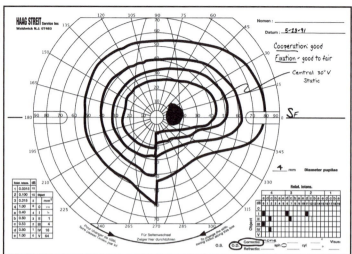

Figure 10-11b. Visual fields are improved, showing no overall constriction, although a lower right incongruous quadrantanopia was still found.

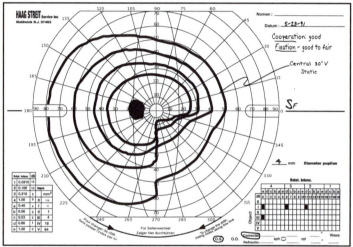

SUMMARY

This is an important case as it is consistent with the symptomology generally encountered in the traumatic brain injury population. It is also interesting to note that treatment was initiated 2½ years after injury, eliminating spontaneous recovery as an explanation for improvement in this patient's visual system deficits.

Case Two

Charles, a 55-year-old male, was referred by his physical therapist. Charles was diagnosed with a brainstem bleed that caused significant motor and visual dysfunction. Charles was told by his physician in the hospital to patch one eye full-time in order to eliminate double vision. The physical therapist, who was trying to help Charles improve walking skills, was concerned with his full-time patching and head tilting. If Charles patched his left eye, he would show a significant head turn to the left, which had a negative effect on balance. If he patched his right eye, he would straighten his head (which improved his balance). However, the left eye showed constant nystagmus, creating symptoms of nausea and dizziness when Charles tried to use that eye.

Visual Acuity, Refraction, Eye Health

Visual acuity was 20/20 both at distance and at near with current glasses for myopia (nearsightedness), astigmatism, and presbyopia. Eye health was unremarkable, except for pupil abnormality of the right eye.

Visual Efficiency Testing

Eye movement dysfunctions were apparent. Charles showed full, unrestricted movement of the left eye, although constant nystagmus was present. His right eye could only move laterally, indicating paresis of the third and fourth nerves of the right eye. He showed no nystagmus of the right eye. Binocular testing revealed constant double vision and no fusion ability. Accommodation was deficient because of age (presbyopia).

Visual Fields

Full visual fields were measured.

Assessment and Diagnosis

1. Eye movement dysfunction (paresis of third and fourth nerves of right eye; nystagmus of the left eye)
2. Binocular dysfunction
3. Pre-existing refractive condition, adequately compensated for with current prescription

Treatment Plan

Vision therapy was initiated. The goal was to improve left eye functioning so that Charles could use his left eye especially with walking tasks. Body balance improved when he did use his left eye because the head tilt was eliminated. Binocular fusion was not obtainable with prism, vision therapy, or strabismus surgery. Therefore, occlusion of one eye was known to still be necessary.

Eye movement techniques were initiated in addition to visual biofeedback techniques. After 4 months of weekly vision therapy sessions, Charles could now use his left eye comfortably. Nystagmus had significantly reduced. There was no change in right eye movement patterns.

Summary

This case demonstrates the severity of eye movement dysfunction after brain injury. Even though binocular fusion was never deemed to be a goal, vision therapy was successful in improving the eye movement status, which thereby allowed the patient to improve walking and mobility skills.

Case Three

Bertha, a 90-year-old cerebrovascular accident patient living in a long-term facility, was referred by her occupational therapist. Since her cerebrovascular accident 4 months previously, Bertha has not been able to do most of the activities of daily living skills she previously could perform independently. She could not dress or feed herself. Bertha sat in her wheelchair, with no eye contact and little interest in interacting with others.

Visual Acuity, Refraction, Eye Health

No visual acuity could be obtained. Light perception was noted. Bertha had previously worn glasses for moderate hyperopia and presbyopia. However, she had not worn them since arriving at the facility. Bertha's visual history and records revealed end-stage glaucoma and cataracts. She had been evaluated by her ophthalmologist 6 months prior to this evaluation. The ophthalmologist was monitoring her glaucoma medications and did not feel cataract surgery was appropriate. Neither visual acuity nor visual fields had been obtainable by the ophthalmologist for several years prior to her cerebrovascular accident, however, Bertha was still able to feed and dress herself at that time.

VISUAL EFFICIENCY TESTING

No results obtained because of decreased visual acuity. Bertha would not respond to pursuit or saccade testing.

VISUAL FIELDS TESTING

Previous visual records showed significant visual field loss from glaucoma. Bertha seemed to show some visual awareness in her lower right field.

ASSESSMENT AND DIAGNOSIS

1. Pre-existing glaucoma, cataracts monitored by ophthalmologist
2. Significant visual acuity, visual field loss
3. Pre-existing hyperopia, presbyopia

TREATMENT PLAN

Bertha's family and therapist wanted to try to help Bertha gain some independence. They wanted her to feed herself.

Our initial treatment plan included a recommendation that Bertha wear her previous glasses. Even though Bertha presented with significant visual loss from ocular disease and neurologic insult, a farsighted adult of her age cannot see well without glasses. Bertha's occupational therapist noticed an improvement in Bertha's alertness once she started wearing glasses again.

Eye movement techniques were initiated by the occupational therapist under optometric supervision. Auditory cues were added to the visual activities so that Bertha would know where to look. The therapy was emphasized more in Bertha's lower right field, as her awareness seemed better in that location. The occupational therapist was also providing sensory integration techniques that included massage and vestibular movement. Recommendations were given for changing the contrast of Bertha's place setting when eating. The food tray was also placed in her lower right field.

After 3 weeks of vision therapy, Bertha was able to feed herself as long as the food tray was placed in her lower right field.

SUMMARY

This is an interesting case in that significant ocular pathology was present in addition to a cerebrovascular accident. Often patients with this type of condition are merely told that nothing can be done. Even though the prognosis for improving the vision is poor in this patient, improvement in activities of daily living can be obtained by using basic visual guidance. When patients present without glasses, improvement can often be immediate by just wearing appropriate glasses. Contrast and lighting changes can help a patient. This patient did not receive in-office vision therapy. She was given treatment by her occupational therapist at her facility, under optometric supervision.

Case Four

Jeff, a 27-year-old male, suffered a severe traumatic brain injury secondary to a motor vehicle accident 6 months prior to his visual evaluation. He was referred by his neuropsychologist. Jeff complained of frequent frontal headaches and was frequently observed squinting or closing one eye when viewing. Jeff recently had a complete neurologic work-up including magnetic resonance imaging. His visual history was unremarkable except for wearing soft contact lenses for myopia and astigmatism. Since his accident, Jeff no longer wore his contact lenses and did not have glasses.

VISUAL ACUITY, REFRACTION, EYE HEALTH

Visual acuity was 20/200 with each eye at distance and 20/60 at near. Myopia (nearsightedness) and astigmatism were measured. Internal and external ocular structures were unremarkable.

Visual Efficiency Testing

Eye movement skills were adequate. Binocular functioning was adequate. Accommodation was found to be inadequate.

Assessment and Diagnosis

1. Uncorrected myopia and astigmatism
2. Accommodative dysfunction

Treatment Plan

Glasses for the refractive condition were prescribed for full-time wear. A bifocal was given, as Jeff needed a different prescription for distance than for near. No vision therapy was initiated because Jeff was moving out of town.

Headache frequency and severity decreased immediately after wearing the glasses.

Summary

This case emphasizes the importance of appropriate glasses for refractive conditions. Jeff presents with brain injury and his other physicians had concluded the headaches were sequelae of the injury, which is often the case. However, uncorrected refractive error may also contribute to the headaches. This is a case where the simple, obvious solution may have been overlooked.

Case Five

Alan, a 48-year-old male, had just been diagnosed with multiple sclerosis. He had been referred by his occupational therapist. His symptoms included dizziness, balance problems, and intermittent double vision. He was wearing an invisible no-line bifocal prescribed 1 year prior to this vision evaluation. Alan had been comfortable in his glasses.

Visual Acuity, Refractive, Ocular Health

Visual acuity with glasses was 20/20 at distance and at near. Hyperopia (farsightedness) with astigmatism similar to current glasses prescription was measured. Internal ocular evaluation revealed mild pallor of the right optic nerve head. No other ocular pathology was noted.

Visual Efficiency Testing

Binocular testing revealed moderate exophoria at near and poor fusion ranges both at distance and at near. Accommodation was deficient because of age (presbyopia). Eye movement skills were full and unrestricted, although endpoint nystagmus was apparent.

Assessment and Diagnosis

1. Optic nerve pallor
2. Nystagmus
3. Convergence insufficiency
4. Pre-existing hyperopia, astigmatism, presbyopia

Treatment Plan

Although Alan's current glasses prescription was adequate, I was concerned with the type of bifocal lens he was wearing. The invisible bifocal sometimes can cause peripheral distortion. Most people learn to adapt to that. However, since Alan now had balance problems, I was concerned as to the effect of his glasses on balance. Therefore, a new prescription for glasses was given for distance only. Alan and his occupational therapist saw immediate improvement in balance when wearing his new glasses.

Vision therapy was initiated. The goals were to improve binocular functioning.

Summary

This case demonstrates how a lens design may positively or negatively affect balance. Multiple sclerosis symptoms may vary, which is more reason why these patients should be visually evaluated on a regular basis. If a patient shows double vision during multiple sclerosis attacks, Fresnel prisms may be useful to compensate temporarily as the double vision may subside. Multiple sclerosis patients are frequently relatively young and are still productive in society. These patients appreciate anything that may be of assistance visually.

Summary

Overall, visual function is based on the development and function of a hierarchy of skills. Skills at the basic level form the foundation for higher level skills. In order to make complex visual decisions necessary for tasks including activities of daily living, reading, math, driving, and vocations, integration of lower skills (tactile, vestibular, proprioceptive, visual) is critical. Therefore, determining the cause of the deficit requires understanding of the brain injury and its effect on the entire visual process from input to output.

Patients who have suffered neurological insult are quite a complex clinical challenge. In the rehabilitation process, a patient comes in contact with numerous physicians and therapists who play a vital role in the rehabilitation process. The occupational therapist is often in the best position to observe functional visual problems either via a visual screening process or merely by observation. The optometrist is the most qualified professional to assess and rehabilitate the visual efficiency and visual perceptual system. Vision, being our dominant sense for gathering information, needs to be evaluated early in the rehabilitation process. It is important that all patients who have suffered a traumatic brain injury/stroke have a complete vision evaluation by an optometrist who has extensive experience in vision rehabilitation and functional vision care. Consultation with an optometrist by the rehabilitation team is crucial so that all health care providers have a good understanding of the patient's visual deficits and functional results. Treatment strategies can then be established, utilizing a multidisciplinary approach. Vision treatment should be concurrent with speech, physical, and/or occupational therapy. Improved visual functioning often will help speed the progress in other rehabilitative areas.

The commonalities between the models of human performance used by optometry and occupational therapy create a natural interaction between optometrists and occupational therapists.[73-76] Educational and clinical interactions between these two groups have grown at an impressive rate. Collaboration and sharing provides increased learning for the therapists and optometrists resulting in a more complete and successful treatment program for the patient.

References

1. Direnfeld G. Traumatic brain injury and case management. *Cogn Rehabil.* 1990;5:20-24.
2. Suter PS. A quickstart in post-acute vision rehabilitation following brain injury. *J Optom Vis Devel.* 1999;30:73-82.
3. Margolis NW, Lederer PJ. Issues concerning the evaluation of closed head injury. *J Opt Vis Devel.* 1999;30:55-57.
4. Kadet TS. Vision rehabilitation in traumatic brain injury. In: Forkiotis CJ, Kadet TS, Shankman AL, et al, eds. *Essays on Vision.* Santa Ana, CA: Optometric Extension Program Foundation; 1990:13-20.
5. Suchoff I, Gianutsos R. Rehabilitative optometric interventions for the adult with acquired brain injury. In: Grabois M, Garrison SJ, Hart KA, Lemkuhl LD, eds. *Physical Medicine and Rehabilitation.* Malden, MA: Blackwall Science; 2000:608-621.
6. Kaplan M. *Seeing Through New Eyes.* Philadelphia, PA: Jessica Kingsley Publishers; 2006.
7. Kaplan M, Edelson SM, Seip JL. Behavioral changes in autistic individuals as a result of wearing ambient transitional prism lenses. *Child Psychiatry and Human Development.* 1998;29:65-76.
8. Padula WV, Argyris S. Post trauma vision syndrome and visual midline shift syndrome. *NeuroRehabilitation.* 1996;6:165-171.

9. Bowers AR, Keeney K, Peli E. Community-based trial of a peripheral prism visual field expansion device for hemi-anopia. *Arch Ophthalmol.* 2008;126(5):657-664.

10. Giorgi RG, Woods RL, Peli E. Clinical and laboratory evaluation of peripheral prism glasses for hemianopia. *Optom Vis Sci.* 2009;86:492-502.

11. Politzer TA. Case studies of a new approach using partial and selective occlusion for the clinical treatment of diplopia. *NeuroRehabilitation.* 1996;6:213-217.

12. Waiss B, Soden R. Head trauma and low vision: clinical modifications for diagnosis and prescription. *J Am Optom Assoc.* 1992;63:559-563.

13. Scheiman M, Scheiman M, Whittaker SG. *Low Vision Rehabilitation: A Practical Guide for Occupational Therapists.* Thorofare, NJ: SLACK Incorporated; 2007.

14. Berne SA. Visual therapy for the traumatic brain-injured. *J Optom Vis Devel.* 1990;21:13-16.

15. Hellerstein LF, Dowis RT, Maples WC. Optometric management of strabismus patients. *J Am Optom Assoc.* 1994;65:621-625.

16. Cohen AH, Soden R. An optometric approach to the rehabilitation of the stroke patient. *J Am Optom Assoc.* 1981;52:795-800.

17. Gianutsos R, Ramsey G. Enabling rehabilitation optometrists to help survivors of acquired brain injury. *J Vis Rehab.* 1988;2:37-58.

18. Hellerstein LF, Freed S. Rehabilitative vision therapy for a traumatic brain injury patient: case report. *J Behav Optom.* 1994;5:143-148.

19. Hinrichs CA. Vision rehabilitation for the multiply challenged child. *J Optom Vis Devel.* 1992;23:9-13.

20. Aksinoff EB, Falk NS. Optometric therapy for the left brain injured patient. *J Am Optom Assoc.* 1992;63:564-568.

21. Cohen AH. Optometric management of binocular dysfunctions secondary to head trauma: case reports. *J Am Optom Assoc.* 1992;63:569-575.

22. Ludlam WM. Rehabilitation of traumatic brain injury with associated visual dysfunction—a case report. *NeuroRehabilitation.* 1996;6:183-192.

23. Valenti CA. Optometric vision therapy for head trauma. *J Optom Vis Devel.* 1999;30:67-72.

24. Raymond MJ, Bennett TL, Malia KB, Bewick KC. Rehabilitation of visual processing deficits following brain injury. *NeuroRehabilitation.* 1996;6:229-240.

25. Ciuffreda KJ, Suchoff IB, Marrone MA, et al. Oculomotor rehabilitation in traumatic brain-injured patients. *J Behav Optom.* 1996;7:31-38.

26. Cohen AH. Optometric rehabilitative therapy. In: Press LJ, ed. *Applied Concepts in Vision Therapy.* St. Louis, MO: Mosby. 1997:278-286.

27. Hillier CG, Rosenow EL. Optometric vision therapy rehabilitation in hospitals. *J Optom Vis Devel.* 1999;30:83-85.

28. Scheiman M, Gallaway M. Vision therapy to treat binocular vision disorders after acquired brain injury: factors affect-ing prognosis. In: Suchoff IB, Ciuffreda KJ, Kapoor N, eds. *Visual and Vestibular Consequences of Acquired Brain Injury.* Santa Ana, CA: Optom Extension Program, 2001:89-113.

29. Han Y, Ciuffreda KJ, Kapoor N. Reading-related oculo-motor testing and training protocols for acquired brain injury in humans. *Brain Res Protoc.* 2004;14(1):1-12.

30. Hillier CG. Vision rehabilitation following acquired brain injury: a case series. *Brain Injury/Professional.* 2005;2:30-32.

31. Kapoor N, Ciuffreda KJ, Han,Y. Oculomotor rehabilitation in acquired brain injury: a case series. *Arch Phys Med Rehab.* 2005;1667-1678.

32. Ciuffreda KJ, Han Y, Kapoor, Ficarra AP. Oculomotor rehabilitation for reading in acquired brain injury. *NeuroRehabilitation.* 2006;21(1):9-21.

33. Ciuffreda KJ, Rutner R, Kapoor N, Suchoff IB. Vision therapy for oculomotor dysfunctions in acquired brain injury. *Optom J Am Optom Assn.* 2008;79:18-22.

34. Scheiman M, Wick B. *Clinical Management of Binocular Vision: Heterophoric, Accommodative, and Eye Movement Disorders.* 3rd ed. Philadelphia, PA: Lippincott Williams & Wilkins; 2008.

35. Ciuffreda KJ, Ludlam, Kapoor N. Clinical oculomotor training in traumatic brain injury. *Optom Vis Dev.* 2009;40(1):16-23.

36. Hellerstein LF, Winkler PA. Vestibular dysfunction associated with traumatic brain injury: collaborative optometry and physical therapy treatment. In: Suchoff IB, Ciuffreda KF, Kapoor N, eds. *Visual and Vestibular Consequences of Acquired Brain Injury.* Santa Ana, CA: Optometric Extension Program; 2002.

37. Rinehart MA. Strategies for improving motor performance. In: Rosenthal M, ed. *Rehabilitation of the Adult and Child With Traumatic Brain Injury.* Philadelphia, PA: FA Davis Co; 1990.

38. Shumway-Cook A, Horak FB. Rehabilitation strategies for patients with vestibular deficits. *Neur Clin.* 1990;8:441-457.

39. Shumway-Cook A, Horak FB. Vestibular rehabilitation: an exercise approach to managing symptoms of vestibular dysfunction. *Seminars in Hearing.* 1989;10:196-209.

40. Ciuffreda KJ, Suchoff IB, Marrone MA, Ahmann E. Oculomotor rehabilitation in traumatic brain injured patients. *J Behav Optom.* 1996;7:31-38.

41. Dennison PE, Dennison GE. *Brain Gym.* Glendale, CA: Edu-kinesthetics Inc; 1986.

42. Levine KJ. *Fine Motor Dysfunction.* Tucson, AZ: Therapy Skill Builders; 1991.

43. Warren M. A hierarchical model for evaluation and treatment of visual perceptual dysfunction in adult acquired brain injury, part 1. *Am J Occup Ther.* 1993;47:42-54.

44. Scheiman M, Rouse M. *Optometric Management of Learning Related Vision Problems.* 2nd ed. St Louis, MO: CV Mosby Elsevier; 2006.

45. Warren M. A hierarchical model for evaluation and treatment of visual perceptual dysfunction in adult acquired brain injury, part 2. *Am J Occup Ther.* 1993;47:55-66.

46. Lane KA. *Developing Your Child for Success.* Lewisville, TX: Learning Potential Publishers; 1991.

47. Lyons E. *How to Use Your Power of Visualization.* Red Bluff, CA: Lyons Visualization Series; 1980.

48. Forrest E. *Visual Imagery: An Optometric Approach.* Santa Ana, CA: Optometric Extension Program; 1981.

49. Prokopich L, Pace R. Visual rehabilitation in homonymous hemianopia due to cerebral vascular accident. *J Vis Rehab.* 1989;3:29-35.

50. Kasten E, Wust S, Behrens-Baumann W, et al. Computer-based training for the treatment of partial blindness. *Nat Med.* 1998;4:1083-1087.

51. Kasten E, Muller-Oehring E, Sabel BA. Stability of visual field enlargements following computer-based restitution training—results of a follow-up. *J Clin Exp Neuropsychol.* 2001;23:297-305.

52. Kasten E, Poggel DA, Muller-Oehring E, et al. Restoration of vision II: residual functions and training-induced visual field enlargement in brain-damaged patients. *Restor Neurol Neurosci.* 1999;15:273-287.

53. Horton JC. Disappointing results from Nova Vision's visual restoration therapy. *Br J Ophthalmol.* 2005;89:1-2.

54. Horton JC. Vision restoration therapy: confounded by eye movements. *Br J Ophthalmol.* 2005;89:792-794.

55. Reinhard J, Schreiber A, Schiefer U, et al. Does visual restitution training change absolute homonymous visual field defects? A fundus controlled study. *Br J Ophthalmol.* 2005;89:30-35.

56. Gianutsos R, Suchoff IB. Visual fields after brain injury: management issues for the occupational therapist. In: Scheiman M. *Understanding and Managing Visual Deficits: A Guide for Occupational Therapists.* 2nd ed. Thorofare, NJ: SLACK Incorporated; 2002.

57. Scheiman M, Scheiman M, Whittaker S. *Low Vision Rehabilitation: A Practical Guide for Occupational Therapists.* Thorofare, NJ: SLACK Incorporated; 2007.

58. Trobe JD. *The Neurology of Vision. Contemporary Neurology Series.* Vol 60. Oxford: Oxford University Press; 2001:451.

59. Zoltan B. *Vision, Perception and Cognition: A Manual for the Examination and Treatment of the Neurologically Impaired Adult.* 3rd ed. Thorofare, NJ: SLACK Incorporated; 1996:211.

60. Gianutsos R. *Computer Programs for Cognitive Rehabilitation: Software Tools for Use with Persons Emerging from Coma into Consciousness.* Vol 5. Bayport, NY: Life Science Associates; 1988.

61. Gianutsos R, Vroman GS, Matheson P, Glosser D. *Computer Programs for Cognitive Rehabilitation: Further Visual Imperception Procedures.* Vol 2. Bayport, NY: Life Science Associates; 1983.

62. Gianutsos R, Klitzner C. *Computer Programs for Cognitive Rehabilitation: Further Visual Imperception Procedures.* Vol 2. Bayport, NY: Life Sciences Associates; 1981:116.

63. Gianutsos R, Cochran EE, Blouin M. *Computer Programs for Cognitive Rehabilitation: Therapeutic Memory Programs for Independent Use.* Vol 3. Bayport, NY: Life Science Associates; 1984.

64. Heikki HA, Julkunen LA. Treatment of visual field deficits after a stroke. *Advances in Clinical Neuroscience and Rehabilitation.* 2004;3(6):17-18.

65. Pedretti W, Zoltan B, eds. *Occupational Therapy: Practice Skills for Physical Dysfunction.* Philadelphia, PA: Mosby; 1996.

66. Niemeier JP. The Lighthouse strategy: use of a visual imagery technique to treat visual inattention in stroke patients. *Brain Inj.* 1998;12(5):399-406.

67. Marshall RS. Rehabilitation approaches to hemineglect. *Neurologist.* 2009;15:185-192.

68. Redding GM, Wallace B. Prism adaptation and unilateral neglect: review and analysis. *Neuropsychologia.* 2006;44(1):1-20.

69. Rossetti Y, Rode G, Pisella L, et al. Prism adaptation to a rightward optical deviation rehabilitates left hemispatial negect. *Nature.* 1998;395:166-169.

70. Saevarsson S. Unilateral neglect: a review of causes, anatomical localization, theories and interventions. *Laeknabladid.* 2009;95:27-33.

71. Shiraishi H. Long-term effects of prism adaptation on chronic neglect after stroke. *NeuroRehabilitation.* 2008;23:137-151.

72. Park WL, Unatin J, Herbert A. A driving program for the visually impaired. *J Am Optom Assoc.* 1993;64:54-59.

73. Hellerstein LF, Fishman BI. Vision therapy and occupational therapy: an integrated approach. *J Behav Optom.* 1990;1:122-126.

74. Schnell R. An innovative connection between rehabilitation optometry and occupational therapy: solving visual problems associated with brain injury. *J Cognit Rehab*. 1992;July/Aug:34-36.

75. Suchoff IB. Occupational therapy and optometry: a developing relationship. *J Behav Optom*. 1991;2:170-171.

76. Collaboration between occupational therapists and optometrists. *OT Pract*. 1999;June:22-30.

Chapter Eleven

Oculo-Visual Disorders Associated With Developmental and Sensory Disabilities

Sarah D. Appel, OD, FAAO and Elise B. Ciner, OD, FAAO

Overview of the Problem

In 1977, there were 29,403 school-aged children who were registered with the American Printing House for the Blind.[1] In 2007, that number almost doubled to 57,696.[2] This increase is due, at least partly, to significant advances in medical pre- and post-natal care that increase the chance for survival of very young and/or very sick premature infants. Many pediatric syndromes have associated ocular abnormalities. Intrauterine infections such as rubella, syphilis, and cytomegalovirus are frequently associated with significant visual impairment. Syndromes and disorders such as Down syndrome, Hallermann-Streiff syndrome, Bardet-Biedl syndrome, Crouzon syndrome, and Leber's congenital amaurosis are associated with a host of ocular disorders. Children born to drug- and alcohol-addicted mothers as well as children who suffer the tragic consequences of shaken baby syndrome and other forms of child abuse are also often left with multiple impairments. As medical technology enables these infants to survive, they often exhibit lasting handicapping conditions, such as hearing loss, cerebral palsy, learning disabilities, and visual impairment. This trend of increasing numbers of children with special needs is not likely to reverse in the near future.

It is unfortunate that, while medicine is increasingly able to save these children, many still do not receive appropriate vision-related services during the critical first few years of life. This is due to the perception that developmentally delayed or sensory-impaired children are unresponsive and therefore untestable. This misconception is prevalent among health care providers who are unable to interpret these children's nonverbal responses. Some eye care providers have even labeled children with usable vision as blind because they were not responsive to the standard vision testing procedures. The key element in developing appropriate vision interventions for developmentally and visually impaired children is adequate and accurate information about visual status and the nature of any visual disorders. The following discussion explores the types and nature of the vision disorders that are associated with developmentally delayed and sensory-impaired children.

Scheiman M
Understanding and Managing Vision Deficits: A Guide for Occupational Therapists, Third Edition (pp 233-252)
© 2011 SLACK Incorporated

Types of Disorders

Refractive Error

There is a high correlation between significant refractive error and developmental disabilities (Table 11-1). Premature birth resulting from intrauterine trauma, infection, or fetal abnormality is frequently associated with an ocular disorder known as retinopathy of prematurity. This condition is associated with a high magnitude of myopia that often prevents affected children from seeing objects that are located beyond arm's reach. A child with retinopathy of prematurity and significant myopic refractive error greater than 10 diopters will experience visual blur at distances greater than 4 inches unless the appropriate spectacle or contact lens correction is worn. Significant myopia can also occur in individuals with Down syndrome[3] (trisomy 21), Stickler syndrome, Pierre Robin syndrome, and microcornea.[4]

Significant hyperopia is a commonly found refractive error in children with developmental disabilities.[5] Children with conditions such as cerebral palsy, fragile X syndrome, hydrocephalus, and brain malformations (ie, septo-optic dysplasia) frequently manifest hyperopic refractive error. Hyperopia is also a common finding in visually impaired children with disorders such as albinism and microphthalmia. Conditions such as Marfan syndrome that are associated with the displacement of the eye's lens create a situation where only part of the pupillary region is occupied by the lens. In this type of disorder, significant myopic refractive error coexists with significant hyperopic refractive error in the same eye. Children with special needs who have uncorrected hyperopia may experience visual fatigue, especially after tasks requiring a close viewing distance. Significant uncorrected hyperopic refractive error may also result in strabismus and amblyopia.

Conditions that involve corneal disorders are typically associated with significant amounts of astigmatism. These include conditions such as keratoconus, keratoglobus, congenital syphilis, and microcornea. Any surgical procedure involving the cornea, such as corneal transplantation or removal of a cataract, may result in significant astigmatism. Astigmatism may also be found in children with congenital nystagmus. Congenital nystagmus is associated with ocular disorders, such as retinal and optic nerve colobomas, aniridia, albinism, retinopathy of prematurity, as well as Leber's congenital amaurosis. Syndromes associated with significant facial and lid deformities such as Treacher Collins syndrome may also be accompanied by significant astigmatic refractive error.

Intrauterine infections such as rubella and congenital syphilis, chromosomal anomalies such as Down syndrome and Turner syndrome, as well as metabolic disturbances such as homocystinuria are associated with congenital cataracts. Surgical removal of the cataracts results in a refractive disorder known as aphakia. If an aphakic refractive error is uncorrected by a spectacle, contact lens, or intraocular lens correction, the child experiences blur both at distance and near. The nature of the refractive error is typically high hyperopia unless the child had a significant myopic refractive error before removal of the cataracts. In that situation, the child may be mildly myopic or hyperopic depending on the magnitude of the original myopic refractive error. The child with aphakia cannot change focus for varying distances due to the absence of a lens. These children therefore, typically require bifocals to enable them to view objects at arm's length or closer.

During the course of the evaluation, a frequently asked question is whether to prescribe a correction to a child who manifests significant developmental disabilities. The impression held by some professionals is that the developmentally delayed child will be unresponsive to the visual enhancement provided by the corrective lenses. In many cases, even a child who appears to be totally withdrawn and unresponsive to his or her environment may, in time, exhibit changes in visual behaviors after adapting to corrective lenses.

Case One

An 8-year-old girl with a history of autism, developmental disability, and a degenerative neuropathy presented for evaluation of her visual status. She had previously been evaluated at other

Table 11-1	
Refractive Error and Developmental Disabilities	
Refractive Error	*Conditions or Syndromes*
Myopia	Retinopathy of prematurity
	Stickler syndrome
	Microcornea
	Marfan syndrome
Hyperopia	Marfan syndrome (in aphakia pupillary sector)
	Microphthalmos
	Cerebral palsy
	Albinism
Astigmatism	Albinism
	Keratoglobus
	Congenital pendular nystagmus
	Treacher Collins syndrome

eye care facilities. No ocular pathology had been noted. No corrective lenses had ever been prescribed. During the course of the evaluation, we found the girl to be minimally responsive to any visual or sensory stimuli. She exhibited minimal movement except for occasional head movements. During the refractive component of the evaluation, we found significant myopia, coupled with a high degree of astigmatism. We prescribed corrective lenses with instructions to slowly habituate the child to the correction. When she returned for a follow-up evaluation 2 months later, the mother reported that the child's teachers had noted increased eye contact and an overall increase in attention. The child's mother also reported that her daughter cried at night when the glasses were removed. During the course of the evaluation, we found an increase in overall response to visual stimuli. We were pleased to see the presence of brief visual tracking behaviors. We also witnessed a significant negative reaction when we removed the corrective lenses from her face.

This 8-year-old child had been without an essential correction during a critical time of her development due to the mistaken belief that she was too developmentally delayed to benefit from corrective lenses.

Case Two

A 16-year-old girl with a history of developmental disability, hearing impairment, and bilateral retinal colobomas was evaluated at a school for the blind. Due to her hearing impairment, her teachers communicated with her by signing. They wanted information on how to adapt their signing (position and distance) to ensure that it was appropriate for her visual status. The student was unresponsive and generally uncooperative for any of the acuity measurement testing procedures that were appropriate for her developmental age. During refraction, we found a significant hyperopic refractive error. Her teachers were uncertain if she would wear a spectacle correction due to her significant tactual defensiveness and her resistance to wearing her hearing aids. When a trial prescription was placed on her face, the student grabbed the frame and, instead of removing it as had been expected, she pushed it higher up on her bridge. Her use of vision while walking increased significantly while wearing the correction. We also observed her use of vision during her workshop activity, which consisted of feeding paper into a shredding machine. With the spectacle correction, she was able to visually guide the paper to the appropriate slot for shredding. Her teachers reported that she had previously performed the same activity solely by touch. We issued a prescription for the corrective lenses.

This 16-year-old girl's previously uncorrected refractive error had interfered with her ability to learn, communicate, and effectively perform activities of daily living. She adapted well to the new correction.

Visual Efficiency

EYE MOVEMENTS

Developmentally delayed and visually impaired children frequently manifest abnormalities in eye movements. Children with significant gross and fine motor delays, as is the case in children with cerebral palsy, often manifest eye movements that are choppy when visually tracking a target. They will typically manifest difficulty in maintaining long-term fixation as well as in scanning their environment for visual targets accurately. They overshoot or undershoot the visual target frequently. It is important to note that overall postural issues frequently have an impact on a neurologically impaired child's visual responsiveness. For example, if a child with cerebral palsy is physically stressed due to lack of postural and head support during a visual activity, that child will manifest more significant impairment in visual skills than if he or she is not in postural distress. The occupational therapist's role in ensuring appropriate positioning is, therefore, critical. Overall fatigue, emotional distress, as well as discomfort or illness can also further degrade the eye movements of these children.

Children with significant visual field defects will also manifest pronounced eye movement disorders. Children with central scotomas resulting from macular degeneration or dystrophy may exhibit frequent losses in fixation as they track a visual target. The losses in fixation may lead to the erroneous diagnosis of intermittent nystagmus. These children will also be inaccurate during visual scanning activities, as the visual targets are often obscured by the central blind spot. Children with peripheral visual field constriction will also exhibit losses of fixation when tracking a visual target, especially if the target is moved quickly. They will also have a very difficult time initiating accurate saccadic eye movements (shifts in fixation from one target to another) during visual scanning activities. Children who manifest hemianopic visual field defects will typically have more difficulty with visual search activities in the defective visual field area than in the intact visual field area.

Neurological defects may eliminate all eye movements or eye movements in a certain direction. Vertical gaze palsies result in an inability of both eyes to fully look up or down. This may be caused by encephalitis, trauma to the midbrain region, and degenerative neurological disease. Horizontal gaze palsies result in the inability of both eyes to look to the right or left. The eyes are affected symmetrically, thereby eliminating double vision. Such disorders may result from brain tumors, brain lesions secondary to head trauma, and congenital conditions such as congenital ocular motor apraxia.

Children who have significant eye movement disorders will typically combine head movements with eye movements in order to increase the range and efficiency of their eye movements. Children with restrictions in gaze will typically adapt head turns to the involved area in order to bring their eyes into the involved visual region.

Case Three

A 7-year-old developmentally disabled girl with a history of head trauma presented to the special populations service for a vision evaluation. In her educational setting, she had been undergoing a vision stimulation program that involved eye movement activities. These activities included both vertical and horizontal tracking of objects. Her mother reported that she was very frustrated during these activities and that the vision teacher was frustrated by her lack of cooperation, especially during vertical tracking activities. During testing, we found that the child manifested pupillary abnormalities. We also noted a marked vertical gaze palsy that prevented her from initiating and maintaining vertical gaze movements. She had been asked to perform an activity that was impossible for her to successfully accomplish as a result of neurological damage most likely to the midbrain region. We shared our findings with the mother and the teacher, and the vertical tracking activities, the source of the child's frustration, were eliminated. We recommended that she be allowed to use head movements to enable her to carry out vertical tracking and scanning activities efficiently.

NYSTAGMUS

Nystagmus is a common finding in both neurologically impaired and visually impaired children. Nystagmus is associated with hydrocephalus, meningitis, and cerebral palsy, as well as other neurological disorders. A child with congenital nystagmus will experience degradation in visual images due to retinal smearing of the visual targets. The child will not, however, see any motion associated with the visual target. Neurologically based nystagmus may manifest in several ways. It most commonly presents as a jerk-type nystagmus, but may also present as a rotary nystagmus or a downbeat nystagmus. Jerk-type nystagmus often has a null point. This is the eye position in which the nystagmus is significantly reduced or eliminated. Some children will adapt a head turn or tilt in order to consistently achieve the null-point region. This becomes especially evident during visually challenging activities.

Sensory nystagmus resulting from significant congenital visual deprivation is typically pendular in nature. Pendular nystagmus is associated with conditions such as albinism, aniridia, and congenital cataracts. Pendular nystagmus typically does not have a true null point. It may dampen significantly, however, during convergence to near targets.

Other forms of nystagmus found in developmentally disabled children include latent and end-point nystagmus. Latent nystagmus is only present when one eye is covered. Children with latent nystagmus will not respond as expected to patching activities, as their visual acuity and efficiency may be significantly degraded by the latent nystagmus. Endpoint or gaze-evoked nystagmus will occur when a child's eyes shift to the limits of his or her range. This type of nystagmus may be associated with a paretic muscle, with cerebellar or cerebral disorders, or with internuclear ophthalmoplegia. Endpoint nystagmus may also be precipitated by anti-seizure medications. Pharmacologically induced nystagmus will disappear after discontinuation of the medication. Table 11-2 summarizes the most common forms of nystagmus.

Table 11-2	
Common Forms of Nystagmus	
Type of Nystagmus	*Description*
Pendular	Horizontal congenital nystagmus may become jerk type on extreme lateral gaze
	Dampens on convergence
	Typically does not have true null point
	Associated with congenital macular and optic nerve abnormalities
Jerk	Horizontal rhythmic jerky eye movements
	Characterized by slow component in one direction followed by fast component in opposite direction
Rotary	Nystagmus characterized by rotary oscillations
Latent	Nystagmus that occurs when one eye is covered
Endpoint	Nystagmus that occurs at the extremes of gaze
	Tends to be a jerk-type nystagmus

CONVERGENCE

Accurate convergence for a near visual target is essential for the establishment of stereopsis as well as for the elimination of diplopia (double vision). Strabismus and accommodative disorders can have a significant negative impact on accurate and efficient convergence responses. Convergence may also be affected by neurological disorders. Brain trauma and encephalitis may result in convergence palsy. Another condition that may result in convergence insufficiency is hypertelorism, or abnormally widely spaced eyes, which is typically found in syndromes like Crouzon syndrome that are associated with skull deformity. These associated syndromes frequently include developmental disability as well. The child with hypertelorism has a greater convergence demand and will be more likely to experience convergence fatigue and diplopia. These children may experience fatigue and diplopia so frequently that they may give up trying to converge for any near target and simply adopt a head turn or an eye closure to eliminate the need for convergence. They essentially function monocularly. Medications such as phenobarbital, which are used to control seizure activity, may also decrease convergence. It is essential to identify convergence difficulties in children in order to ensure that proper interventions are implemented so that the child can function effectively during near visual activities.

Case Four

A 4-year-old boy with a history of hyperactivity, hearing impairment, developmental disability, and hypertelorism had a history of reduced visual attention and head turning behaviors when viewing objects at reduced distances. During our evaluation, we noted that, while there was no evidence of any gaze restriction, he was not able to converge his eyes for objects that were presented at a reduced distance. When asked to look at a near object, he would turn his head to the right or left of the object in order to view it monocularly. In order to provide him with binocularity for near targets, we introduced bilateral base-in prisms in a spectacle correction. With the prisms, he was able to view the object without any head-turning behaviors. We were able to elicit a brief convergence response as we brought the object closer to him. He also demonstrated better eye-hand coordination while wearing the correction. We issued a prescription for the prismatic correction with instructions to use it for activities that required a reduced viewing distance. Table 11-3 summarizes the causes of accommodative and convergence abnormalities.

Table 11-3

Causes of Accommodative and Convergence Problems

Problem	Causation
Accommodation	Medications
	Gross and fine motor delays
	Aphakia
	Visual fatigue caused by significant uncorrected hyperopic refractive error
	Neurological disorders
Convergence	Hypertelorism
	Neurological disorders
	Medications
	Accommodative disorders
	Strabismus

Strabismus

Strabismus is often associated with developmental disabilities and is commonly seen in various syndromes. The lack of binocularity or eye alignment associated with strabismus results in decreased or absent stereoscopic vision. This may negatively affect activities that necessitate accurate eye-hand coordination and compromise the child's safety during mobility-related activities that require accurate depth perception such as negotiating curbs and stairs. The prevalence of strabismus in the general population is approximately 2% to 4%.[6-8] In contrast, the prevalence of strabismus in the developmentally disabled is often much higher, depending on the diagnosis.[9] Therefore, a careful assessment of binocular status should be completed in all of these individuals. Strabismus can occur for a variety of reasons. For example, strabismus can result from decreased visual acuity in one or both eyes, or it can be secondary to brain trauma or damage resulting in conditions such as cortical visual impairment. Strabismus is also frequently found in children with poor muscle tone, such as children with cerebral palsy. Significant uncorrected refractive error can also cause an exotropia or esotropia depending on the type of problem. Strabismus can be present as a direct result of a craniofacial anomaly characteristic of a particular syndrome. Often, however, strabismus may be present in individuals with developmental disabilities without any specific etiology for its presence.

Strabismus Secondary to Decreased Visual Acuity

Strabismus frequently occurs secondary to an early onset long-term reduction of visual acuity in one or both eyes. An example would be congenital cataracts, especially when the cataract is present in one eye only. Even when the cataract is removed and the eyes are optically corrected, there is a very high prevalence of strabismus and rarely is any type of binocularity present.[10-12]

Strabismus Secondary to Poor Muscle Tone

Strabismus is a common feature in conditions in which poor muscle tone is present, such as cerebral palsy. Studies have shown the prevalence of strabismus to be between 31% and 60% in individuals with cerebral palsy.[13-15] This strabismus can either be esotropia, exotropia, hypertropia, or hypotropia. Often, however, it is variable in nature, changing from an exotropia to esotropia periodically. Children with cerebral palsy also show a high prevalence of limitations of gaze ranging from 4% to 18%.[14,16] Both the variability of the strabismus and the gaze paresis make the management of binocular vision anomalies in children with cerebral palsy much more challenging.

Strabismus Secondary to Significant Refractive Error

Because many children with developmental disabilities have high hyperopia, it is not uncommon for there to be an accompanying accommodative esotropia secondary to the uncorrected hyperopia. For example, children with albinism are predisposed to significant hyperopia and astigmatic refractive errors. This can, in turn, contribute to the development of esotropia.

Strabismus Secondary to Craniofacial Anomalies

Facial structure can contribute to the development of strabismus. An example is hypertelorism, which is an abnormally wide separation between the eyes. This anatomical feature can result in the presence of exotropia, especially at near distances, due to the increased demand on convergence.

Strabismus of Unknown Etiology

No specific etiology may be associated with a strabismus other than its known association with a particular syndrome or condition. An example of this would be Down syndrome (trisomy 21) in which the prevalence of strabismus is 23% to 44%.[17] Fragile X syndrome is another frequently encountered, inherited genetic disorder that results in mental retardation. It is highly associated with strabismus (either esotropia or exotropia).[14] Several other chromosomal abnormalities also highly associated with the presence of strabismus include syndromes associated with the duplication, trisomy, and deletion of various chromosomes.[18]

A wide range of developmental disabilities is associated with the presence of some type of strabismus. The type and magnitude of the strabismus is as variable as the presenting condition and the child who is being examined. The prognosis for achieving ocular alignment or normal binocular functioning depends upon many factors, including the type, magnitude, and frequency of the strabismus present, the nature of associated eye disorders, as well as the visual acuity, age, and cognitive functioning of the developmentally disabled child. Most importantly, an accurate assessment of both the child's motor (how the eyes look) and sensory (what the child sees) functioning should be attempted in each case.

CONTRAST SENSITIVITY

A reduction in contrast sensitivity will compromise a child's ability to see low contrast objects in the environment. Although this aspect of vision is often overlooked during the standard eye examination, it plays a significant role in the use of vision during activities of daily living and mobility as the majority of objects in our environment tend to be of low contrast. A child with reduced contrast sensitivity will have difficulty seeing curbs, stairs, facial detail, or educational materials such as low contrast drawings or text. Any clouding of normally transparent ocular structures arising from internal eye inflammation, cataracts, corneal disease, or vitreous abnormalities will result in reduced contrast sensitivity. Eye disorders that are associated with damage to the optic nerve or central retina will also result in reduced contrast sensitivity. Contrast-enhancing strategies such as the use of high contrast markings on stairs or curbs as well as the use of high contrast educational materials such as bold-lined paper and broad-tipped soft graphite pencils will enhance the use of vision in children with reduced contrast sensitivity. Reduction of ambient glare and the use of glare-free task lighting will also enhance the contrast of educational materials.

ACCOMMODATION

Accommodative disorders in children with developmental disabilities can interfere with their fine motor development as well as with overall learning. There are a number of causative factors for accommodative disorders in developmentally delayed as well as visually impaired children. Significant uncorrected hyperopic refractive error can create visual stress that reduces the efficiency and stability of a child's accommodation. Correcting the refractive error ensures that the visual stress is eliminated, thereby facilitating accommodation. Children with gross and fine motor delays, as is the case in cerebral palsy, will often display inaccurate or poorly maintained accommodation for near visual tasks.[19] Children with low vision often have accommodative disorders. Accommodation may also be reduced by systemic medication used to control seizures, reduce depression, and hyperactivity. Accommodation is totally absent in children with aphakia or pseudophakia who have undergone cataract surgery. It is important to establish the presence of accommodative disorders in order to prescribe appropriate corrective lenses or implement appropriate accommodative therapy.

FLUCTUATIONS IN VISION

Many caregivers report that they are concerned about fluctuating levels of visual attention. This is often interpreted to be a result of fluctuating vision. Systemic conditions may cause changes in visual acuities. Diabetes and hypoglycemia will create fluctuations in visual acuity due to fluctuating sugar levels, which create changes in refractive error. Multiple sclerosis can also result in fluctuating acuity depending on energy, stress, and even temperature levels. Medication may create accommodative fluctuations that result in visual acuity changes. In some situations, however, mild or focal seizure activity is misinterpreted as changes in visual acuity or visual attention. It is important to observe if there are consistent changes in facial expressions, ocular deviations, increases in nystagmoid eye movements, or if there are subtle postural changes that may indicate the possibility of seizure-related activity. In such situations, prompt referral back to a neurologist is indicated.

Low Vision

In working with children who are visually impaired, it is important to note that only a small percentage (approximately 15%) of visually impaired individuals are functionally or totally blind.[20] The majority of visually impaired children have residual vision, or low vision, that is useful for educational activities as well as for activities of daily living. It would take an entire textbook to adequately explore all of the conditions that result in low vision. The following discussion will explore the more common low vision conditions, as well as their implications for overall visual functioning.

ACHROMATOPSIA

Individuals with achromatopsia have no color vision. This condition is most commonly caused by a hereditary disorder called rod monochromatism. In this disorder, the cone photoreceptors of the retina that are responsible for processing fine detail, color vision, and adaptation to brightly illuminated environments do not develop properly. Children with this condition tend to be very photophobic or sensitive to light. They experience enhanced vision with a reduction in ambient illumination and visual acuity actually improves under dimmer illumination. Visual acuity is typically in the range of 20/100 to 20/200. These children will not have any color vision. No visual field defects are associated with this condition. Retinal and optic nerve appearance is typically normal. Nystagmus is frequently associated with rod monochromatism. Interventions typically recommended by the low vision rehabilitation optometrist to improve visual functioning include light filtration, magnification, and contrast enhancement, especially for visual targets with poorly contrasting colors. Dark red contact lenses and sunlenses have been found to significantly reduce outdoor light sensitivity.

Case Five

A 5-year-old boy with a history of Leber's congenital amaurosis presented to our special populations service. His parents reported that he demonstrated significant difficulty maintaining visual attention, especially outdoors. He tended to walk with his head down and consistently held on to someone's hand when he walked. His parents reported that he preferred dimly lit environments. During testing, we found that his visual fields were full. Visual acuities were approximately 20/120. Retinal and optic nerve appearance was normal. We noted the presence of a pendular nystagmus. We found that he had significant color vision defects and that he was very photophobic. We evaluated his response to a dark red sunlens while outdoors under sunny conditions and found that he was able to walk with his head up. He also was able to walk without holding his mother's hand. Indoors, he demonstrated excellent responses to a 32% gray tint. We suggested that he undergo testing for rod monochromatism. Rod monochromatism was confirmed during electrodiagnostic testing. His parents were educated about low vision rehabilitative options and were advised to return for a magnification evaluation in 1 year. His parents reported during a follow-up telephone conversation that the sunlenses significantly improved his visual attention and his independence.

ALBINISM

This hereditary disorder results from an inability or a reduced ability to produce the melanin that is necessary for pigmentation of the skin, hair, and eyes. Individuals with the full manifestation of this condition, oculocutaneous albinism or OCA 1, typically have very pale skin as well as white to yellow-white hair. Eye color is typically light blue due to the lack of iris pigmentation.

Individuals with milder forms of oculocutaneous albinism (OCA 2, OCA 3, and OCA 4) are able to produce some pigment and may have darker pigmented hair and eyes. Pendular nystagmus is associated with a hypoplastic or underdeveloped macular region. Optic nerve hypoplasia may also be present and be a contributing factor. Astigmatic refractive error is common. Strabismus and lack of stereovision is also common in individuals with albinism due to the abnormal crossing pattern of neural fibers at the optic chiasm. Visual acuity ranges from 20/200 to 20/400. Children with albinism tend to be very sensitive to brightly illuminated environments, as there is minimal pigmentation in the iris to absorb the excess light. The visual disability as well as the sensitivity to light is less severe in OCA 2, OCA 3, and OCA 4. Another form of albinism, ocular albinism, is restricted solely to the eye. Children with ocular albinism tend to have higher levels of vision and more ocular pigmentation. Some forms of albinism have associated systemic disease. Hermansky-Pudlak syndrome is associated with oculocutaneous albinism, a bleeding disorder, and pulmonary fibrosis. The disorder has a higher incidence in individuals of Puerto Rican descent but is found in other nationalities as well. Chédiak-Higashi syndrome is associated with oculocutaneous albinism and blood cell abnormalities resulting in prolonged bleeding, recurrent infection, and early death. Children with albinism respond well to low vision rehabilitation. Interventions typically recommended by the low vision rehabilitation optometrist include light filtration and magnification devices.

Aniridia

Aniridia is a hereditary developmental disorder that results in an absent or rudimentary iris (Figure 11-1). As the iris provides the mechanism for light control in the eye through the constriction and dilation of the pupil, these individuals tend to be very photophobic. The constant incidence of uncontrolled light levels on the retina results in an underdevelopment of the macular region. Visual acuity typically is between 20/100 and 20/200. Pendular nystagmus is highly associated with this condition. There is also a marked association with cataracts, as well as a late-onset corneal disorder that results in corneal clouding. No visual field defects are associated with aniridia unless there is a secondary glaucoma as a result of defective angle formation. In cases of aniridia in which no previous family history of the condition exists, there is an increased chance of developing a

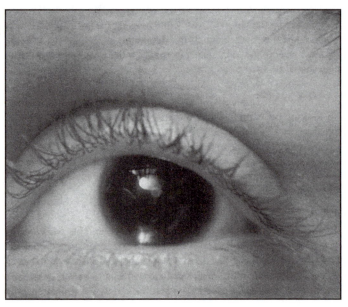

Figure 11-1. Aniridia is a hereditary developmental disorder that results in an absent or rudimentary iris.

metastatic kidney tumor, called Wilms' tumor, within the first decade of life. Children with this sporadic form of aniridia must be monitored for this tumor during the first decade of life, as prognosis is excellent if the tumor is removed during the early stage of its development. Interventions for visual enhancement recommended by a low vision rehabilitation optometrist include light filtration devices, magnification devices, and reduced aperture contact lenses.

CATARACTS

Cataracts are associated with a number of syndromes including rubella, retinopathy of prematurity, Down syndrome, and Hallermann-Streiff syndrome. Cataracts may be caused by trauma to the child's orbital region or by systemic medications, such as cortisone. Cataracts may also be associated with congenital glaucoma or present as an isolated finding in children with inherited congenital cataracts. Congenital cataracts typically result in visual impairment and nystagmus unless they are removed early in the child's visual development. Long-standing congenital cataracts result in amblyopia due to significant sensory deprivation during the critical period of the eye's development. The removal of the cataracts results in aphakia. It is necessary to correct the significant refractive error induced by surgical aphakia through the use of corrective spectacle lenses, contact lenses, or intraocular lenses. If the child has an associated visual impairment, intervention typically consists of magnification, contrast enhancement, and illumination control.

CEREBRAL PALSY

Cerebral palsy is a disorder of movement and posture resulting from brain injury that has occurred before the brain has matured or a nonprogressive developmental abnormality of the brain. The defect in this disorder is in the brain's control of muscle and nerve function and not in the actual nerve and muscle fibers.[21] The most common form of cerebral palsy, spastic cerebral palsy, consists of a tightening or stiffening of muscles. Less common forms are dyskinetic cerebral palsy, which consists of uncontrolled movements of arms, legs, and head and ataxic cerebral palsy, which results in coordination and balance issues.[22] Cerebral palsy may be caused by pre- and peri-natal causes, such as intrauterine infections, drug abuse by pregnant women, developmental abnormalities, birth trauma, prematurity, and lack of oxygen. Post-natal causes include severe malnutrition, meningitis, head trauma, and lead poisoning. Ocular defects may include strabismus, nystagmus, and optic atrophy. Eye movements are typically choppy and poorly controlled. Accommodative dysfunction is common.[19,22,23] Many children will have a refractive error with a greater proportion demonstrating a hyperopic error.

COLOBOMA

Colobomas are developmental disorders that result in the segmental absence of normal ocular structures (Figure 11-2). A choroidal coloboma results in the absence of normal retinal and choroidal layers in the lower ocular region. Frequently, the optic nerve and macular region is involved. This inferior colobomatous defect translates into a significant upper visual field loss. Children with this type of defect are prone to injury from objects such as tree branches, the corners of cabinets, and shelving that are undetected in their defective upper visual field region. Colobomas may also be found in the iris and the lens. Iris colobomas will result in a misshaped or displaced pupil that is poorly reactive or unreactive to light. Intervention consists of the prescription of protective lenses to prevent ocular injuries. Magnification devices should be introduced in cases where the coloboma involves the macula and/or optic nerve and has resulted in visual acuity loss. The child should be referred to an orientation and mobility professional who will teach the child how to use residual vision for travel. A discussion should also occur with the child's caregivers about repositioning visual targets into the lower field region in order to reduce visual fatigue and enhance visual attention. Reduced aperture contact lenses may be used for correction of a misshaped colobomatous pupil.

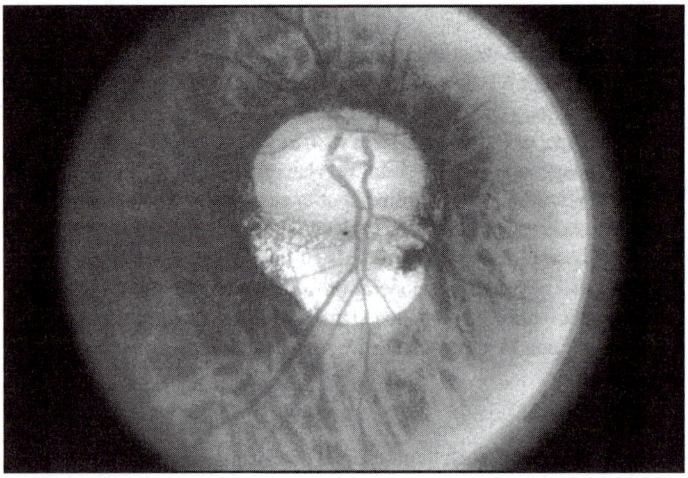

Figure 11-2. Colobomas are developmental disorders that result in the segmental absence of normal ocular structures.

Cone and Cone-Rod Degenerations

Cone and cone-rod dystrophies are typically hereditary disorders. This group of disorders is characterized by the progressive degeneration of the retinal photoreceptors, cones, that are responsible for fine detail central acuity, color vision, and adaptation to light. As a result, children with a progressive disorder of the cone photoreceptors typically have central blind spots, reduced visual acuity, reduced color vision, and significant light sensitivity. Children who have progressive cone-rod dystrophies also experience a degeneration of the rod photoreceptors later in the course of the disorder. They will develop progressive peripheral visual field loss as well as dark adaptation difficulties. This group of disorders may also be associated with a systemic disorder, spinocerebellar ataxia (SCA7), that results in both visual and progressive neurological impairment. Children with cone and cone-rod dystrophies benefit from magnification devices, contrast enhancement, sunlenses, and orientation and mobility services.

Glaucoma

Glaucoma is caused by intraocular pressure that is too high to maintain the normal physiology of the eye. The most common finding in glaucoma is a damaged optic nerve, which results in visual field loss. Visual field loss may initially be isolated to a small area of the visual field but, if uncontrolled, may progress to significant visual field constriction and eventual total blindness. In the late stages of the disease, visual acuity is significantly reduced. Contrast sensitivity is also significantly reduced as the damage to the optic nerve progresses. Congenital glaucoma is associated with many syndromes involving developmental disability. These include rubella, trisomy 13, Lowe syndrome, and Pierre Robin syndrome. The associated significant elevation in intraocular pressure present at such a critical time in the eye's development may result in severe corneal opacification, as well as in enlargement of the cornea and, possibly, of the entire eye. Pharmacological, as well as surgical, interventions are used to reduce the intraocular pressure and control the progression of the disease. In cases of severe corneal damage, corneal transplantation may be an option. Interventions to improve visual functioning typically recommended by vision rehabilitation optometrists include field enhancement devices, contrast enhancement, reading guides, as well as orientation and mobility instruction.

Leber's Congenital Amaurosis

Leber's congenital amaurosis is a hereditary retinal dystrophy associated with severe visual impairment. Keratoconus and cataracts are frequently associated with this condition. Children with

Leber's congenital amaurosis prefer higher levels of illumination, although they have a difficult time adapting to glare. Mobility is frequently affected because significant peripheral visual field loss is a common finding. Children with Leber's congenital amaurosis with associated peripheral field constriction have a very poor awareness of where their eyes are in relation to their visual environment. These children will typically have wandering eye movements that do not fall into any particular pattern, as is the case in congenital pendular or jerk-type nystagmus. They also typically have a very poor sense of directionality. Early intervention involving a comprehensive program of basic visual skills enhancement (see Chapter Twelve) provides the best prognosis for developing higher levels of visual functioning in children with severe visual impairment like Leber's congenital amaurosis.

Children with severe visual impairments are more likely to exhibit a behavior called the oculodigital reflex during which they press on the globe or generalized orbital region. Pressing on the globe in this manner may be visually stimulating, as raising the intraocular pressure will precipitate pressure phosphenes or scintillating lights and multicolored visual phenomena. When this behavior is observed, however, it is important to determine the cause. Other possible etiologies for this behavior should be ruled out. These include pain in the orbital region resulting from injury, infection, elevated intraocular pressure, or stress-related factors. If appropriate, behavior modification programs may be implemented to eliminate the problem. Such eye-poking behavior may result in retinal tears or detachments in children with previous history of detachment, as well as in children with high myopia or other conditions that are highly associated with retinal detachment.

MACULAR DEGENERATION

There are many types of macular degenerations. The most common form of macular degeneration, age-related macular degeneration, typically occurs after age 60. Some less common forms, like Best vitelliform degeneration and Stargardt's maculopathy, are hereditary and occur during the first two decades of life. Others may result from ocular trauma, systemic medications, or infectious agents such as toxoplasmosis. While some macular degenerations such as Best's vitelliform degeneration may result in relatively mild central vision loss, the majority of macular degenerative conditions result in a central blind spot or scotoma and significant central vision loss. In order to compensate for the loss of central vision and the presence of a central blind spot, children with this condition will adopt an eccentric viewing strategy (see section on central field defects). Children with macular degenerations or dystrophies typically have a difficult time adapting to glare and experience difficulty successfully accomplishing fine detail visual tasks such as reading. As the peripheral visual field area is typically not involved in macular degeneration, children with this group of disorders will not experience difficulty in negotiating crowded visual environments. They may, however, experience difficulty negotiating curbs and stairs due to associated contrast sensitivity as well as depth perception issues. An orientation and mobility evaluation would determine if the child demonstrates any visually based orientation and mobility issues. Interventions to enhance visual efficiency should include magnification, glare reduction, exploration of and instruction in appropriate eccentric fixation strategies (see Chapter Twelve), and overall contrast enhancement.

OPTIC ATROPHY/OPTIC NERVE HYPOPLASIA

Optic atrophy may be a result of a hereditary condition, such as autosomal dominant optic atrophy, or may result from other causative factors. These include intrauterine infections, inflammatory conditions, maternal drug or alcohol abuse, hydrocephaly, as well as congenital structural malformations of the brain. Optic atrophy presents with a wide range of visual disorders ranging from minor visual acuity reduction to severe reductions in visual acuity and visual fields. Reductions in contrast sensitivity are often associated with optic atrophy, as well as with color vision defects, typically red-green in nature. Congenital brain malformations, such as septo-optic dysplasia (de Morsier's syndrome) and holoprosencephaly, are often associated with an underdeveloped optic nerve (optic nerve hypoplasia). Children who are diagnosed with septo-optic dysplasia should be monitored for associated endocrine disorders. Optic nerve hypoplasia manifests in a range of visual disorders. The most common visual manifestation of optic nerve hypoplasia is peripheral visual field contraction. In its most severe forms, optic nerve hypoplasia is associated with severe to total loss of visual functioning. Interventions by the vision rehabilitation optometrist may include magnification, visual field enhancement, contrast enhancement, and recommendations for orientation and mobility instruction in the case of significant visual field involvement.

Case Six

A 10-year-old girl presented to the low vision service with a history of optic nerve hypoplasia. She had been monitored for her eye condition since infancy, and her mother had been told that her visual status was stable. Her mother reported that she tended to be clumsy and that she exhibited reduced visual attention while traveling. This resulted in many bumps and bruises incurred during mobility-related activities. Upon questioning, her mother reported that the most typical site of injury was on top of her head or in the forehead region. During the evaluation, visual fields revealed a constriction in the upper visual field area to approximately 5 degrees above fixation. Such altitudinal visual field defects are not uncommon in optic nerve hypoplasia. The cause for the "clumsiness" was actually an upper visual field impairment. A referral was made for orientation and mobility services, and protective eyewear was prescribed. Her mother reported back to us that her daughter had experienced a significant reduction in her mobility-related injuries after she was taught how to effectively and consistently scan her upper visual field region.

PHOTOPHOBIA

Photophobia is characterized by extreme sensitivity to illuminated visual environments. Children with photophobia experience significant stress when they are in brightly illuminated environments. Photophobia may be caused by retinal disorders such as rod monochromatism and cone dystrophies. It may also be caused by conditions such as aniridia and albinism. These hereditary disorders result in an inability of the eyes to adequately screen out excessive light due to inadequate pigmentation or a lack of pupillary light control. Photophobia is one of the most common side effects of systemic medications used to control seizures and depression. These medications may cause pupillary dilation, which reduces the eye's ability to screen out extraneous light. Children with photophobia benefit significantly from light-filtration devices such as light-absorptive lenses and contact lenses. Children who will not tolerate frames may benefit from head-worn visors.

RETINOPATHY OF PREMATURITY

Retinopathy of prematurity has a strong association with premature birth and low birth weight. Although high levels of ambient light and supplemental oxygen therapy have been proposed as causative factors in the emergence of retinopathy of prematurity, more recent studies have disproven that association.[24,25] Associated findings include high myopia, scarring of the retina and vitreous, retinal detachment, and cataracts. Visual status ranges from normal vision to no light perception. Children with the advanced stages of this condition may have residual vision but will manifest reductions in visual acuity as well as in visual field. Interventions include magnification, light filtration to control the scatter of light through a cloudy media, correction of significant myopia with spectacles or contact lenses, and orientation and mobility instruction if there is significant peripheral visual field loss.

RETINITIS PIGMENTOSA (ROD-CONE DEGENERATION)

This hereditary retinal disorder is characterized by the progressive degeneration of the retinal photoreceptors. Initially, the disease affects only the rods, which mediate adaptation to reduced light levels and provide peripheral visual information. At the end stage of this disorder, there is progressive degeneration of the cone photoreceptors as well. Retinitis pigmentosa may present solely as an ocular condition or may be part of a multisensory syndrome such as Usher syndrome, which is associated with hearing impairment. Rod-cone degeneration may also be associated with generalized systemic disorders, such as Bardet-Biedl syndrome, which includes polydactyly (extra digits), learning disability, obesity, and disorders of the kidney and genital system (in males), and a similar syndrome, Laurence-Moon syndrome, which does not include polydactyly or kidney disorders but does include ataxia. Children with retinitis pigmentosa will initially experience a reduction in adaptation to reduced light levels or "night blindness." They will then experience significant midperipheral visual field impairments, which typically present as a "ring scotoma." This ring-shaped blind region will gradually progress to total peripheral visual field loss until they are left with the characteristic "tunnel vision" associated with retinitis pigmentosa. At this stage, progressive degeneration of the central visual region's cone photoreceptors leads to total blindness. Low vision interventions for enhancing the use of residual vision include field-expanding devices (image minifiers), field-enhancing devices (prismatic scanning devices), illumination devices, night vision enhancers, orientation and mobility instruction, and contrast enhancement.

Visual Field Disorders

CENTRAL VISUAL FIELD DEFECTS

Central visual field defects are most typically associated with macular diseases or disorders. Central defects may present as areas of distortion or metamorphopsia. Metamorphopsia causes a bending or warping of visual detail so that it becomes difficult to identify the target. An individual with metamorphopsia who views a grid pattern will notice a bending or bowing of the lines or may notice that a section of the grid may be foggy or missing. Metamorphopsia is commonly present in the early stages of macular degeneration. People with metamorphopsia will complain that words appear to run together while reading. The other type of central visual field defect is characterized by a central scotoma. This is the type of visual field defect found in individuals with toxoplasmosis or with late-stage macular degeneration. The blind spot is typically at fixation, resulting in an obscuration or deterioration of visual detail in the central visual region. The blind spot corresponds to an area of damaged retina in the affected macular region. Magnification can reduce the portion of the visual target that is obscured or distorted, by enlarging the image size, thereby placing a greater portion of the image outside of the damaged region.

Viewing with a retinal point that is outside of the damaged macular region (eccentric fixation) further reduces the impact of the area of visual deterioration by shifting the damaged retinal region out of the line of fixation. Individuals with central scotomas increase their visual efficiency when they eccentrically fixate. Despite societal pressures to "look someone in the eyes" while conversing, the child with macular degeneration should be encouraged to shift fixation to the side of the visual target (eccentric fixation) in order to obtain optimal visual information. Some children may adapt a head turn in order to more easily achieve and sustain a large-angle eccentric fixation position.

PERIPHERAL VISUAL FIELD DEFECTS

Peripheral visual field constriction is most typically associated with retinitis pigmentosa and with end-stage glaucoma. Children with this type of visual field impairment will have a very difficult time with independent mobility. Developmentally delayed individuals with such significant visual field loss will be very fearful of unfamiliar locations. Tactile compensatory behaviors, such as dragging their feet while walking or trailing a wall with their hand, provides essential feedback that reduces the chances of mobility-related mishaps.

Hemianopic defects associated with brain injury or disease can also significantly compromise mobility-related activities. Individuals with such defects will frequently adapt head turns to the direction of the impaired visual field region. During mobility-related activities, children with hemianopic defects tend to gradually veer toward the intact visual environment. They also attempt to obtain tactile feedback from the missing visual field environment. Children with hemianopic visual field defects will consistently miss objects in the affected visual field region unless they learn to scan their visual environment effectively and efficiently. Orientation and mobility evaluation and instruction is the key to safe and independent mobility for children with peripheral visual field loss. The use of a long cane or auditory biofeedback mobility aids provides essential information about the unseen visual region. Optical devices such as minifiers, prisms, and mirrors, when developmentally appropriate, provide the visually impaired child with an image of the missing visual environment.

Case Seven

A 7-year-old girl had a long-standing history of bilateral hemianopic lower field loss. Her mother reported that her daughter was unable to read or write for extended periods of time. This was due to postural discomfort created by the severe downward head tilt that was necessary for her to see objects in the lower visual field region. Her daughter also experienced significant mobility-related issues especially with stairs and curbs. We evaluated base-down prismatic lenses for reading and found that the upward image shift created by the prismatic lenses significantly reduced her downward head tilt. When we coupled the prismatic spectacles with a slant board, she was able to achieve a comfortable head position while reading and writing. A prescription was issued for prismatic spectacles, which were to be used for reading and writing activities at school and at home. Due to her reported mobility issues, we discussed the use of a mobility cane and referred her for an orientation and mobility evaluation.

Summary

Individuals with developmental and physical disabilities frequently have accompanying visual problems. We have discussed some of the common visual deficits that are associated with syndromes or disorders (Table 11-4). These visual problems can reduce responsiveness to therapeutic programs and interfere with overall progress. This results in the loss of valuable time in the rehabilitative process as well as in frustrations for both therapists and children. In order to develop and implement an effective habilitative or rehabilitative program, therapeutic techniques and activities must be individualized for the visual capabilities of the disabled child. It is therefore essential that programming be a collaborative effort between occupational therapists and eye care practitioners. A comprehensive evaluation of ocular health and visual skills is crucial before the implementation of any therapy. Findings from the optometric evaluation may be helpful in explaining observed behaviors, postural deviations, movement-related problems, as well as lapses in attention. Information from the evaluation may be used to establish the size, color, and contrast of visual targets used during therapy as well as to develop visual activities and environmental modifications that would enhance responsiveness to therapy. Collaboration between optometrists and occupational therapists is also crucial in order to maximize information obtained during the optometric evaluation. The occupational therapist can provide valuable information on positioning, observed behaviors, and sensory integrative issues that would enhance responsiveness during the evaluation process. This interdisciplinary rehabilitative model provides the necessary tools for members of both professions to function effectively and efficiently in the care of children with special needs.

Table 11-4

Ocular Manifestations of
Syndromes With Multiple Impairments

Classification	Criteria
Aicardi syndrome	Chorioretinitis, microphthalmia, optic disc anomalies
Apert syndrome	Antimongoloid slant of lids, strabismus, exophthalmos, optic atrophy, cataracts, congenital glaucoma, retinal hypopigmentation
Bardet-Biedl syndrome	Rod cone dystrophy, strabismus, cataract
Cerebral palsy	Optic atrophy, strabismus, refractive error (typically hyperopia), accommodative dysfunction, eye movement abnormalities, nystagmus
CHARGE syndrome	Coloboma, microphthalmia
Cornelia de Lange syndrome	Strabismus, optic atrophy, ptosis, prominent eyebrows
Crouzon syndrome	Optic atrophy, hypertelorism, exotropia, exophthalmos, cataracts, convergence abnormalities
Cytomegalovirus (congenital)	Chorioretinitis, optic atrophy, microphthalmia, cataracts
Dandy-Walker syndrome	Optic atrophy, nystagmus, strabismus, visual field defects, gaze palsies, pupillary abnormalities
Fetal alcohol syndrome	Optic nerve hypoplasia, ptosis, strabismus, refractive error
Fragile X syndrome	Refractive error, strabismus, accommodative abnormalities, convergence abnormalities, amblyopia, ptosis, eye movement abnormalities
Hallermann-Streiff syndrome	Microphthalmia, cataracts, blue sclera, nystagmus
Hydrocephalus	Optic atrophy, strabismus, nystagmus, visual field defects, gaze palsies
Joubert syndrome	Pigmentary retinopathy, optic nerve pallor, nystagmus, eye movement dysfunction
Lowe syndrome	Congenital cataracts, glaucoma
Marfan syndrome	Lens dislocation, glaucoma, retinal detachment, sectoral myopia in pupillary area occupied by lens
Peters plus syndrome	Corneal opacity, cataract, iris adhesions, glaucoma, microphthalmia
Pierre Robin syndrome	Myopia, retinal detachment, microphthalmia, cataract, glaucoma
Reiger's syndrome	Glaucoma, pupillary abnormalities, corneal opacity, microcornea, iris adhesions

(continued)

Table 11-4

Ocular Manifestations of
Syndromes With Multiple Impairments (continued)

Classification	Criteria
Rubella (congenital)	Cataracts, pigmentary retinopathy, microphthalmia, glaucoma, keratitis
Septo-optic dysplasia (de Morsier's syndrome)	Optic nerve hypoplasia, visual field defects, amblyopia
Shaken baby syndrome	Retinal hemorrhages, retinal detachment, optic atrophy, eye movement disorders, pupillary asymmetry, cataracts, dislocated lenses
Spina bifida	Optic atrophy, strabismus, visual field defects, gaze palsies
Stickler syndrome	Myopia, retinal detachment, glaucoma
Syphilis (congenital)	Chorioretinitis, uveitis, interstitial keratitis, corneal scarring, astigmatic refractive error associated with corneal scarring, optic atrophy, nystagmus
Toxoplasmosis (congenital)	Chorioretinitis, microphthalmia, cataracts, uveitis, optic atrophy
Trisomy 18	Short palpebral fissures, coloboma, epicanthal folds, ptosis, cataract, microphthalmia
Trisomy 21 (Down syndrome)	Strabismus, nystagmus, keratoconus, cataract, myopia, Brushfield spots (iris flecks), epicanthal folds, mongoloid slant to lids
Treacher Collins syndrome	Antimongoloid slant to lids, coloboma of lower lid, astigmatic refractive error
Turner syndrome	Cataract, ptosis
Usher syndrome	Retinitis pigmentosa, cataracts

The preceding table describes the ocular manifestations of the syndromes that we have encountered in our Special Populations Clinic (SPARC). For a more detailed discussion of both systemic and ocular manifestations of syndromes resulting in multiple impairments, there are several texts that may be consulted.[26-28]

References

1. Scholl GT. What does it mean to be blind? Definitions, terminology, prevalence. In: Scholl GT, ed. *Foundations of Education for Blind and Visually Handicapped Children and Youth*. New York, NY: American Foundation for the Blind; 1986:23-33.
2. American Printing House for the Blind Inc. *2007 Annual Report*. www.aph.org/about/ar2007.html.
3. Pesch RS, Nagy DK, Caden B. A survey of the visual and developmental abilities of the Down syndrome child. *J Am Optom Assoc*. 1978;49:1031.
4. Maino D. *Diagnosis and Management of Special Populations*. Optometric Extension Program Foundation, 2001.

5. Manley JM, Schuldt WJ. The refractive state of the eye and mental retardation. *American Journal of Optometry and Archives of American Academy of Optometry.* 1970;47:236.

6. Friedman L, Biedner B, David R, et al. Screening for refractive errors, strabismus, and other anomalies from age 6 months to 3 years. *J Ped Ophthalmol Strabismus.* 1977;17:315.

7. Graham PA. Epidemiology of strabismus. *Br J Ophthalmol.* 1974;58:224.

8. Nixon RB, Helveston EM, Miller K, et al. Incidence of strabismus in neonates. *Am J Ophthalmol.* 1985;100:798.

9. Ciner EB, Macks B, Schanel-Klitsch E. A cooperative demonstration project for early intervention vision services. *Occup Ther Pract.* 1991;3(1):42-56.

10. Beller R, Hoyt CS, Marg E, Odom JV. Congenital monocular cataracts: good visual function with neonatal surgery. *Am J Ophthalmol.* 1981;91:559-567.

11. Gelbart SS, Hoyt CS, Jastrebski G, Marg E. Long-term visual results in bilateral congenital cataracts. *Am J Ophthalmol.* 1982;93:615-621.

12. Maurer D, Lewis TL. Visual outcomes after infantile cataract. In: Simons K, ed. *Early Visual Development, Normal and Abnormal.* New York, NY: Oxford University Press; 1993.

13. Duckman R. The incidence of visual anomalies in a population of cerebral palsied children. *J Am Optom Assoc.* 1979;50:1013-1016.

14. Wesson MD, Maino DM. Oculovisual findings in children with Down syndrome, cerebral palsy, and mental retardation without specific etiology. In: Maino DM, ed. *Diagnosis and Management of Special Populations.* St. Louis, MO: Mosby; 1995.

15. Miller F, Bachrach SJ. *Cerebral Palsy. A Complete Guide for Caregiving.* 2nd ed. Baltimore, MD: The John Hopkins University Press; 2006.

16. Scheiman MM. Optometric findings in children with cerebral palsy. *Am J Optom Physiol Opt.* 1984;61:321-333.

17. Committee on Practice and Ambulatory Medicine. Vision screening and eye examination in children. *Pediatrics.* 1986;77:918-919.

18. Punnett HH, Hatley RD. Genetics in pediatric ophthalmology. In: Harley RD, ed. *Pediatric Ophthalmology.* Philadelphia, PA: WB Saunders; 1983.

19. Duckman R. Accommodation in cerebral palsy: function and remediation. *J Am Optom Assoc.* 1984;4:281.

20. Kirschner C. *Data on Blindness and Visual Impairment in the United States.* New York, NY: American Foundation for the Blind; 1985:82.

21. Scheiman M. Assessment and management of the exceptional child. In: Rosenbloom A, Morgan M, eds. *Principles and Practice of Pediatric Optometry.* Philadelphia, PA: JB Lippincott; 1990:388-419.

22. McClelland JF, Parkes J, Hill N, Jackson AJ, Saunders KJ. Accommodative dysfunction in children with cerebral palsy: a populations-based study. *Invest Ophthalmol Vis Sci.* 2006;47:1824-1830.

23. Leat SJ. Reduced accommodation and in children in cerebral palsy. *Ophthalmic Physiol Opt.* 1996;16:385-390.

24. The STOP-ROP Multicenter Study Group. Supplemental therapeutic oxygen for prethreshold retinopathy of prematurity (STOP-ROP): a randomized, controlled trial. I: primary outcomes. *Pediatrics.* 2000;105:295-310.

25. Kennedy KA, Fielder AR, Hardy RJ, Tung B, Gordon DC, Reynolds JD, for the LIGHT-ROP Cooperative Group. Reduced lighting does not improve medical outcomes in very-low-birth-weight infants. *J Pediatrics.* 2001;139:527-531.

26. Taylor D, ed. *Pediatric Ophthalmology.* Boston, MA: Blackwell Scientific Publications; 1990.

27. Nelson LB, ed. *Harley's Pediatric Ophthalmology.* Philadelphia, PA: WB Saunders; 1998.

28. Maino DM, ed. *Diagnosis and Management of Special Populations.* St. Louis, MO: Mosby; 1995.

Chapter Twelve

Management of Vision Problems for Children With Special Needs

Elise B. Ciner, OD, FAAO; Sarah D. Appel, OD, FAAO; and Marcy Graboyes, ACSW, LSW

The development and implementation of an individualized management plan that addresses each child's vision issues is based upon information gathered before, during, and after the actual optometric examination. Prior to the evaluation, information may be gathered from sources including the parent/caregiver, teachers, rehabilitation therapists, as well as eye care specialists. Observations and concerns raised by family and team members; historical information regarding the child's visual, health, and developmental status; and educational and rehabilitation plans and goals are elicited during the case history. This information is combined with visual information that is gathered and analyzed during the optometric examination to develop an appropriate management plan that addresses the child's vision problems within the framework of the medical, functional, and educational needs of the child. The management plan typically includes a series of recommendations that address each of these areas.

Medical Recommendations

This type of recommendation closely mirrors those made during any routine eye exam. It may include treatment for ocular problems such as conjunctivitis or chronic blepharitis (inflammation of the eyelids). Referral to other health care providers, such as retinal or glaucoma specialists, pediatric ophthalmologists, or neurologists is also often necessary. Further evaluations, such as electrodiagnostic testing for a visual evoked potential test (VEP) (also called a visual evoked response [VER]) or electroretinogram (ERG) to aid in determining the etiology, diagnosis, and extent of the visual impairment may also be indicated. It is important for the occupational therapist to understand why a referral is being made and how soon the child needs to be seen. An occupational therapist who accompanies the child and parent(s) to the optometric examination may provide valuable information about positioning that often enhances the child's responsiveness during testing.

Scheiman M
Understanding and Managing Vision Deficits: A Guide for Occupational Therapists, Third Edition (pp 253-276)
© 2011 SLACK Incorporated

Because occupational therapists often see children with special needs on a regular basis, they can play a critical role in facilitating any additional appointments or referrals and ensure that appropriate care is received in a timely manner.

Functional Recommendations

These types of recommendations relate directly to the child's developmental needs, including the implementation of communication devices and visual interactions in an educational or residential environment. A typical eye exam report might state that the child has normal ocular health, good eye alignment, minimal refractive error, and 20/80 visual acuity. Functional recommendations, however, go significantly beyond these statements in meeting the visual needs of the children with developmental disabilities. For example, it is not only important for the therapist to know that a child sees 20/80 but also how efficiently that child is using that level of vision in his or her activities of daily living. While children with 20/20 would not want to read a book with 20/20 print for long periods of time, those with reduced visual acuity often need to use print that is larger than the actual level measured during an exam. It is important for the therapist to also understand what 20/80 means at various distances and under various levels of illumination. Excessive or reduced lighting, for example, can impede functional use of best visual acuity.

Beyond the actual description of a child's functional level of vision, recommendations may be made regarding prognosis for improvement as well as guidelines for how appropriate vision stimulation programs should be developed and implemented. The following is a discussion of functional vision recommendations that might be made depending on the results of the evaluation and the needs of each child.

Optometric Treatment Methods Using Lenses and Optical Devices

An optometrist might prescribe various types of lenses and optical devices for a child with special needs. The decision to prescribe is made by the optometrist with appropriate input from other members of the rehabilitation team that include consideration as to whether the child has the ability to use the devices effectively. The occupational therapist can be very helpful in assessing the behavioral and functional changes demonstrated by the child when these treatments are implemented.

PRESCRIBING GLASSES FOR MANAGEMENT OF REFRACTIVE ERROR

It is well known that refractive error is a common visual problem in children with special needs.[1,2] The presence of a refractive error, however, does not automatically necessitate prescribing glasses. When glasses are prescribed, polycarbonate lenses should always be used in children to avoid injury from the lenses. The polycarbonate lenses also afford ultraviolet protection from the sun. There are several factors that the optometrist takes into account when deciding when to prescribe. These include the factors below.

Age of the Individual

The age of the child is one of the first areas that should be considered. This is because significant refractive error may be normal at certain ages and may disappear on its own with time as the child matures. This is especially true during the first few years of life. An example is astigmatism, which is very common during infancy, but often decreases or disappears by age 3 or 4.[3] In general, the younger the child, the more common it will be to find a significant refractive error and the more likely it will be that the optometrist may want to monitor it for a period of time before correction. There are many instances, however, in which the refractive error will be corrected right away. In general, this would occur in a child who has a significant amount of refractive error, beyond that typically seen for his or her age or in the presence of an eye misalignment that may improve with the application of lenses. In any case, it is important to understand that each refractive error has its own developmental timeline, which will have an impact on the decision to prescribe. The optometrist should be aware of these changes and discuss them with the rehabilitative team.

Magnitude of Refractive Error

The amount of refractive error present is the next consideration when prescribing. Although it is very common for children with a developmental disability to have some refractive error, in some cases the magnitude is low, is considered within a normal range, and has no impact on the child's ability to see or on other aspects of the visual system. An example of this is moderate hyperopia, which is common during the preschool years and is often not necessary to correct unless there is an accompanying binocular vision problem.[4] Glasses might even be contraindicated if the child is tactually defensive or has a limited visual field, which might be further impeded by the presence of a frame. In contrast, when a high amount of refractive error is present (greater than 5 D), glasses and sometimes contact lenses are often indicated regardless of the age, cognitive level, or degree of visual impairment.[4] The correction of significant refractive error may have a profound effect on the attention level of children with developmental disabilities.[2,5] It is important to always consider prescribing even moderate levels of refractive error as it is not always known in advance what type of impact it will have on the child's responsiveness to his or her rehabilitative and/or educational program. The decision to prescribe, however, rests not only with the child's age and magnitude of the refractive error, but with several other factors as well.

Level of Visual Impairment

The decision to prescribe also depends on the type and level of visual impairment of the child. In general, there are three levels of visual impairment that can be considered when prescribing.

No Light Perception. In these cases, the child is not responding to any type of illuminated targets under any conditions. It is unlikely that any level of refractive correction would provide improved ability to see lights. Correction of any magnitude is, therefore, often contraindicated, other than polycarbonate lenses for protection if indicated.

Light Perception Only. If the child is only responding to illuminated targets, correction of moderate or low refractive errors would be unlikely to provide better light perception or to allow patterned vision. Unless the refractive error is exceedingly high, it is often advisable to hold off on prescribing until the child becomes more visually responsive through a program of vision stimulation. Prescribing glasses in these cases may give parents or caretakers a false sense of hope that glasses will cure the disability. An exception to this guideline is a child who either has or is working on independent mobility in which case protective polycarbonate lenses should be prescribed to prevent eye injury.

Pattern Vision Present. When the child shows even a minimum level of responsiveness to pattern vision (ie, 20/1200 with Teller Acuity Cards) and a high amount of uncorrected refractive error is present, a trial period with lenses is often attempted as long as the child is responding to patterned objects. When a child has higher levels of visual acuity (ie, 20/400 or better with Teller Acuity Cards), moderate amounts of refractive error might be corrected in order to improve the visual acuity, provide magnification, reduce the effort to sustain focus at near, and optimize the level of visual functioning. If a child's level of pattern vision is within a normal range for his or her age (ie, 20/60 or better with Teller Acuity or Lea Symbols Cards), consideration can be given to correcting lower amount of refractive error that might result in blurred vision or visual discomfort at near.

Developmental Level

The child's developmental level is an important factor when prescribing refractive lenses. Specific areas that must be considered include cognitive level, communication abilities, and needs including the type of communication device being used or considered, the type of educational and rehabilitation materials that are used, and the working distance at which these are being implemented. An example would be a child with a moderate amount of hyperopia who is functioning at a 6-month developmental level and is only responding to large, illuminated objects. Corrective lenses would not be indicated because this child's visual demands are not at a sufficiently high level to benefit from correction. In contrast, a child who is functioning at a higher level and who is learning to use a communication device that requires visual attention at near might very well benefit from correction of even a moderate amount of hyperopia. Correction would allow the child to see detailed objects at a near distance with decreased accommodative effort, increased comfort, and magnification.

Refractive Error and Other Aspects of Vision

Often the decision to prescribe is based primarily on the impact of correction on visual skills other than visual acuity. These can include the effect of refractive error on binocularity, accommodation, magnification, or visual fields. An example would be a child with a low degree of hyperopia and normal visual acuity for whom corrective lenses would not normally be prescribed. A child with an intermittent esotropia (a tendency for one eye to turn in) might benefit from correction of lower amounts of hyperopia to control the eye turning. In contrast, if a child has an intermittent exotropia (tendency for one eye to turn out), along with a moderate degree of hyperopia, the actual prescription for hyperopia might be decreased in order to provide optimal visual acuity without causing the eye to turn out more as a result of the corrective lenses.

Another example would be a child who is using his or her vision primarily for near work. If this child was found to have a moderate degree of myopia and cortical visual impairment resulting in reduced visual acuity, corrective lenses would be specifically contraindicated. This is because the optical correction would result in a greater accommodative demand at near through the lenses along with a minification of the image. Both of these effects would place more demand on the child's visual system, making it more difficult to sustain focus at near with myopic lenses. The result might be a child who either refuses to wear the glasses or who is less attentive for near tasks.

PRESCRIBING SUNLENSES

It is not uncommon for children with special needs to have enhanced sensitivities to external stimuli. For example, a child may demonstrate photosensitivity or photophobia in brightly lit rooms or outdoors. Photosensitivity may be secondary to medications that result in pupillary dilation or in heightened sensitivity to glare. Photosensitivity is also associated with congenital disorders, such as rod monochromatism, congenital cataracts, albinism, and aniridia. If photosensitivity or photophobia is reported during the history or observed during the examination, the optometrist may prescribe various filters or absorptive lenses (Figure 12-1). Recommendations will include a specific tint and percentage of light transmission. The addition of side or top shields to prescribed sunlenses will filter light that comes into the visual system at an angle and may cause discomfort from glare. A tactually defensive child may not tolerate a frame but may accept a visor that can provide relief from a glare-filled environment.

PRISM LENSES

In addition to lenses for correction of refractive error and photosensitivity, a third type of lens that may be prescribed is one that incorporates prism into the prescription. Prism bends light and moves the image onto a specific part of the retina (see Chapter Seven). An optometrist might prescribe prism for several reasons as described below.

Prism to Improve Binocularity

Prism may be prescribed in order to allow a child with a strabismus to achieve fusion and stereopsis. In general, low amounts of prism can be ground into the actual lenses of the child's

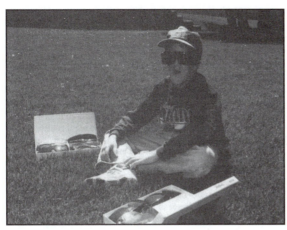

Figure 12-1. Various filters or absorptive lenses used by the optometrist for light sensitivity. (Photograph by Ron Davidoff.)

glasses. If higher amounts of prism are indicated, the use of removable Fresnel or press-on prism, may be recommended (see Chapter Seven). An example would be a child with cerebral palsy who also has an eye that intermittently turns in. While the child might have some control over the eye turning, the reduced muscular control may prevent him or her from achieving binocularity much of the time. The application of a small amount of prism might be enough in this case to allow the child to avoid diplopia and have more comfortable binocular vision on a regular basis without the need for surgical intervention.

Prism to Improve Visual Fields

The second reason prism is prescribed is to allow greater access to all areas of the visual environment for children with peripheral visual field loss. This prism functions as an enhancer of peripheral field awareness. A Fresnel prism is placed on a segment of a spectacle lens that corresponds to the missing visual field area. When the child scans into the region where the prism is placed, the prism shifts visual information from that region onto the child's undamaged visual area so that it becomes visible. Without the prism, the child would have to initiate extreme eye and head movements in order to reposition visual targets on a retinal location that corresponds to an area of residual vision. Visual field disorders that respond well to Fresnel prism intervention include hemianopic and altitudinal visual field defects that arise from brain injury as well as concentric constriction that typically arises from retinal degenerations such as retinitis pigmentosa and optic nerve damage resulting from glaucoma (see Chapter Eleven).

Prism to Improve Head Posture and Balance

Prism can also be useful to improve a head turn or tilt. A child with an extraocular muscle palsy might position his or her head in a manner that moves the image he or she is viewing into the visual field of the affected muscle. This adaptation helps to reduce the incidence of diplopia that that might otherwise occur as a result of ocular misalignment. The strategic placement of a prism could move the image so that the child is able to achieve binocularity in spite of the paretic muscle. This would allow him or her to continue to use the vision from each eye and avoid diplopia.

Yoked prisms (see Chapter Seven) can also be used to improve a head turn or tilt in a child who has a field loss. For example, prism can be used for a child who responds to a missing inferior field by adapting a downward head tilt during activities like eating or typing so that visual scanning can occur more efficiently in the lower visual field region. This could result in an awkward head posture. Placement of a vertical prism in front of each eye would have the effect of raising the visual field so that the child will not have to assume a downward head tilt in order to see objects in the lower visual hemisphere. Full-field vertical prism is not appropriate, however, for mobility-related activities as it shifts the position of potential obstacles such as stairs or curbs and may confuse a child who must maneuver safely around them. (The long cane is the most effective traveling tool for children with significant inferior visual field defects. Use of the cane while in motion enables the child to maintain a normal head posture while detecting obstacles efficiently and effectively.)

Yoked or ambient prisms have also been used to alter visual space for children with autism and thereby affect their behavior.[6] The occupational therapist can provide valuable insights as to whether a child with special needs is showing significant and consistent head turns or tilts or exhibits behaviors that might warrant a trial of yoked or other prisms. Once prescribed, the occupational therapist's observations are critical to monitoring compliance and efficacy of these types of glasses.

LOW VISION DEVICES

Children with visual impairments may benefit from magnification devices for enhancement of vision during near point activities. Conditions such as macular degeneration result in a central blind spot that significantly interferes with the identification of small targets. Magnification increases the image size of small targets sufficiently so that the child with a visual impairment is able to identify them. The magnification requirements depend on the difference between the child's visual acuity and the visual requirements of the activities in which the child is involved.

The strategy frequently used by visually impaired children is to view targets at a very close distance, as close as 1 to 2 inches from their eyes. They do this because getting close to an object magnifies the image of that target on the retina. Long-term viewing of visual targets at such a reduced distance can, however, result in visual fatigue. Hand-held magnifiers enlarge the visual target so that the child can view it at a greater, more comfortable distance. Children respond well to a variety of stand magnifiers that are placed directly on pictures or letters. They especially enjoy dome stand magnifiers, as they can easily incorporate the magnifier into playtime activities as a "crystal ball" that magically makes things easier to see (Figure 12-2). Children can also be introduced at an early age to closed-circuit television (CCTV) magnification systems. Such CCTV systems provide high contrast and variable magnification, as well as an enhanced field of view and comfortable viewing distance (Figure 12-3). Technologies that provide screen magnification options as well as text-to-speech capability are also of significant value when developmentally appropriate. Magnification can also be introduced by enlargement of print and visual targets. It is also essential to discuss nonvisual reading options such as braille or speech output devices when the child's visual status is so compromised that visual reading will interfere with educational progress. In these situations, the child may choose to use vision for short-term reading and nonvisual educational media for extended reading tasks.

Children also enjoy looking through low-powered telescope binoculars that magnify distant objects on a television screen, across the room, or across the street (Figure 12-4). These telescopic devices magnify visual targets without necessitating a reduced viewing distance. Telescopic devices may also be mounted onto spectacle lenses so that the child's hands are free for other activities. Head-worn telescopes significantly reduce fatigue and prolong viewing sessions. Such devices are ideal for long-term stationary visual activities, such as watching a movie or television. The key is to make visual activities fun so that the child is motivated to use the magnifier. For all magnification devices, rehabilitative instruction is critical to ensure proper usage and facilitate adaptation. Recommendations for appropriate lighting, high-contrast lined paper, and writing implements as well as the use of reading stands and other non-optical devices will further facilitate the use of vision with or without recommended devices.

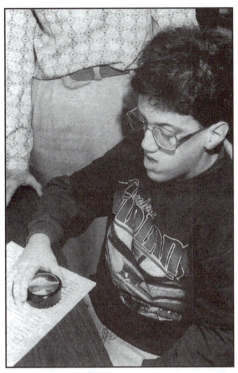

Figure 12-2. A dome stand used to enlarge the visual target so that the child can view at a greater, more comfortable distance.

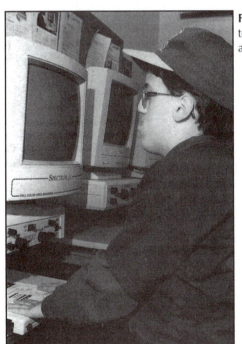

Figure 12-3. Closed-circuit television magnification systems provide variable, high-contrast magnification as well as an enhanced field of view.

Figure 12-4. Low-powered telescope binoculars that magnify distant objects on a television screen, across the room, or across the street.

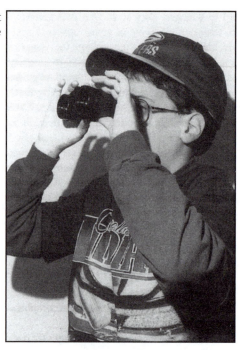

Occupational Therapy Evaluation of Lens and Device Effectiveness

Once lenses or devices are prescribed, the occupational therapist plays an important role in determining their effectiveness. This is most easily accomplished by answering a number of questions and reporting this information back to the optometrist:

1. Are the glasses being worn on a regular basis?
2. Are the glasses sitting comfortably on the child's face?
3. Does the child seem annoyed with the glasses?
4. Are there marks on the child's nose, temples, or behind the ears when the glasses are removed indicating the need for adjustment?
5. Are the glasses cleaned regularly and free of smudges and smears, which can reduce clarity and increase glare?
6. Are the glasses sitting flush against the face or do they slide down the child's nose?
7. Does the child seem to look over the top of the glasses to view?
8. Does the child seem more attentive, smile more, or make better eye contact with the glasses?
9. Does the child appear to see things better?
10. Do the child's eyes appear straighter?
11. Does the child hold his or her head straighter or more upright?
12. Is the child more or less aware of peripheral objects?
13. Are the facial muscles more relaxed with the glasses?
14. Is mobility better with the glasses?
15. Does wearing the glasses make the child seem less irritable?
16. Is there more or less squinting with the glasses?

17. Do the glasses make the child seem more confident of him- or herself?

18. Are there other changes in behavior noted when the child wears his or her glasses?

Binocular Vision Disorders

The high prevalence of binocular vision disorders in children with special needs[1,7] presents a unique challenge and opportunity for occupational therapists to work closely with optometrists during rehabilitation. There are several alternatives to treatment for strabismus and other binocular vision disorders in nonverbal children. Unfortunately, children with limited cognitive and communication skills are often unable to describe or communicate what they are seeing and may be unable to complete formal therapeutic interventions such as a vision therapy program in an optometric office. While this significantly narrows the various approaches, there may still be several alternatives to treatment. These include, but are not limited to, the following:

SURGERY

Surgery is performed by an ophthalmologist and involves a procedure whereby one or more extraocular muscles are shortened or lengthened to prevent the eye from physically turning. Surgery may be successful in providing cosmetically straighter eyes and is often recommended when the eye turn is constant or very large. When a child has an eye turn (esotropia or exotropia) and is nonverbal, the therapist, educators, and family members may not always be able to determine if the child is "on task" during rehabilitative or other activities as each eye is "pointing" in a different direction. Surgically aligning the eyes may allow a better understanding by the child's caregivers as to when the child is attending and encourage increased eye contact with the child. While surgery has benefits for children with special needs and may result in better ocular alignment, there is not necessarily an accompanying improvement in functional binocular vision and stereopsis. This is especially true when there is poor vision in one eye or the eye turn was constant for an extended period of time prior to surgery.

REFRACTIVE CORRECTION

As mentioned earlier, correction of refractive error often results in a change in a child's binocular vision along with a change in visual acuity. Correction of hyperopia when the eye is turned in (eso) results in better alignment of the eyes, while correction of hyperopia when an eye is turned out (exo) could result in an increase in the exodeviation. Similarly, correction of myopia when the eye is turned in (eso) may result in an increase in the deviation, while correction of myopia when the eye is turned out (exo) may result in better alignment of the eyes. The optometrist may consider eye alignment when deciding when and how much to prescribe.

PRISMATIC CORRECTION

Application of prism can result in an improvement in eye alignment, allowing for better binocularity and stereopsis. Prism is also sometimes prescribed in order to allow for a better cosmetic appearance of the eyes even though no improvement in binocularity is expected.

PARTIAL OCCLUSION

Partial occlusion in the form of bitemporal or binasal occlusion is sometimes used to provide the child with feedback about eye alignment. An example is a child with an intermittent exotropia. Application of partial occlusion to the temporal aspect of each lens might increase the child's visual awareness of when the eye actually drifts outward (Figure 12-5).

VISION THERAPY

Vision therapy or orthoptics has been shown to be effective in the treatment of many types of binocular vision, accommodative, and ocular motor disorders. Generally, vision therapy is

Figure 12-5. Bitemporal occlusion used with intermittent exotropia.

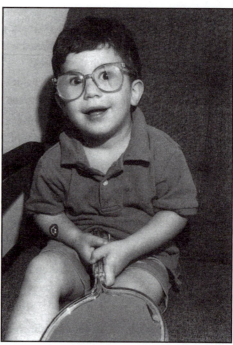

conducted at the optometrist's office using specially developed lenses, prisms, anaglyphic, Polaroid, and computerized equipment. This in-office therapy is often supplemented with short periods of home-based exercises each day that may also be computerized. In general, a child would need to be cognitively at approximately 5 years of age in order to benefit from in-office therapy, although decisions need to be made on an individual basis most of the time. There are many times when in-office therapy is not practical or possible. For example, a child who is developmentally delayed may not be able to tolerate a therapy program for more than a few short minutes at a time throughout the day or may not be able to understand the instructions. In the former case, the occupational therapist, teacher, and other members of the rehabilitation team can be invaluable in providing a more limited type of vision therapy program through more frequent and regular rehabilitation sessions. Providing this type of therapy can also alleviate the burdens on the parent or caregiver who is often already overloaded with day-to-day responsibilities for the child with special needs. The following are examples of the types of therapies that can easily be administered by an occupational therapist in a school or rehabilitation setting.

Vision Therapy Recommendations

Convergence Therapy

Short periods of convergence therapy each day can be helpful for children with either a convergence insufficiency or intermittent exotropia. In either case, the child has difficulty converging his or her eyes to objects up close. As a detailed object is brought close to the eyes, one eye actually drifts outward (temporally), and double vision may be reported. The occupational therapist can generally administer convergence exercises when prescribed by the optometrist in the rehabilitation setting. The following procedure can be used by occupational therapists to assist the optometrist with convergence therapy.

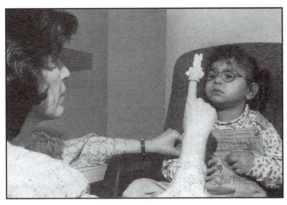

Figure 12-6. Convergence exercise is performed by slowly moving the target in toward the eyes until one eye no longer fixates on the target or one eye appears to drift outward.

CONVERGENCE EXERCISES
Objective

The objective of convergence exercises is to increase and maintain the ability for near point convergence.

Equipment Needed
• Several appropriate targets based upon the results of the vision exam and recommendations of the optometrist. Targets will be a specified size, such as 1-inch stickers or 2-inch finger puppets, and may have specific recommendations for contrast.

Appropriate targets are recommended that are as small and as detailed as possible, yet large enough so the child can see them. Scratch-and-sniff stickers are often ideal because they provide visual as well as olfactory input to the child. Hold the target in front of the child along the midline and approximately 20 inches from the face. Slowly move the target in toward the child's eyes along the midline and watch for equal movements of both eyes toward the nose. The endpoint occurs when one or both eyes are no longer fixating on the target or when one eye appears to drift outward. Record the closest distance at which the child is able to converge. Repeat several times. Change targets as needed or when the child loses interest (Figure 12-6).

Antisuppression Therapy

This therapy can be useful for children who have the ability to develop normal binocular vision but who are unable to do so because they are actively suppressing the information from one eye. Antisuppression therapy is useful in certain cases of amblyopia or intermittent strabismus.

This type of therapy should only be instituted upon the recommendation of the optometrist. The use of antisuppression therapy with children who do not have the potential to develop normal binocular vision could result in the development of untreatable and permanent double vision.

Antisuppression therapy can take many forms. Generally, it requires the child to wear anaglyphic (red and green) glasses with a red filter over one eye and a green filter over the other. When viewing appropriately colored red and green objects, the eye with the red filter will see the objects that are red in color while the eye with the green filter will see the objects that are green in color. If one eye is being suppressed or not used, the objects with the same color will appear black. Two examples of antisuppression activities follow.

TV TRAINER: ANTISUPPRESSION THERAPY
Objective

The objective of the TV trainer is to allow the child to be passively aware of when the eyes are not working together as a team.

Figure 12-7. TV trainer: Antisuppression therapy. An acetate sheet is placed directly over the TV screen.

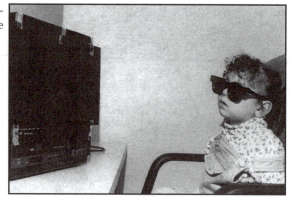

Equipment Needed
- Red and green acetate sheets
- Red and green anaglyphic glasses

This is a passive type of therapy technique whereby the child simply watches television with the red and green filter glasses. Two acetate sheets, one red and one green, are placed side by side, (touching, but not overlapping) and directly over the TV screen. The child simply watches television. If one eye is not being used, half of the screen will darken. If the side of the television with the red filter darkens, then the eye with the red filter is not being used. If the side of the television with the green filter darkens, then the eye with the green filter is not being used (Figure 12-7).

BEAR FAMILIES: ANTISUPPRESSION THERAPY
Objective
The objective of the Bear Families activity is to increase awareness of when the two eyes are working together as a team through a playful sorting activity.

Equipment Needed
- Red, green, and black 1-inch bears or other similar objects
- Red and green anaglyphic glasses

This technique uses small, 1-inch bears or other similar objects that are red, green, and black in color. The child wears the red and green filter glasses. In this variation, if one eye is not being used, the bears of that color will darken, and the child will be unable to distinguish them from the black bears. The goal of this game is to sort the bears by color into piles of red, green, and black. Another variation is to make "bear families" with a specified number of each color bear in each group (Figure 12-8).

Computer-Based Vision Therapy

There are several computer-based vision therapy programs available to treat accommodative, binocular, and visual processing deficiencies as well as amblyopia that are designed for use in the home. These programs can also be used or shared in the rehabilitation or educational setting by the occupational therapist with guidance from the optometrist. As with other types of vision therapy, the optometrist will determine when and if this type of vision therapy program would be of benefit and work with the occupational therapist to determine optimal setting, positioning, and on task time for the child.

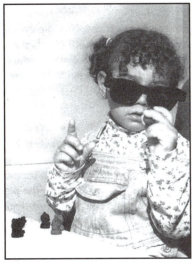

Figure 12-8. Bear families: Antisuppression therapy. The goal of this game is to sort the bears by color into piles of red, green, and black.

Amblyopia

Optometrists often prescribe amblyopia therapy for developmentally delayed children and adults who have a loss of vision in one eye due to refractive error or strabismus. This type of therapy can often be implemented by the occupational therapist under the guidance of the optometrist. Traditional amblyopia therapy requires simply patching the good eye for a specified period of time each day in order to force the weaker, amblyopic eye to be used. Consideration needs to be made by the optometrist in consultation with the educational and rehabilitation team as to whether the possible benefit of improved vision for a poorly seeing eye through several hours of patching outweighs the loss of educational and rehabilitative time for the child when using his or her better seeing eye. When patching is recommended, the following need to be kept in mind:

CHOOSING THE APPROPRIATE PATCH

This is generally done by the optometrist in consultation with the members of the rehabilitation team. The main goal here is to determine the type of occlusion that will be tolerated by the child, be of benefit in the treatment of the amblyopia, and also prevent peaking. While patching is not contraindicated when ocular disease or macular scarring is present, the prognosis for success may be modified in these cases. There are many choices for patches available, among them a pirate patch with strap, decorative bootie patches that slide over glasses, and adhesive patches that can either be placed directly on the eye or on the glasses (Figure 12-9). In some children, the

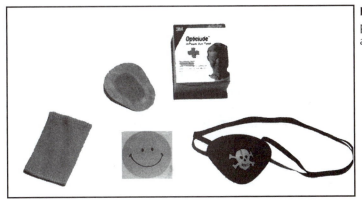

Figure 12-9. Various forms of patches used for occlusion with amblyopia.

patch may also be in the form of a "fogging lens" in front of the better seeing eye. This might be recommended when a nystagmus emerges when the better seeing eye is totally occluded (latent nystagmus). This can be done by either prescribing a very strong lens, which in effect blurs out any useful visual information, or by the application of special fogging stickers, which have the same effect. At times, the use of a contact lens occluder may be used to achieve compliance. This contact lens, which is worn only in the nonamblyopic eye, is either a very high powered lens that blurs the vision in that eye or a lens with the center blackened to prevent any significant light from reaching that eye while it is worn.

MONITORING EFFECTIVENESS OF PATCHING

This can be accomplished jointly by both the occupational therapist and optometrist. The optometrist will periodically measure actual changes in visual acuity and other visual functions during amblyopia therapy using Teller Acuity Cards, Lea Symbols Cards, or standard Snellen Charts. The occupational therapist can provide valuable information of behavioral changes noted during therapy sessions. Signs of effective patching include decreased objections to wearing the patch, increased alertness when the patch is on, increased ability to detect objects in the environment with the patch on, and improved awareness of depth and enhanced eye-hand coordination skills with the patch off.

It is also important for the occupational therapist to assess whether there is compliance with patching. Indications of noncompliance include the following:
* A child who is agitated and upset when the patch is on
* A child who is constantly trying to remove the patch or turning his or her head to one side when wearing the patch, which often indicates that the child might be peeking out the side of the patch

Based upon these observations, the optometrist will make further recommendations for either an increase or decrease in patching time, changes in the type of patch worn, as well as modifications in the actual activities performed during patching or amblyopia therapy.

DROPS AS AN ALTERNATIVE TO PATCHING

Recent research[8,9] has shown that dilating the pupil of the better seeing eye with drops used only on the weekends but lasting throughout the week is an effective alternative to wearing a patch. Atropine drops, which blur the better seeing eye for near tasks by preventing the eye from focusing and therefore forcing use of the amblyopic eye, may be prescribed by the optometrist. This alternative to patching is contraindicated in some children with special needs who may have increased sensitivity to the drops. The occupational therapist can be helpful in observing any difficulties the child has due to the drops. Since one eye is dilated, the child may experience reduced depth perception which can impact mobility and eye-hand coordination tasks. In addition, increase sun sensitivity and photophobia often necessitates the use of sunlenses outdoors.

VISION EXERCISES

Incorporation of specific activities based upon the visual skills of the amblyopic eye and level of cognitive and motor functioning of the child are often recommended. Because an amblyopic eye has both reduced visual acuity and poor visual functioning, amblyopia therapy is designed to work on all aspects of visual functioning. Aside from patching, activities to improve other areas of visual functioning, such as tracking, and figure ground activities are equally beneficial in improving the visual skills of the amblyopic eye. Examples of these activities follow.

Flashlight Tag
Objective. The objective of flashlight tag is to work on the development of accurate pursuit eye movements of the amblyopic eye.

Equipment Needed.

- Two flashlights with a colored filter over one light
- Eye patch over the better seeing eye

The therapist holds one flashlight, and the child holds the other, if possible. Room illumination is initially kept to a minimum but is sufficient enough for the therapist to watch the child's eyes. If a child is unable to hold a flashlight, he or she is encouraged to simply follow the therapist's light with his or her eye. Positive reinforcement in the form of verbal praise or other behavior-motivating techniques is used. The therapist shines the light in various and random patterns on the wall, ceiling, and floor. The child is to keep the beam on the assistant's beam as much as possible. Once this is easily achieved, a second method is to have the child keep the light about 2 feet behind the leading light as he or she "follows the leader."

Lollipop Licks Tag

Objective. The objective of Lollipop Licks is to work on the development of accurate pursuit eye movements of the amblyopic eye.

Equipment Needed.

- One lollipop in a flavor the patient enjoys and of a size he or she is able to see
- Eye patch over the better seeing eye

A lollipop is held approximately 16 inches in front of the child's face. He or she is encouraged to keep his or her eyes on the lollipop at all times. The therapist moves the lollipop back and forth and up and down while the child follows it with his or her eyes. Periodically, the child is allowed to lick the lollipop as positive reinforcement for good visual attention and eye tracking skills.

Figure Ground Play Activity

Objective. The objective of figure ground play activity is to help develop age-appropriate perceptual skills in the amblyopic eye.

Equipment Needed.

- Assorted objects of a size that can be seen by the amblyopic eye
- Eye patch over the better seeing eye

Assorted objects are placed in front of the child. The patch is placed over the better seeing eye. Among the objects laid out can be a favorite picture, toy, or food (such as Cheerios). Depending on the visual acuity level and visual skills, the background upon which the objects are placed can be either high or low contrast. The child is encouraged to find the object of interest. If the high interest object is food, the child can be allowed to eat it for further reinforcement. The objects are "shuffled" when the child is not looking, and the activity is repeated.

Eye Tracking

The optometrist often recommends eye tracking exercises for children with poor skills in this area. These can include pursuit (smooth tracking movements), saccades (moving eyes from place to place), searching, and scanning exercises. The actual size, color, and illumination of the target used will depend on the visual and cognitive skills of the child. Tracking exercises can be done in conjunction with amblyopia therapy (described above) or as a primary vision therapy activity. Examples of these activities follow.

SMOOTH PURSUIT TRACKING

Objective

The objective of smooth pursuit tracking is to encourage the child to maintain fixation on a target into all positions of gaze.

Equipment Needed
- Flicker bulb, large hand puppet, small finger puppet, or colorful sticker, depending upon the visual skills of the child

An appropriate visual target is used based on the recommendations of the optometrist. For children with severe visual deficits, this is often a flicker bulb, glow worm, flashlight, or hand puppet. Horizontal tracking is often initiated first. Place the target at approximately 15 inches from the child's eyes, and move it back and forth slowly. Keep in mind that there may be a time delay in responses. If a flicker bulb or flashlight is used, periodically turn the light off and then on again in order to enhance the child's interest in the task. If the child enjoys music, it may also be helpful to initially use a tape recorder or pleasing sounds coupled with the moving objects. Reinforcement using auditory or tactile feedback is also recommended. This can be done by using objects such as a shining ball, a bell, or a tactually pleasing toy. Eventually, the child should be able to initiate visual tracking without any other sensory reinforcement. The goal is to bring about a consistent and repeatable visual tracking response.

VISUAL SCANNING ACTIVITIES
Objective
The objective of visual scanning is to develop the child's ability to search for important and useful visual information in the environment.

Equipment Needed
- Objects and toys of interest
- A flashlight

Several objects of high interest are placed in front of the child. These can be favorite toys, pleasing food, or other special objects. The child should be asked to look from one object to another in the horizontal plane initially, and then vertically and diagonally. Positive reinforcement and motivating targets are essential for success. Training techniques can also include shining a flashlight on various objects in a visual area close to the child and encouraging him/her to look at each object as it is illuminated. This can initially be done in a dimly lit room in order to eliminate other visual distractions and to emphasize the contrast between the illuminated target and the background.

VISUAL REACH ACTIVITIES
Objective
The objective of visual reach activities is to encourage the child to begin to tactually interact with objects in the environment using appropriate eye-hand coordination skills.

Equipment Needed
- Objects and toys of interest and finger foods

Place a favorite toy, object, or food just beyond the child's reach and encourage him or her to find it, first with the eyes and then with the hands. This should be done in different quadrants of the visual environment. When doing this exercise, it is important to use toys or objects that do not "blend" into the background. For example, placing a red ball on a white rug or a vanilla cookie on a black felt background improves contrast and enables the child to see and grasp the object or food more readily. Initially, these activities may be coupled with sound to motivate visual attention (eg, swatting at a ball that chimes when hit).

PERIPHERAL AWARENESS THERAPY
Objective
This type of therapy is most useful for children who are unaware or neglectful of surroundings. It is designed to increase the ability to detect and then look at objects in the peripheral visual field.

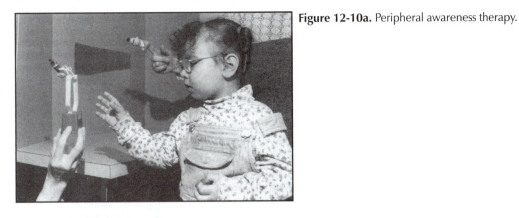

Figure 12-10a. Peripheral awareness therapy.

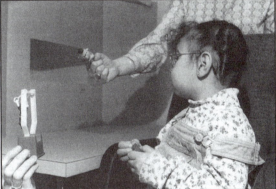

Figure 12-10b. Peripheral awareness therapy.

Equipment Needed

- Toys and objects with bright colors and high contrast that are of high interest to the child. These items should not have any sounds associated with them. The order of presentation of objects should be as follows: flickering lights (ie, flicker bulb); glowing toys (ie, glow worm); large, high-contrast hand puppets; large, low-contrast hand puppets; small, high-contrast finger puppets; and then small, low-contrast finger puppets.

The child's gaze should be directed straight ahead at an appropriate high-interest target, such as the television or a friendly face that is positioned directly in front of him or her at the beginning of this exercise. Other possible targets include a favorite toy, mirror, tape recorder, or even another person, such as the teacher. Toys and objects with bright colors are slowly and quietly brought in from the periphery until the child indicates that he or she can detect it by either initiating a head turn or by looking at it. Positive reinforcement is essential for optimal performance. Begin with lights or toys that are easy to see and gradually change to objects that are smaller and of lower contrast (Figures 12-10a and 12-10b).

Contrast Awareness

A reduction in contrast sensitivity can have a significant impact on independent mobility, as well as on visual tasks relating to activities of daily living. Poor contrast awareness can also reduce visual responsiveness during educational activities. A dual approach should be used to compensate for reduced contrast sensitivity. The strategies are to enhance the contrast of targets in the child's environment, as well as to increase the child's awareness of poorer contrast targets as long as they are within the limits of his or her contrast sensitivity.

Enhancement of Contrast in the Environment

The following environmental modifications will increase contrast:

- High-contrast stripes on stairs, curbs, and other areas of drop-off that impact mobility.
- Bold primary colors or black-on-white figures for all visual targets.
- Use of contrasting backgrounds to offset the visual target (eg, use of a white plate on a black placemat at mealtime).
- Reduce glare as much as possible by using task lighting that is directed toward the visual target and not toward the child's face, covering windows and shading lights.
- Explore the use of colored filters to enhance contrast (eg, evaluate the use of yellow filters for printed materials with reduced contrast).
- Provide bold-lined paper and high-contrast pencils for writing activities.

Enhancing Reduced Contrast Awareness

Objective

The objective of this activity is to increase the child's awareness of reduced contrast visual targets.

Equipment Needed

- High-contrast visual symbols that are meaningful and appropriate for the child's developmental level.
- Reduced-contrast visual symbols identical in size and shape to the high-contrast symbols that are within the contrast threshold of the child.
- High-contrast border of identical size and shape to be placed around the lower contrast targets. This can be obtained by cutting out the symbol from contrasting construction paper. Target sizes should be appropriate for the child's level of visual acuity based upon the results of the optometric evaluation.

High-contrast targets are placed before the child who is asked to point to the named targets or match to a duplicate target. If successful, low-contrast targets are then placed before the child who is asked to point to the named targets or match to a duplicate high-contrast target. If the child is unable to find the targets, the contrasting borders are placed on the lower contrast symbols, and the child is asked to point to the named symbols or make a match to another high-contrast sample. The contrasting borders are then removed, and the child is again asked to point to the named symbols. The child is then asked to participate in a scavenger hunt for specific poor-contrast targets. These can be scattered throughout the visual environment on backgrounds of varying contrast. The child is rewarded for bringing back the targets.

Central/Eccentric Fixation

This type of therapy is useful for children who are not using fixation strategies that are appropriate for their visual status. It is designed to increase the ability to efficiently and accurately identify targets in the visual environment.

Central Fixation Therapy

Objective

This technique is only for children who inappropriately view objects at an eccentric viewing angle. It is not appropriate for children with central macular disorders who need to eccentrically fixate in order to obtain optimal visual information about the environment. It is also not appropriate for children with a diagnosis of strabismus and a small angle of eccentric fixation. This therapy is directed toward children without ocular pathology or central visual field defects who will only respond to targets that are presented eccentrically and who have poor central fixation strategies.

Equipment Needed

- Toys and objects with bright colors and high contrast that are visually stimulating.
- High- and low-contrast pictures that are developmentally age appropriate.
- Frames with lenses.
- Construction paper cut out in the shape of the lenses.
- A 5-mm diameter round aperture cut from the construction paper template at the anatomical pupillary distance of the child. The construction paper template is taped onto the spectacle lenses, and the frames are placed on the child.

Children should be positioned so that visual targets are presented at the postural midline. Avoid any head turns during visual activities that enable them to view the target eccentrically. Present varying targets at midline and ask the child to touch or grab for the targets. Present pictures of varying contrast and size, and ask him or her to identify the pictures. If the child enjoys watching television, have him or her wear the glasses while watching a favorite show.

ECCENTRIC FIXATION THERAPY

Objective

A child with central vision loss will typically benefit from using retinal points eccentric to the damaged macular region while fixating on visual targets. Such eccentric fixation strategies, when combined with magnification of the target, will enhance the visual image. Many children with long-term central vision defects develop eccentric fixation strategies themselves. This type of therapy is directed toward embedding an appropriate eccentric viewing strategy in a child with a recent-onset visual impairment who has not yet adopted an eccentric fixation strategy.

Equipment Needed

- Toys and objects of varying sizes and with bright colors and high contrast are visually stimulating. Some targets should have auditory output capability. Children should be able to focus at the testing distance either through corrective lenses or by accommodation.

The child's fixation should be orientated toward a large, high-contrast target that is presented at postural midline. He or she is told that the puppet is expecting visitors, and he or she should announce the visitors to the puppet. The child is asked to look at the puppet. A different puppet that the child can identify is then brought in from behind the child in an arc until he or she is able to identify it. The child is then asked to look at the visiting puppet and ask if the puppet looks the same. In the presence of a central scotoma, central fixation, especially on a smaller target, should significantly reduce visual detail. The activity is continued in the other three visual quadrants to determine if the child is able to identify the incoming targets more easily or more consistently at these other eccentric viewing positions. Activities are then concentrated in the optimal eccentric viewing angle that provides optimal visual discrimination. Visual targets are placed at the appropriate visual angle, and the child is asked to identify them while looking straight ahead. Always allow the child to fixate centrally on the target in order to demonstrate that vision is reduced when a central fixation strategy is employed.

Educational Recommendations

The optometrist will be able to provide information as to whether the child is considered "legally blind" (ie, the child cannot read any of the letters on the 20/100 line of the acuity chart after correction with the better seeing eye or if residual visual field diameter in the better seeing eye is 20 degrees or less [Federal definitions as of 2/20/2007]).[10] The guideline for visual impairment that is not considered to be legal blindness is a visual acuity of 20/70 to 20/100 in the corrected better seeing eye. For children, visual impairment, including blindness, means an impairment in vision that, even with correction, adversely affects a child's educational performance. The term includes both partial sight and blindness. Each state or school district may have additional guidelines for providing services for children with visual diagnoses.

The optometrist is often also asked provide input to assist in determining educational recommendations (to make appropriate recommendations regarding educational needs and placement based upon the results of the visual evaluation). The occupational therapist can be helpful in this process by documenting behavioral observations and by preparing a list of questions to be brought to the vision evaluation. The following information is a list of possible questions that can be presented to the optometrist. The optometrist can provide answers to these questions that may be useful for educational planning purposes:

- What is the appropriate level of lighting?
- Does the child have increased sensitivity to glare or brightness?
- What level of contrast should materials have?
- What is the appropriate positioning of the child that will maximize visual responsiveness?
- What size materials will the child best respond to?
- Where in the visual field should objects or materials be placed?
- Are there any colors that the child is most responsive to?
- Is there a need for clutter reduction in the work area?
- Does visual information need to be spaced in any particular way?
- What is the child's level of visual processing?
- Is the level of visual skills presenting potential concerns with mobility and orientation?

Case Studies

Case One

A 7-year-old girl presented with a history of encephalocele and developmental delays. She had a wide bridge and an ocular diagnosis of hypertelorism, which is a wider than average distance between the two eyes. Her occupational therapist and teachers noticed that she would turn her head to one side whenever she was required to look at objects up close (Figure 12-11). An optometric evaluation indicated that she had an intermittent alternating exotropia that was only present at distances closer than approximately 15 inches. Her visual acuity was 20/30 with preferential looking, and she demonstrated poor tracking and scanning skills.

Treatment Plan

1. Optometric treatment: A small amount of base-in prism to decrease the demand on convergence.
2. Occupational therapy intervention: Home-based convergence exercises reduce visual clutter; present her with large objects at distances greater than 12 inches; reaching activities to improve scanning and grasping.
3. Educational compensation techniques: Holding material further away than 15 inches.

Outcome of Treatment

1. Improved ability to maintain eye alignment.
2. Decreased head turning at near (Figure 12-12).
3. Increased visual attention for near objects.
4. Follow-up—continuing to do well with prism and able to view without head turn at near.

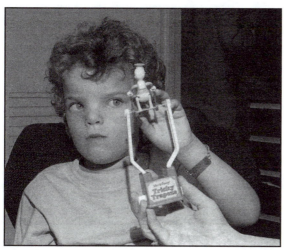

Figure 12-11. The individual turns her head to one side whenever she looks at objects up close.

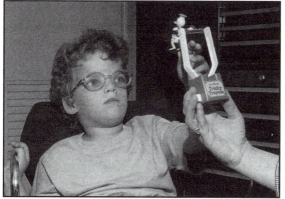

Figure 12-12. Decrease in head turning at near.

Case Two

A 4-year-old girl was born at 28 weeks of gestation with a history of retinopathy, prematurity, and cerebral palsy. She had light perception in her right eye and 20/60 vision in her left eye. She was receiving occupational therapy and vision stimulation. Her parents brought her for an optometric evaluation because they were unsure of what she could see and also wanted to understand how she interpreted what she saw.

TREATMENT PLAN

1. Optometric treatment: Small stand magnifier that she can use to view small pictures in books; in-office optometric visual perceptual therapy.
2. Occupational therapy intervention: Fine motor coordination techniques; visual perceptual therapy (see Chapter Five).
3. Educational compensation techniques: Decrease clutter; larger materials; allow her to walk up to the board at school.

OUTCOME OF TREATMENT

1. Increased ability to find visual objects in books and on paper.
2. Significant increase in visual perceptual skills.
3. Improved prereading skills in school.

Figure 12-13. Glasses with special frames adapted for his ears are necessary to correct astigmatism in a child diagnosed with Treacher Collins syndrome.

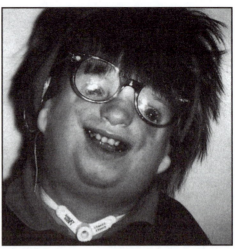

Case Three

A 4-year-old boy was diagnosed with Treacher Collins syndrome. In this rare syndrome, lid and ear deformities, along with hearing impairment, are present. The specific lid malformation is a downward slant of the eyelids. He had been previously diagnosed with myopia in both eyes but never wore corrective lenses due to the difficulty in finding appropriate frames that would fit over his ears. The primary concern of his parents and therapists was that he required a very close working distance for all his activities, including the signing he used to communicate. He also exhibited a significant head tilt. An optometric evaluation indicated that he has a high amount of astigmatism that corresponded to the orientation of his eyelids. His visual acuity was reduced to 20/100, and he had a tendency to move his head, rather than his eyes, in order to view objects. He was also sensitive to sunlight.

TREATMENT PLAN
1. Optometric treatment: Glasses to correct his astigmatism with special frames adapted for his ears (Figure 12-13); sunlenses for outdoors.
2. Occupational therapy intervention: Tracking and scanning exercises to reduce head movement.
3. Educational intervention: Total communication program geared toward vision, speech, and language stimulation.

OUTCOME OF TREATMENT
1. Increased attentiveness.
2. Developing better communication skills.
3. Holding books at a comfortable working distance.
4. Notices his surroundings more.

Summary

Vision plays a key role in the education and rehabilitation of children with special needs. The management of these visual needs can be a rewarding experience when the optometrist and occupational therapist work together as a team. The areas of vision that were discussed along with the techniques given in this chapter are only a few examples of how this cooperative effort can benefit the child with special needs. Most important is that each professional provides the knowledge and expertise of the respective discipline. The optometrist, whose knowledge lies in a complete understanding of the visual system, can guide the occupational therapist in providing the most appropriate services in education and rehabilitation settings along with the type of vision services that are needed for the child.

Resources for Children With Visual Impairment

American Council of the Blind

www.acb.org

Organizational listing of resources for parents and teacher of children who are blind and visually impaired.

American Foundation for the Blind

www.afb.org

Offers resources on issues related to children with visual impairment including publications and local agencies.

Blind Children's Fund

www.blindchildrensfund.org

Mission: "to encourage the development, education and welfare of children with visual and/or multiple impairments" through the provision of information and resources.

National Association for Parents of Children with Visually Impairments

www.spedex.com/napvi

"NAPVI is a national organization that enables parents to find information and resources or their children who are blind and visually impaired including those with additional disabilities."

National Federation of the Blind

www.nfb.org/nfb/Default.asp

National Organization of Parents of Blind Children.

References

1. Ciner EB, Macks B, Schanel-Klitsch E. A cooperative demonstration project for early intervention vision services. *Occup Ther Pract.* 1991;3(1):42-56.
2. Maino D. *Diagnosis and Management of Special Populations.* Optometric Extension Program Foundation, 2001.
3. Gwiazda J, Scheiman M, Mohindra I, Held R. Astigmatism in children: changes in axis and amount from birth to six years. *Invest Ophthalmol Vis Sci.* 1984;25:88-92.
4. Ciner EB. Management of refractive error in infants, toddlers and preschool children. *Problems in Optometry.* 1990;2(3):204-219.
5. Bader D, Woodruff ME. The effectiveness of corrective lenses on various behaviors of mentally retarded persons. *Am J Optom Physiol Opt.* 1980;57:447-459.
6. Kaplan M, Edelson SM, Seip JL. Behavioral changes in autistic individuals as a result of wearing ambient transitional prism lenses. *Child Psychiatry and Human Development.* 1998;29(1):65-76.
7. Miller F, Bachrach SJ. *Cerebral Palsy. A Complete Guide for Caregiving.* 2nd ed. Baltimore, MD: The John Hopkins University Press; 2006.
8. Repka MX, Kraker RT, Beck RW, et al. Treatment of severe amblyopia with weekend atropine: results from 2 randomized clinical trials. *J AAPOS.* 2009;13(3):258-263.
9. Scheiman MM, Hertle RW, Kraker RT, et al. Patching vs. atropine to treat amblyopia in children aged 7 to 12 years: a randomized trial. *Arch Ophthalmol.* 2008;126(12):1634-1642.
10. Disability Evaluation Under Social Security (Blue Book-October 2008). *2.00 Special Senses and Speech–Adult.* www.ssa.gov/disability/professionals/bluebook/2.00-SpecialSensesandSpeech-Adult.htm#2.04%20Loss%20of%20Visual%20Efficiency.

Chapter Thirteen

Low Vision:
Overview and Review of
Low Vision Evaluation and Treatment

Paul B. Freeman, OD, FAAO, FCOVD

Introduction

Definition of Low Vision

Low vision can be defined based on either a limitation of visual acuity, visual field, or visual function. The World Health Organization recommends that low vision be defined based on a Snellen acuity of 20/70 to 20/160 for moderate low vision, 20/200 to 20/400 or visual field of 20 degrees or less for severe low vision, 20/500 to 20/1000 or visual field of 10 degrees or less for profound low vision, and worse visual acuity or less visual field for severe blindness (Table 13-1).[1] Others define low vision functionally as, for example, the inability to read conventional size print[2] or simply "vision that is not adequate for the person's needs."[3] Faye expands the definition to incorporate the concept that "the visual acuity cannot be corrected to normal performance levels with conventional spectacle, intraocular, or contact lens refraction."[4]

Another system of defining low vision was developed for the primary purpose of administering financial aid to those who qualify under Title X of the Social Security Act of 1935.[5] The term *legal blindness* was developed for this purpose and is defined as 20/200 or worse in the best conventionally corrected eye or a visual field diameter of 20 degrees or less in the better eye. The concept of legal blindness came about due to the perceived socioeconomic disadvantage of individuals with this level of vision loss.[5] This definition is still used today to qualify those who are legally blind to receive funding for vocational training, rehabilitation (with some carriers), schooling, and sometimes optical and nonoptical devices. As an aside, in 1934, the American Medical Association Section on Ophthalmology developed a definition that only included total and near-total blindness. While this definition addressed total or near-total blindness, the thought then was that it was harmful for a visually impaired person to use remaining vision for any activity.[5] Therefore, even those with some form of useful or residual vision were encouraged to not use their vision and were considered totally blind. We know today that this concept is incorrect, and, in fact, visually impaired individuals are encouraged to use their vision in order to enhance and stimulate that vision.

Scheiman M
*Understanding and Managing Vision Deficits: A Guide for
Occupational Therapists, Third Edition* (pp 277-300)
© 2011 SLACK Incorporated

Table 13-1

World Health Organization Level of Visual Impairment

Classification	Criteria
Moderate visual impairment	Snellen visual acuity = 20/70 to 20/160
Severe visual impairment	Snellen visual acuity = 20/200 to 20/400 or visual field of 20 degrees or less
Profound visual impairment	Snellen visual acuity = 20/500 to 20/1000 or visual field of 10 degrees or less

---

Unfortunately, none of the current definitions allow any of the ophthalmic professionals who must be integral to the evaluation and management process an easily agreed upon definition. While this does not necessarily impact on the care of the patient with visual impairment, it does impact on the perceived numbers of individuals suffering from low vision. This is important for policy making and funding considerations.

To accurately determine the visual acuity and visual field of patients requires very specific testing by a licensed eye care practitioner. The results of labeling a patient "legally blind" can have a dramatic effect on a person's life. This connotation can lead to psychosocial issues of depression, loss of independence, loss of income, or lowered self-esteem.[6-8] Although there are many goals an individual who is legally blind can achieve with the use of various optical and nonoptical devices, the greatest negative impact generally is the inability to drive a car, thereby curtailing independence and modifying self-esteem. State laws or regulations often dictate this after a person is found to be legally blind.

Prevalence of Visual Impairment

Visual impairments can be due to many causes including the aging process, trauma, heredity, congenital causes, neurological insult, ocular or systemic disease, or nutrition. Because the definition of visual impairment can be so varied, accurate data about the numbers of people who suffer vision loss are challenging to obtain. However, we can still identify the leading causes of visual dysfunction. In the aged population (ie, those age 55 and older), the leading causes of visual impairment are macular degeneration (general decrease in central sight and contrast), diabetic retinopathy (general decrease in central and peripheral sight and contrast, as well as multiple areas of sight loss), inoperable cataracts (general decrease in light, contrast, and resolution and increase in glare), and glaucoma (general decrease in central and peripheral sight and contrast). In fact, it is estimated that one out of every six individuals older than 65 is visually impaired and that one out of every four individuals older than 85 is visually impaired.[9] In the very young population (ie, starting at birth), visual impairment can be caused by any number of eye pathologies or cortical deficits (leading to the frequently used term *cortical visual impairment*).[10] Trauma at any age is also a cause of visual impairment, with the leading dysfunction being a field loss, usually in the form of a hemianopic loss. In fact, there are some statistics to suggest that "as many as one-third of stroke survivors in rehabilitation have either homonymous hemianopia or hemineglect."[11]

The Vision Rehabilitation Team

The optometrist/occupational therapist rehabilitation team is in many respects similar to the physiatrist/occupational therapist team.[12] In both situations, the occupational therapist is given

---

Table 13-2

Optometric Low Vision Evaluation

- Case history
- Distance visual acuities
- Near visual acuities
- Amsler grid testing
- Color vision testing
- Visual/mobility field testing
- Contrast sensitivity testing
- Refraction
- Eye health evaluation
- Magnification evaluation

---

information about the patient's status and then must integrate that information into a rehabilitative hierarchy with the emphasis on overall functional improvement. When working with an optometrist, the information the occupational therapist should expect includes the patient's sight (central and peripheral), visual physiological (accommodation, convergence, divergence, eye movements), and visual perceptual status (see Chapters Three through Five) and those optical and nonoptical devices and basic rehabilitative activities that can be used to help the patient functionally. In addition, the cause of the decrement is usually shared and reviewed with the therapist and other members of the health care team.

The rest of this chapter will present information about the optometric low vision evaluation; the sight, optical, and nonoptical considerations; and some basic low vision rehabilitative activities that are important for occupational therapists to be aware of, understand, and/or implement. Proceeding with rehabilitation of a patient with visual impairment without this critical information or without the proper prescriptive devices necessary to achieve maximum sight is a disservice to the patient with visual impairment.

Optometric Examination

It is imperative for occupational therapists involved in low vision rehabilitation to be familiar with the low vision examination. Table 13-2 is a description of the optometric low vision evaluation. This evaluation can be performed in a variety of settings, including a professional office, rehabilitative facility, or personal care facility.

Case History

The history of a patient with visual impairment, as with any other history, is a snapshot of the patient up to the time of questioning. The general areas that this history should cover are listed in Table 13-3. This information may be obtained from a number of sources including the patient, family, friends, caregivers, therapists, and doctors. Among the most common chief visual complaints of visually impaired patients is the inability to see conventional size print and the inability to drive.

It is always important to determine the date and results of the last eye examination. In many cases, individuals who believe they are visually impaired may simply require an eye examination and conventional eyeglasses. This was demonstrated in the Baltimore Eye Survey, which found that "the acuity of about three-fourths of the visually impaired caucasians and two-thirds of the visually impaired African-Americans could have been corrected to better than 20/40 with only eyeglasses."[13]

<table>
<tr><td colspan="2">

Table 13-3

Case History Components

</td></tr>
</table>

- Chief complaint
- Last eye examination
- Visual/ocular history
- Distance visual abilities (present and past)
- Independent travel
- Near visual abilities (present and past)
- Social/emotional review
- General health review
- Environmental challenges (present and past)
- Education and/or vocation and avocation (present and past)
- Specific visual goals and desires in a prioritized order

Once it is established, however, that the patient has a legitimate decrement in visual acuity that cannot be corrected by conventional eyewear, the remaining questions explore the impact of this visual deficit on the patient's ability to visually interact with the environment and the challenges faced. During the case history, the doctor can obtain information about the patient's understanding of the impact of the visual impairment, cognitive level, motivation, support systems, and previous attempts at vision rehabilitation.

Distance Visual Acuities

Distance visual acuities are performed to establish the patient's baseline ability to see at a specific distance. Specially designed charts (which allow for better quantification of reduced acuity levels) other than the standard Snellen chart can be used, but when doing so, the specific chart used and the actual testing distance should be noted (Figure 13-1). Other factors that should be considered when assessing visual acuity at distance are listed in Table 13-4. Expressive and receptive language skills and cognitive functioning can also affect this measurement.

There are occasions when a person cannot recognize, identify, or match symbols. In these instances, there are other ways the practitioner can establish what a patient can see. In these cases, a more functional approach can be used. For instance, the patient's ability to fixate and follow a light and/or localize a specific sized target (without the actual ability to identify it) at a specific distance can be used to indirectly assess visual acuity.

Visual acuity is generally communicated as a fraction, which can be in either Snellen (feet) or metric notation. The numerator signifies the actual or calculated testing distance and the denominator the actual or calibrated target size. For example, 10/200 should be written if the physical testing distance was 10 feet and the smallest target size correctly identified was a 200-size letter. Included should be any of the modifiers listed in Table 13-4, if there is anything unusual or pertinent about the manner by which the acuity was measured. These findings are typically obtained for each eye independently, if possible, both with and without the patient's current eyeglass prescription.

Near Visual Acuities

The vast majority of activities for which patients require assistance revolve around near work; therefore, a measure of visual acuity should be done at near as well as distance. This information will not only help the occupational therapist when trying to determine an appropriate-sized target with which to work, but it also helps the optometrist to evaluate the consistency between

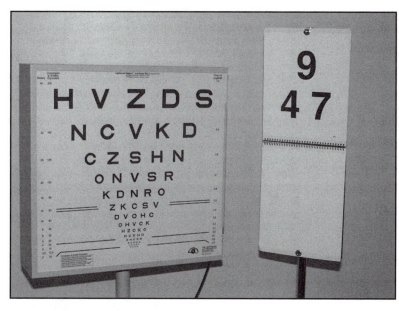

Figure 13-1. Specially designed charts for testing visual acuity in visually impaired patients. (Reprinted with permission from John Graves, University of Houston College of Optometry, Houston, TX.)

Table 13-4

Factors to Be Considered When Assessing Visual Acuity

- Lighting
- Contrast
- Specific chart used
- Numbers of targets at each acuity level
- Spacing of the targets
- Difficulty of the targets being identified (ie, letters, numbers, pictures, etc)
- Single letter versus reading acuity
- Type of letters (ie, block, serif, etc)
- Ease with which the targets are identified
- Expressive as well as receptive language skills
- Cognitive functioning
- Eccentric viewing (body positioning, eye/head posture)

---

distance and near acuity measurements. As with distance visual acuity measurement, all pertinent information about the test (see Table 13-4) should be made available to anyone reviewing the data. Additionally, knowing whether the target size was based on identification (discrimination) acuity or actual reading acuity is important, as there can be a difference. The ability to recognize a letter does not always equal the ability to actually read. Figure 13-2 illustrates some of the commonly used near visual acuity charts.

Amsler Grid Testing

Using an Amsler grid (Figure 13-3) can help to determine whether a patient is experiencing distortion or has (multiple) areas of scotoma. A scotoma is defined as "an isolated area of absent vision or depressed sensitivity in the visual field, surrounded by an area of normal vision or of less depressed sensitivity."[14] The Amsler grid measurement can provide information used to identify the onset of a pathology, monitor a pathology, or modify the ultimate optical device(s) that might be

Figure 13-2. Commonly used near visual acuity charts. (Reprinted with permission from John Graves, University of Houston College of Optometry, Houston, TX.)

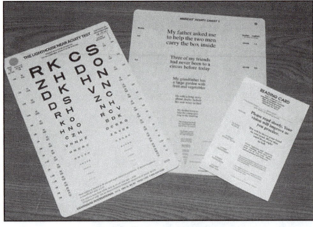

Figure 13-3. Amsler grid. (Reprinted with permission from John Graves, University of Houston College of Optometry, Houston, TX.)

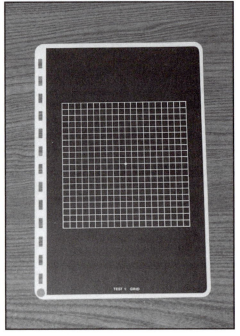

needed by a patient for a specific task. Functionally, the results can also give guidance as to whether a patient eccentrically views or needs to learn to do so. Figure 13-4 illustrates the distortion of the Amsler grid experienced by a patient with macular degeneration.

Color Vision Testing

Several tests are available for color vision testing (Figure 13-5). The results of color vision testing can be used to identify the onset of a pathology, monitor a pathology, or alert a therapist to color deficits that might impact a therapeutic regimen for the patient. Color vision deficits are generally not as detrimental to functioning as other losses such as visual acuity, visual field, or contrast; however, knowing the color vision status of the patient can be important in educational, vocational, and social planning or training.

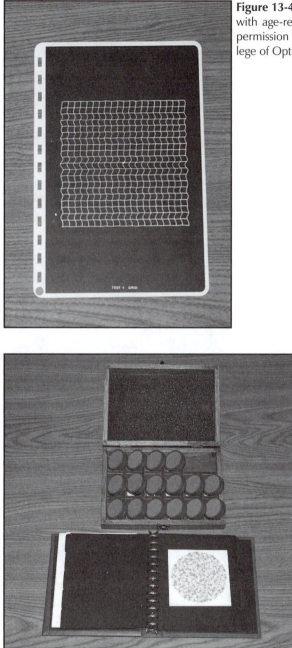

Figure 13-4. Distortion of Amsler grid typical of a patient with age-related macular degeneration. (Reprinted with permission from John Graves, University of Houston College of Optometry, Houston, TX.)

Figure 13-5. Several tests available for color vision testing. (Reprinted with permission from John Graves, University of Houston College of Optometry, Houston, TX.)

Visual/Mobility Field Testing

Visual field testing is designed to evaluate the intact depth and breadth of an individual's peripheral vision. Visual field loss can be either absolute or relative. An absolute visual field loss is one for which no matter how large and bright the target is, it will not be seen within the blind area. A relative visual field loss, on the other hand, is dependent on the size, brightness, and contrast of the target relative to the environment. This translates functionally into variations of visual field consistency based on environmental conditions. For example, a person with a relative peripheral visual field loss might function better under bright illumination than under dim lighting conditions

Figure 13-6a. Illustration of confrontation field testing. (Reprinted with permission from John Graves, University of Houston College of Optometry, Houston, TX.)

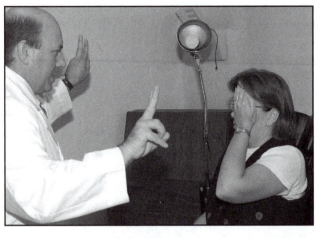

Figure 13-6b. Illustration of confrontation field testing. (Reprinted with permission from John Graves, University of Houston College of Optometry, Houston, TX.)

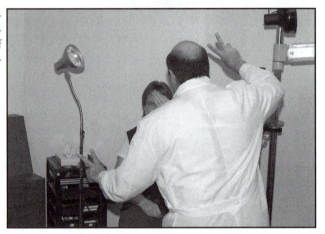

or at night. There are several instruments that can formally quantify the extent of the visual field. However, for initial screening, confrontation field testing (Figures 13-6a and 13-6b) is the method of choice. It is typically carried out by the doctor sitting opposite the patient, each covering the eye on the same side, and having the patient then demonstrate awareness of when the doctor's (or a third person's) hands (or object) are brought in from the periphery. As in other testing, environmental notations should be made (see Table 13-4). This type of testing will uncover gross peripheral visual field deficits and is very important for determining the presence of a hemianopia. Confrontation field testing is not as sensitive for subtle peripheral field loss or central visual field disturbances.

To accurately quantify visual field loss, a formal visual field study must be performed. Typically, a computerized visual field apparatus is used for this purpose. However, for purposes of determining visual disability from a medical-legal standpoint, a manual Goldmann visual field test is required (Figure 13-7).[15]

Contrast Sensitivity Testing

Contrast sensitivity testing determines the patient's ability to distinguish borders (ie, a gray car against a foggy background or coffee in a dark cup). It is a method of assessing the qualitative aspects of visual functioning. This is particularly important when following a patient's progress over multiple visits. Patients sometimes report that their sight has changed, but on a standard eye chart (which has a maximum contrast of black and white) there may be no measured difference.

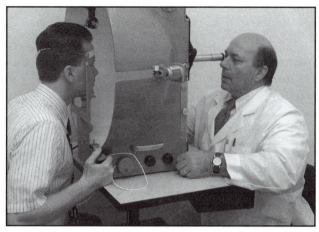

Figure 13-7. Manual visual field apparatus. (Reprinted with permission from John Graves, University of Houston College of Optometry, Houston, TX.)

These are patients who are noticing legitimate functional difficulties, even though their measured visual acuity has not changed. In these cases, contrast sensitivity may demonstrate a qualitative change in vision that confirms the patient's report. This test is also valuable when it is difficult to pinpoint a visual complaint, especially with patients with "good" visual acuities. Proper lighting is integral to this testing.

Refraction

Refraction is the term used to describe the evaluation of the optical system of the eye. We use the term *refractive error* to describe any deviation from emmetropia. When the optometrist performs the refraction, it can be determined whether the individual is emmetropic (absence of refractive error), myopic (nearsighted), hyperopic (farsighted), or astigmatic. The refraction is the examination procedure used to determine if a patient has a refractive error that needs to be corrected, as well as the exact prescription that is appropriate. A phoropter or a trial frame with loose lenses is used to perform the refraction. When a patient is visually impaired, the optometrist must also use information about the refractive error when designing low vision optical devices.

As noted previously, we sometimes encounter patients who appear to be visually impaired or legally blind, but a thorough refraction indicates that the patient simply requires an updated eyeglass prescription to regain normal vision. I cannot emphasize enough the importance of performing a careful refraction before initiating any low vision rehabilitation activity. For example, a patient who needs a bifocal correction and is not wearing it may not be able to see clearly through a "simple" stand magnifier. A misleading conclusion might be that the patient is unable to cognitively handle the task, when in fact it is simply the omission of the appropriate refractive prescription.

Eye Health Evaluation

An eye health evaluation can include but is not limited to the following tests: observation of the external structures of the eye and adnexa, intraocular pressure measurement, evaluation of the anterior structures of the eye, and evaluation of the internal structures of the eye through a dilated pupil (unless contraindicated). The goal of the eye health evaluation is to determine the underlying basis for the visual acuity, contrast sensitivity, and/or visual field loss. There are many good texts available for a detailed description of these procedures.[16,17] An ocular health evaluation is indicated prior to beginning any low vision rehabilitation; if any change in vision or functioning is noticed by the patient, family, or therapist; and periodically as indicated by the patient's primary eye care doctor.

Magnification Evaluation

Determining the magnification necessary for the patient to see desired materials is another prerequisite for beginning a vision rehabilitation program. Magnification of an object can be accomplished using four different methods: relative size magnification, relative distance magnification, angular magnification, or electronic magnification.

Relative Size Magnification

Relative size magnification refers to enlarging the target. This is similar to taking conventional size print and enlarging it to fit on a billboard. When viewing targets at distance, the patient's appropriate refractive correction should always be in place. When viewing objects at closer distances, a compensatory lens for a specific viewing distance must be considered. This concept is reviewed in detail in Chapter Four. Therefore, even when using large print, conventional glasses or bifocals may be needed to see the print clearly even before other forms of optical magnification are considered.

Relative Distance Magnification

Relative distance magnification is accomplished by bringing the object of interest closer. It might be considered similar to "airplane magnification," where at 10,000 feet houses look small, but the closer one gets to the ground, the larger the houses appear. Similarly, a target at 2 inches will give an appearance of being eight times larger than the same target at 16 inches. Remember that when objects are held at a closer working distance, the patient must exert additional muscular effort (if possible) to accommodate (focus). This muscular effort can lead to discomfort and eyestrain after short periods of time. Additionally, many older patients are unable to exert this muscular effort and, along with discomfort, will not see clearly. Thus, an appropriate-powered lens must be used for the target to be seen clearly at that distance. This lens minimizes or eliminates the need for the patient to accommodate (or focus) the eyes.

Angular Magnification

This form of magnification is typical of a stand magnifier or a telescope in which the relationship between lenses in the system creates an enlarged image. Use of a stand magnifier almost always requires close focusing abilities (ie, accommodation, uncorrected refractive error [myopia], or lens power). The amount of focus necessary depends on the optics of the stand magnifier. Likewise, telescopic lenses must be focused properly. To see clearly through a telescope, the refractive error must be corrected or compensated for in some manner. This can be done by using glasses or by adjusting the telescope for the refractive error. It should be noted that focusing the telescope to an uncorrected eye may modify the power of the telescope, even though the image will be clear.

Electronic Magnification

This form of magnification uses electronic equipment and is basically a combination of relative size and relative distance magnification considerations. Once again, the application of lenses for the near focusing demand must be considered. Otherwise, the target may be made big enough to see but will be out of focus. Big and blurry is not as easy to see as big and clear. In some instances, a clearer image can be made smaller, thereby allowing more information to be displayed on the screen.

Magnification Optics

The unit of measurement to determine the power of a lens is a diopter (D). The dioptric power of a lens specifies the bending power of a lens and where it will focus light. Plus lenses converge light, bending parallel light rays so they eventually come together to a focus. For example, a +1 D lens focuses parallel light rays at 1 meter or approximately 40 inches from the lens, a

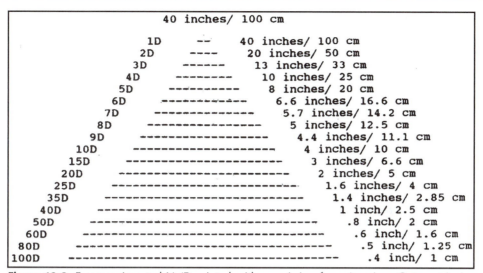

Figure 13-8. Freeman Inverted V. (Reprinted with permission from American Optometric Association. *Self-Study Course for Paraoptometric Certification*. 2nd ed. Boston, MA: Butterworth-Heinemann; 2000:283.)

+2 D lens focuses parallel light at 0.5 meters or approximately 20 inches from the lens, a +3 D lens focuses parallel light at 0.33 meters or approximately 13 inches. This is important information to know when working with magnification, as it will determine the position of the target being viewed in relation to the magnifier and the patient.

By using the Freeman Inverted V (Figure 13-8), one can determine the approximate working distance or power of a particular near lens. To do that, "either divide the focal length or the power of the lens into the apex of the inverted V to arrive at the complementary information. The other option is to simply look opposite to the number you have been given, that is, 20 D = 2 inches/5 cm."[18]

This is mostly helpful when using microscope glasses (head/lens to reading material), hand magnifiers (lens to reading material), and electro-optical systems (head/lens to monitor). It is also important but more optically complicated (and beyond the scope of this chapter) for stand magnifiers.

Determining Magnification

When an individual cannot see to perform a task, magnification may be required. Simply stated, magnification is determined by dividing the patient's present acuity by the desired acuity. For example, an individual has 20/200 distance visual acuity and sees the 20/200 near target at 16 inches (with appropriate glasses). We would like that individual to see 20/50 size print at near. That requires magnification of 4X and can be done in a number of ways:

1. Using "billboard" magnification (relative size magnification), the target can be made four times bigger.

2. If the 20/200 target is at 16 inches initially, it can be brought four times closer ("airplane" or relative distance magnification) to approximately 4 inches, which would require a lens of approximately +10.00 D.

3. A combination of relative size and relative distance magnification could be provided with electronic equipment like a closed-circuit television (CCTV). For example, the target can be made physically larger on the CCTV monitor, and the patient can sit closer (or farther) than 16 inches with the appropriate glasses.

If this individual needed to see the 20/50-sized target at a 20-foot measured distance, a 4X telescope or electronic equipment that could magnify four times at distance could be used. The limiting physical and optical factors of these as well as near devices are weight, appearance, field of view, and lighting constraints that these systems impose.

A summary of the general categories may help the reader to understand when and which magnification systems are appropriate. These are generalities and should be reviewed with the optometrist who has prescribed the devices in relation to what the occupational therapist has identified are the visual requirements necessary for the task.

Review of Low Vision Devices

Magnifying Spectacles

These are magnification systems in the form of glasses and can be either in a full diameter lens, half lens, or bifocal (Figure 13-9). The power of the lens compensates for the distance the material to be viewed is held from the face.

The stronger the lens being used, the shorter the focal distance, and therefore the closer the patient must hold the material being viewed. Sometimes, these systems can be binocular, other times monocular. Although these lenses are usually cosmetically acceptable, give practically the largest field of view of any device (in the full diameter form), allow for mobility (in the half eye and bifocal form), allow for hands-free performance, and are very portable, they do have some drawbacks. The short working distance is sometimes difficult for a patient to adjust to, especially for writing. Even when they can be worn full-time (as with half eyes or bifocals), the blur they create inferiorly when the patient is walking is sometimes unsettling.

Telemicroscopes

These are magnification systems that are a modification of a telescopic lens (Figure 13-10). They can be monocular or binocular, spectacle or head mounted, clip-on or hand-held. Their advantage is that materials can be held further from the face than with an equivalent-powered magnifying spectacle. While these can be used for reading, writing, knitting, typing, sewing, etc, the field of view is relatively small, especially compared to magnifying spectacles of comparable power. Cosmetically, these devices generally are obvious, as they are miniature telescopic systems designed for near.

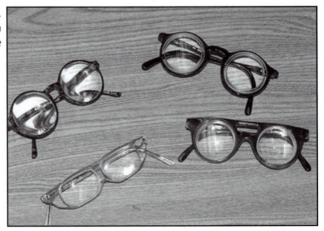

Figure 13-9. Magnifying spectacles. (Reprinted with permission from John Graves, University of Houston College of Optometry, Houston, TX.)

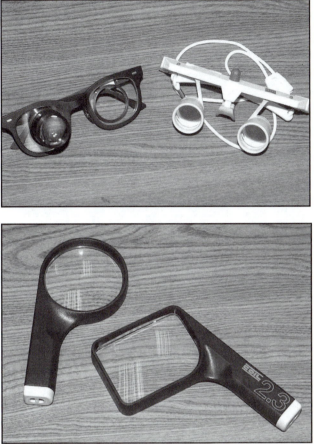

Figure 13-10. Telemicroscopes. (Reprinted with permission from John Graves, University of Houston College of Optometry, Houston, TX.)

Figure 13-11. Hand magnifiers. (Reprinted with permission from John Graves, University of Houston College of Optometry, Houston, TX.)

Hand Magnifiers

These are hand-held magnification systems that are typically used for short-term identification or spotting activities such as reading price tags, menus, etc (Figure 13-11). They are generally used with the distance part of conventional eyeglasses (rather than a bifocal) and can be held at any distance from the spectacle lens, provided the separation between the hand magnifier and the reading material is equal to the focal length of the hand magnifier (see Figure 13-8). The power of the lens and the distance it is held from the face determines the usable field of view of the hand magnifier (ie, the closer the lens-target combination is to the eye, the larger the field of view through the lens). These are very portable and easily fit into a pocket or purse. The downside is that the patient must learn to use the distance part of the eyeglasses with the magnifier to achieve maximum magnification (a challenge for individuals who are accustomed to looking through their bifocals) and must be able to hold the lens steady (tremors can often decrease clarity).

Stand Magnifiers

Stand magnifiers are also used for short-term spotting and reading but most typically require the use of a bifocal, a reading glass, or the patient's own accommodative ability (Figure 13-12). The distance the stand magnifier is held from the eye is dependent upon where the image is projected by the stand magnifier (different for every stand magnifier). Like hand magnifiers, the closer the lens is to the eye, the larger the field of view seen through the lens. However, because of the optical characteristics of the stand design, the image will be clearest at only one specific distance

Figure 13-12. Stand magnifiers. (Reprinted with permission from John Graves, University of Houston College of Optometry, Houston, TX.)

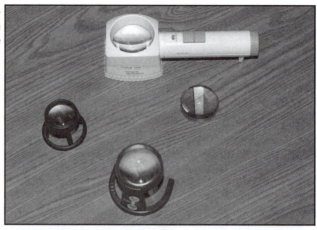

Figure 13-13. Electro-optical magnifiers. (Reprinted with permission from John Graves, University of Houston College of Optometry, Houston, TX.)

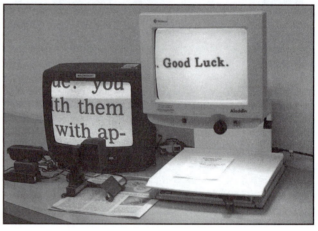

(dependent on the combined power of the stand magnifier and the patient's bifocal). Therefore, it is important to learn from the prescribing doctor what that distance is for a given magnifier/patient lens combination. Although these are very portable, they are a little more bulky than hand magnifiers because of the lens housing; however, both these and hand magnifiers can have their own illumination sources, a benefit when lighting cannot be controlled. Their primary advantage is ease of use, as the stand maintains the proper focal distance with minimal effort.

Electro-Optical Magnifiers

Electro-optical magnifiers come in various forms. A CCTV consists of a display screen, a camera used to magnify, and a platform on which to place materials that can be either stationary or movable (Figure 13-13). Some systems are head-mounted with the display screen in the glasses much the same as a pair of virtual reality glasses, with the camera being hand-held like a computer mouse and moved across a page or on a platform that can be moved across a page. There are also some that can focus for distance as well as near and can change focus between distances automatically. Electro-optical systems have a larger field of view than most optical devices and the capability of changing magnification, contrast, and color. Some now have batteries so that the system is no longer tethered to a wall outlet. The patient's working distance can be modified by altering the magnification and contrast on the display screen. As with all low vision devices, CCTVs require the appropriate refractive and/or near correction for maximum benefit.

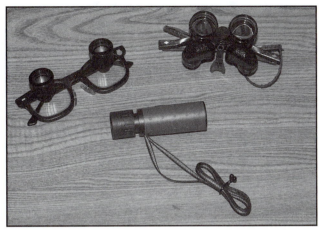

Figure 13-14. Telescopes. (Reprinted with permission from John Graves, University of Houston College of Optometry, Houston, TX.)

Telescopes

Telescopes, as their name implies, are designed for distance viewing. They can be hand-held, clipped onto glasses, or mounted in glasses (Figure 13-14). The field of view of the telescope is dependent on the type (Keplerian or Galilean) and power of the system, as well as how far the telescope is held from the eye. These devices are typically used for distance activities, such as reading chalkboards, bus signs and street signs, and watching television. In some states, individuals are permitted to drive legally using spectacle-mounted telescopes.

Table 13-5 lists the advantages and disadvantages of the low vision devices mentioned previously.

Visual Field Loss Strategies and Optics

Patients with visual field loss require a method of helping them become aware of the "lost space." The challenge is taking a passive system, making it briefly active, only to make it passive again. Peripheral awareness is generally a passive process in a patient with an intact visual system. With peripheral visual field loss, however, the patient must actively turn the eye or head toward the blind side to appreciate what is ordinarily seen without any effort. Once the information is obtained, the eyes are moved back toward straight-ahead gaze, remembering what was seen as either figure or ground. If it is ground, the patient responds to it passively. If it is figure, the patient turns toward it, making it central to the patient's visual processing. The analogy might be to driving and looking in the rear view mirror every so often.

This can be done nonoptically by scanning into the nonseeing area periodically, using visual memory, and making appropriate adjustments to that segment of the environment. "Anchoring" can also be used to establish the parameters of the environment on the nonsighted side by identifying the limits of how far a patient has to look to appreciate the pertinent environment. As an example, a marker, such as a red "spine" for report covers, is a portable anchor that can be placed on a table to define the workspace on the nonseeing side.

To accomplish this field awareness optically, several optical devices can be used. The optics for these devices are challenging to design. The design depends on the amount, type, and location of the visual field loss.[19,20] Placement of the optical device is dependent on the location and extent of the field loss and may need to be modified as the patient gains experience using the device. This is especially true of prism lenses. A summary may help to understand when and which "field awareness" systems are appropriate. These are generalities and should be reviewed with the optometrist who has prescribed them in relation to what the occupational therapist knows are the visual requirements necessary for the task.

Table 13-5

Advantages and Disadvantages of Low Vision Devices

Device	Advantages	Disadvantages
Magnifying spectacles	• Cosmetically acceptable • Largest field of view of any optical device • Allows for mobility (in the half eye and bifocal form) • Allows for hands-free performance • Very portable	• Short working distance • Difficult to use for writing • Creates blur inferiorly when walking
Telemicroscopes	• Longer working distance than magnifying spectacle • Can be used for reading, writing, knitting, typing, sewing, etc	• Small field of view • Cosmetically obvious
Hand magnifiers	• Lightweight and portable • Cosmetically and socially acceptable • Relatively inexpensive • Large variety of designs available	• Patient must learn to use the distance part of the eyeglasses with the magnifier to achieve maximum magnification • Patient must be able to hold the lens steady (tremors can often decrease clarity) • Focal distance must be held constant • Field of view is limited depending on the magnification • One or both hands must be used
Stand magnifiers	• Lightweight and portable • Cosmetically and socially acceptable • Relatively inexpensive • Large variety of designs available • Have their own illumination sources • Easy to use because the stand maintains the proper focal distance with minimal effort	• More bulky than hand magnifiers • Field of view is limited depending on the magnification • One or both hands must be used

(continued)

Table 13-5

Advantages and Disadvantages of Low Vision Devices (continued)

Device	Advantages	Disadvantages
Electro-optical magnifiers	• Allow high magnification • Brightness and contrast can be controlled • Postural fatigue is reduced • Can be used for reading and writing • Can be portable • Working distance can usually be increased	• Expensive • Many systems are not portable • Training is generally required
Telescopes	• Beneficial for distance viewing	• Require specialized instruction for proper use • Hand-held telescopes cannot be used for activities that require two hands • The higher the power, the smaller the field of view • Hand-held devices require good eye-hand coordination

---

Minus Lenses

These are single lenses that are typically hand-held, minifying the image so that more informa-tion fits into the restricted area, thereby expanding the visual field picture. They can be carried or worn on a cord around the neck. The power of the lens and where it is held as well as the accom-modative system or lens worn by the patient determines the maximum usable field of view.

Reverse Telescopes

These are telescopic lenses that are turned around and used closer to the eye than the minus lens system. They can be clipped on or mounted in glasses, as well as hand-held. The concept is much the same as when viewing through a security peephole in a door (ie, the environment is minified so that more information fits into the restricted field of view, expanding the visual field picture). Their use, advantages, and limitations are similar to minus lenses. The challenge to using these optical devices is to perceptually reconcile object relationships in the minified image to the real-world image.

Prisms

Prisms are used to shift targets within the nonseeing area toward the seeing area so that less of an eye movement into the nonseeing field is needed to appreciate the target(s). Their power and position are typically determined by the amount of field loss and the fitting philosophy of the optometrist. Prisms can either be ground into a lens or placed on the lens. The challenge to using these optical devices is to perceptually reconcile object relationships in the shifted image to the real-world image. Critical to success is scanning into and out of the prism as well as adjusting to the rapid jump of the image into and out of the patient's visual world.

Mirrors

Mirrors reflect images of targets from the nonseeing area to the usable visual field. Mirrors are used for visual field loss much like a side-view mirror on a car, except that the patient glances opposite to the field loss to appreciate what is in that field. Mirrors can either be clipped onto glasses or held. The biggest challenge in using mirrors is adjusting to where the object/target is in the environment due to left-right reversal.

Basic Low Vision Therapy

The Role of the Occupational Therapist in the Management of the Patient With Low Vision

The role of the optometrist is to:

- Complete a thorough evaluation of the patient with low vision
- Determine the appropriate optical and nonoptical devices necessary to enhance sight for specific activities
- Review the use of these devices so that the patient recognizes how the devices are to be used, along with their limitations

Once the optometrist has prescribed the optical aids, the use of these devices for activities of daily living needs to be addressed. This is the critical role that the occupational therapist can play. The occupational therapist's assessment of the patient should include what activities were inaccessible due to a decrease in sight. If the optometrist has evaluated and prescribed appropriate devices and the occupational therapist has assessed the activities of daily living that are affected by the sight loss, there should be a seamless transition. The occupational therapist can now teach the patient to use the device(s) for specific activities and not just for the sake of learning to use the device.

Rehabilitative Training With Low Vision Devices

The key to training a patient with visual impairment, with or without low vision devices, is to understand not only the patient's visual limitations, but also the advantages and limitations of the device(s) (see Table 13-5) and how the two are synergistically interwoven.

The following examples will illustrate how an occupational therapist might functionally apply the devices prescribed.

GENERAL ACTIVITIES

Preliminary activities are generally performed before using optical devices. The following are two examples of activities that can prepare a patient for the use of low vision devices.

Eccentric Viewing Without a Device

Remember that normally sighted individuals use their foveas to view and identify objects in the environment. The fovea is that part of the eye capable of the most acute sight. When we look at an object, we must aim the eye so that the image of the object is focused on the fovea. Smooth eye movements (pursuits) and jump eye movements (saccades) are both designed to allow the individual to always use the fovea. In many patients with low vision, the fovea no longer functions normally. In such cases, using an off-foveal point of reference (another point on the retina) sometimes enables patients with central vision loss to better use their remaining sight. To do this automatically, the patient must practice viewing with that off-foveal spot. The following is but one example of techniques used to establish eccentric viewing (modified from *Believing Is Seeing*)[21]:

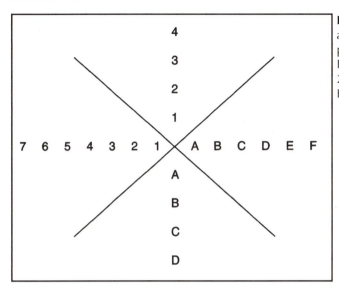

Figure 13-15. The Freeman Functional Near Field Chart. (Reprinted with permission from Freeman PB, Jose RT. *The Art and Practice of Low Vision.* 2nd ed. Boston, MA: Butterworth-Heinemann; 1997.)

1. With the patient seated, place a target larger (target size determined by the doctor) than the central scotoma (as measured by the Amsler grid or formal visual field) 10 feet away.

2. Have the patient look to the right, left, up, and down to determine in which position of gaze the target appears clearest.

3. Once this position is established, have the patient practice placing the scotoma directly on the target, then accurately moving to the eccentric position determined for best seeing. By having control over placement of the scotoma, the patient takes control of his or her reflexive eye movements, something that is critical for consistent eccentric viewing.

4. Once this position is well-established, the patient should walk around in the environment performing this same ocular exercise to establish spatial relationships between off-foveal viewing and coordinated motor movement in space.

5. The above should be performed while the patient reaches for objects in the environment to establish accurate eye-hand coordination with an off-foveal point of reference.

Functional Field of View Through a Low Vision Device

Regardless of the low vision device, whether for distance or near, the usable visual field of that device should be considered. The usable visual field can be considered the size of the physical area that can be seen and used comfortably when viewing through a low vision device. At near, the Freeman Functional Near Field Chart (Figure 13-15) can be used; at distance, the same type of chart can be reproduced, for example, on a chalkboard. The following instructional set is adapted from *The Art and Practice of Low Vision*[22]:

1. Have the patient place the card, whether distance or near, parallel to the patient's face and at the focal length of the low vision device. The print size on the card should be the same size as the patient wants to see and is capable of seeing with the device. All of the conditions for successful viewing (ie, proper refraction, good lighting, etc), along with the low vision device, should be in place.

2. Have the patient view the center dot or where the X would cross if the center dot cannot be seen.

3. Have the patient first tell you how far from the center, both horizontally and vertically, can be seen without moving the eye. Next, with only eye movement, the patient should scan within the field of the low vision device and again tell you the horizontal and vertical extent that can be seen. Outline the extent of what the patient describes, with and without eye movements.

4. Place a word(s), object(s), or task that the patient wants to see in that space. This will help the therapist determine how much of the task at hand can be viewed through the low vision device and what visual physiological and perceptual skills will be needed to maximize what is seen.

Patient With Central Sight Loss

GOALS: READING BOOKS, NEWSPAPERS, MAIL, AND MAGAZINES; SHOPPING; TELEVISION VIEWING

A. For extended reading, the patient might be prescribed a head-mounted microscope or an electro-optical magnification system. After determining the functional visual field and the appropriate distance the materials are to be held from the device, specific tracking exercises can be given to the patient to help maximize the efficient use of that device prior to actually reading. The type of tracking activity will depend upon whether the patient can eccentrically view (use an off-foveal spot) or not.

1. Eccentric viewing instruction and chart (Figure 13-16)
2. Tracking exercise and chart (Figure 13-17)

B. For shopping, either a hand magnifier or stand magnifier is appropriate. These devices are typically used for short-term spotting activities, such as reading labels and price tags.

After determining the functional visual field, specific instruction in the use of the device with conventional eyewear should be reviewed. Typically, for hand magnifiers held at their focal length, the distance prescription (upper part of the glasses for a bifocal wearer) should be used. For stand magnifiers, accommodation or a near lens (the bifocal if the glasses incorporate one) should be used. The patient should then be encouraged to practice the motor movements in coordination with the eye movements to rapidly and accurately locate and identify specific targets through these devices.

C. For watching television, patients have one of three options. The first is to simply move closer to the television, creating a relative distance form of magnification. The second is to use a telescopic lens. Third is to use electro-optical devices in the form of head-borne virtual reality systems. The second and third options require that the patient initially determine the functional visual field of the device. With a telescope, if it is hand-held, repeated eye-hand movements to bring the telescope to the eye smoothly and efficiently should be practiced. This is termed *spotting*. If the telescope is head mounted, raising and lowering the head to view into and out of the telescope should be practiced. With electro-optical systems, most of the activity is in determining the appropriate magnification (which can be controlled electronically by the patient) as well as the contrast and color definition that the systems afford.

Peripheral Vision Loss

GOAL: SAFE MOVEMENT IN THE ENVIRONMENT

A. As was mentioned previously, peripheral vision loss primarily affects the ability to travel safely through the environment. Consequently, both nonoptical and optical considerations must be integrated. Scanning the environment becomes extremely important; the patient should be taught to scan in a systematic and sequential fashion. The smaller the visual field, the more often and the broader the saccadic movement must be to "paint" the landscape.

Individuals with peripheral vision loss can be encouraged to go to safe but busy environments with family and friends and to describe what is around them as they walk. An ideal environment would be an enclosed mall. The patient should describe the environment based on the pieces that are observed while methodically scanning. The person walking with the patient should always be visible to the patient, but should not prompt any observations. It should be evident that, where safety is concerned, the patient should be warned and protected.

Eccentric Viewing I:
12-Point Print with Low Vision Device

You have demonstrated that you are almost ready to begin tracking activities that will help you read print. However, because you cannot use straight-ahead viewing, we have designed materials to help establish the best off-center viewing spot for you.

SELECTING THE BEST ANGLE FOR ECCENTRIC VIEWING
The following exercises will help you select the best angle for eccentric viewing. Three lines of decreasing thickness appear above each letter or word, and three lines of increasing thickness appear below each letter or word. Starting with the single letters, select the line above or below the letter that allows you to see the letter most clearly; that is, you should center your vision on the line that gives the clearest view of the letter in your peripheral visual field. The following few pages of training materials provide lines of the same height to help you learn eccentric viewing.

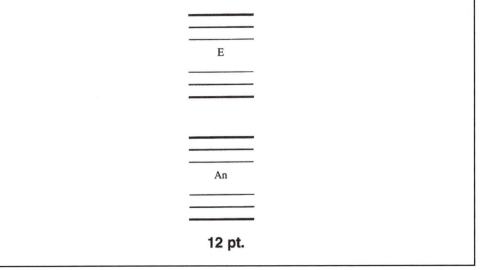

12 pt.

Figure 13-16. Eccentric viewing instruction and chart. (Reprinted with permission from Freeman PB, Jose RT. *The Art and Practice of Low Vision.* 2nd ed. Boston, MA: Butterworth-Heinemann; 1997.)

B. Optical systems can now be added to maximize the information seen in one fixation. For generalized constricted visual fields, viewing through either a reverse telescope or a minus lens and then viewing the natural environment can create some size and spatial relations confusion. More information will now be seen, but will be minified. For selective visual field losses (ie, hemianopic or quadrant losses), prism lenses can be applied to the spectacle lenses, either full diameter or sector placement. The patient is taught to glance into the prism periodically (much like using a rearview mirror when driving) to detect obstacles in the field loss. Perceptual concepts of spatial relations now play a very important role. As before, these patients should be encouraged to describe what is being seen through the optical system and the spatial relationship of those objects to themselves as well as to each other.

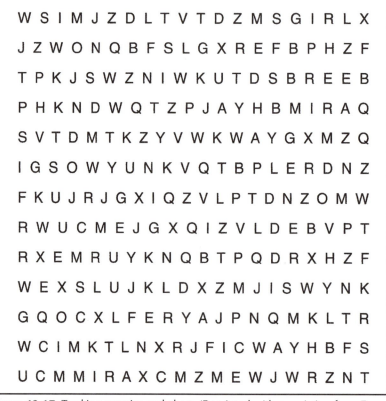

Low Vision
Tracking Exercise—16-Point Print

These tracking sheets are designed to further improve the eye movement skills necessary for reading. The basic sequence begins with single letters followed by two-letter words; three-letter words; four- and five-letter words; six-, seven-, eight-, and nine-letter words; and word columns. When you become proficient with one page, progress to the next page of longer words.

```
W  S  I  M  J  Z  D  L  T  V  T  D  Z  M  S  G  I  R  L  X

J  Z  W  O  N  Q  B  F  S  L  G  X  R  E  F  B  P  H  Z  F

T  P  K  J  S  W  Z  N  I  W  K  U  T  D  S  B  R  E  E  B

P  H  K  N  D  W  Q  T  Z  P  J  A  Y  H  B  M  I  R  A  Q

S  V  T  D  M  T  K  Z  Y  V  W  K  W  A  Y  G  X  M  Z  Q

I  G  S  O  W  Y  U  N  K  V  Q  T  B  P  L  E  R  D  N  Z

F  K  U  J  R  J  G  X  I  Q  Z  V  L  P  T  D  N  Z  O  M  W

R  W  U  C  M  E  J  G  X  Q  I  Z  V  L  D  E  B  V  P  T

R  X  E  M  R  U  Y  K  N  Q  B  T  P  Q  D  R  X  H  Z  F

W  E  X  S  L  U  J  K  L  D  X  Z  M  J  I  S  W  Y  N  K

G  Q  O  C  X  L  F  E  R  Y  A  J  P  N  Q  M  K  L  T  R

W  C  I  M  K  T  L  N  X  R  J  F  I  C  W  A  Y  H  B  F  S

U  C  M  M  I  R  A  X  C  M  Z  M  E  W  J  W  R  Z  N  T
```

Figure 13-17. Tracking exercise and chart. (Reprinted with permission from Freeman PB, Jose RT. *The Art and Practice of Low Vision*. 2nd ed. Boston, MA: Butterworth-Heinemann; 1997.)

Summary

Many references that an occupational therapist can consult for additional information have been listed in this chapter. However, the best source of information is an optometrist who specializes in low vision rehabilitation. The team effort is one that will benefit those patients who most need the integrated services of both the low vision optometrist and the occupational therapist.

Acknowledgments

I would like to thank my wife, Kathleen F. Freeman, OD, for her assistance in the development of this chapter.

References

1. Freeman KF, Cole RG, Faye EE, et al. *Optometric Clinical Practice Guideline: Care of the Patient With Low Vision.* St. Louis, MO: American Optometric Association; 1997:4.
2. Brilliant RL, Graboyes M. Historical overview of low vision: classifications and perceptions. In: Brilliant RL, ed. *Essentials of Low Vision Practice.* Woburn, MA: Butterworth-Heinemann; 1999:6.
3. Nowakowski RW. *Primary Low Vision Care.* Norwalk, CT: Appleton & Lange; 1994:2.
4. Faye EE. Identifying the low vision patient. In: Faye EE, ed. *Clinical Low Vision.* 2nd ed. Boston, MA: Little, Brown and Co; 1984:6.
5. Yeadon A, Grayson D. *Living With Impaired Vision: An Introduction.* New York, NY: American Foundation for the Blind; 1979:9-10.
6. Morse JL. Psychosocial aspects of low vision. In: Jose RT, ed. *Understanding Low Vision.* New York, NY: American Foundation for the Blind; 1983:46-47.
7. Brennan M, Silverstone B. Developmental perspectives on aging and vision loss. In: Silverstone B, Lang MA, Rosenthal BP, Faye EE, eds. *The Lighthouse Handbook on Vision Impairment and Vision Rehabilitation.* New York, NY: Oxford University Press; 2000:409-425.
8. Fischer ML, Cole RG. Functional evaluation of the adult. In: Silverstone B, Lang MA, Rosenthal BP, Faye EE, eds. *The Lighthouse Handbook on Vision Impairment and Vision Rehabilitation.* New York, NY: Oxford University Press; 2000:835.
9. Select Committee on Aging. *Independent Living Services for the Elderly Blind.* Washington, DC: House of Representatives; 1992. Comm. Pub. No. 102-836.
10. Stiles S, Knox R. Medical issues, treatments, and professionals. In: Holbrook MC, ed. *Children With Visual Impairments, A Parents' Guide.* Bethesda, MD: Woodbine House; 1995:25-36.
11. Peli E. Field expansion for homonymous hemianopia by optically induced peripheral exotropia. *Optom Vis Sci.* 2000;77:453-464.
12. Wainapel SF. Low vision in rehabilitation and rehabilitation medicine: a parable of parallels. In: Massof RW, Lidoff L, eds. *Issues in Low Vision Rehabilitation, Service Delivery, Policy and Funding.* New York, NY: American Foundation for the Blind; 2001:56-59.
13. Tielsch JM. Prevalence of visual impairment and blindness in the United States. In: Massof RW, Lidoff L, eds. *Issues in Low Vision Rehabilitation, Service Delivery, Policy and Funding.* New York, NY: American Foundation for the Blind; 2001:16-18.
14. Cline D, Hoffstetter HW, Griffin JR. *Dictionary of Visual Science.* 4th ed. Newton, MA: Butterworth-Heinemann; 1997:617.
15. United States Social Security Administration. *List of Impairments.* Washington, DC: US Department of Health and Human Services; 1992. Code of Federal Regulations, Title 20, Ch. III, Pt. 404, Subpt. P, App.1.
16. Spalton DJ, Hitchings RA, Hunter PA. *Atlas of Clinical Ophthalmology.* London, England: Gower Medical Publishing; 1984.
17. Harley RD. *Pediatric Ophthalmology.* Vols I and II. Philadelphia, PA: WB Saunders Co; 1983.
18. Freeman PB. Low vision examination. In: Jameson M, ed. *Self-Study Course for Optometric Assisting.* 2nd ed. Newton, MA: Butterworth-Heinemann; 1997:283.
19. Nowakowski RW. *Primary Low Vision Care.* Norwalk, CT: Appleton & Lange; 1994:215-229.
20. Cohen JM, Waiss B. Visual field remediation. In: Cole RG, Rosenthal BP, eds. *Remediation and Management of Low Vision.* St. Louis, MO: Mosby-Year Book Inc; 1996:1-26.
21. Freeman PB, Mendelson R. *Believing Is Seeing.* Pittsburgh, PA: Author; 1996:81-82.
22. Freeman PB, Jose RT. *The Art and Practice of Low Vision.* 2nd ed. Newton, MA: Butterworth-Heinemann; 1997:67-68.

Chapter Fourteen

Activities of Daily Living and Individuals With Low Vision

Maureen A. Duffy, MS, CVRT;
Kathleen Mary Huebner, PhD, COMS;
and Diane P. Wormsley, PhD

Overview

The purpose of this chapter is to describe the professional disciplines of teachers of children who are visually impaired (TVIs), orientation and mobility specialists (O&Ms), and vision rehabilitation therapists (VRTs, formerly rehabilitation teachers), specifically in relation to occupational therapists (OTs) and the management of activities of daily living by individuals with visual disabilities. While it is unlikely that an OT will provide services to an individual who is singularly blind or visually impaired (ie, with no additional functional impairments or medical conditions), it is important to note that OTs can occupy a critical role within the interdisciplinary vision-related rehabilitation process. According to Orr and Huebner,[1] OTs can be effective vision-related team members when an additional functional limitation or a physical condition affects the adult or child with low vision; an individual with low vision ages with concomitant sensory and physical age-related functional impairments; or an individual with multiple impairments ages and exhibits functional vision impairments. Kern and Miller[2] concur with this assessment in their exploration of the role of the OT in collaborative service interventions for individuals with low vision.

Definitions of Teachers of Children Who Are Visually Impaired, Orientation and Mobility Specialists, and Vision Rehabilitation Therapists

TVIs acquire the common core of knowledge and skills essential for all beginning special education teachers in addition to the specialized body of knowledge required for teachers of students with visual impairments, as defined by the Council for Exceptional Children.[3] TVIs are prepared to work with blind and visually impaired infants, children, and youth of all ages, including those with multiple disabilities, and the skills they teach encompass those included in the "expanded core

Scheiman M
Understanding and Managing Vision Deficits: A Guide for
Occupational Therapists, Third Edition (pp 301-320)
© 2011 SLACK Incorporated

curriculum," which addresses the unique and special needs of students that result from their visual impairment.[4,5] The curriculum includes the following nine components:

1. Compensatory skills, defined as those that enable the visually impaired student to participate in the regular curriculum and include instruction in such areas as communication skills, braille, use of an abacus, and listening skills

2. Orientation and mobility

3. Social skills, such as nonverbal communication

4. Independent living skills, such as money identification and management

5. Recreation and leisure skills

6. Career education

7. Assistive technology specifically developed for individuals with visual impairments

8. Visual efficiency skills, including the use of low vision devices

9. Self-advocacy skills[6]

TVIs assess, teach, and evaluate students' abilities in all expanded core curriculum areas and are uniquely qualified to teach these specific strategies and techniques. TVIs often operate as itinerant teachers, traveling from school to school to serve children. They often become the child's primary case manager and may solicit the expertise of additional therapists on the transdisciplinary or interdisciplinary assessment team to develop specific goals and objectives that comprise the child's individualized education plan. TVIs may also teach in highly specialized settings where additional therapists may be on staff, and they may function as interdisciplinary team members to meet the needs of children who have visual impairments with additional physical disabilities.

O&Ms are identified as related service personnel in the 2004 Reauthorization of the Individuals With Disabilities Education Act (IDEA). These professionals specialize in teaching travel skills to people who are visually impaired, including the use of sighted guides, canes, and electronic devices. They may also teach skills that will prepare their clients or students to learn to travel with a dog guide (pre-guide dog skills). The goal of O&M instruction is to enable individuals with visual impairments to travel safely, efficiently, confidently, and independently throughout the environment. O&Ms are prepared to work with individuals of all ages, including individuals with multiple disabilities. They work one on one with students in home, school, work, and community settings, and they function as interdisciplinary team members with TVIs and VRTs to provide related services to clients or students. Some O&Ms have additional certification as TVI; others may possess dual O&M/VRT certification.

According to Crews and Luxton,[7]

> *[Vision rehabilitation therapists] constitute a cadre of university-trained professionals who address the broad array of skills needed by individuals who are blind and visually impaired to live independently at home, to obtain employment, and to participate in community life. As a discipline, [vision rehabilitation therapy] combines and applies the best principles of adaptive rehabilitation, adult education, and social work to the following broad areas: home management, personal management, communication and education, activities of daily living, leisure activities, and indoor orientation skills.*

VRTs provide instruction and guidance in adaptive independent living skills, enabling individuals who are blind and visually impaired to confidently carry out their daily activities. They are active members of multidisciplinary and interdisciplinary service teams and provide consultation and referrals through the use of community resources. VRTs provide services in a variety of settings: agencies serving people who are blind and visually impaired, community-based rehabilitation teaching services, centers for people with developmental disabilities, centers for independent living, state vocational rehabilitation services, hospital and clinic rehabilitation teams, residential schools, and local school districts.

Education of Teachers of Children Who Are Visually Impaired, Orientation and Mobility Specialists, and Vision Rehabilitation Therapists

TVIs and O&Ms are prepared in accredited higher education programs and recognized by the Association for Education and Rehabilitation of the Blind and Visually Impaired in the United States, Canada, and New Zealand (O&M only). Most programs are at the graduate level, although there are a limited number of undergraduate programs in both specialties.[8] At present, there are approximately 42 institutions of higher learning offering special education programs for teacher preparation in the area of blindness and low vision and 22 that prepare O&Ms. TVI programs often recommend or require prior degrees or state certification in elementary, secondary, or special education. The majority of O&M programs are at the graduate level and attract students with diverse backgrounds, including the social and physical sciences, art and music therapy, business, and general education. Individuals who possess the necessary prerequisite credentials may choose to earn state certification as a TVI or professional certification as an O&M specialist without earning a complete graduate degree. The certificate or graduate degrees in either specialization may be combined with certification in VRT and/or low vision therapy (LVT). VRTs are also prepared in accredited programs. Presently, 10 colleges and universities in the United States, Canada, Central Europe, and New Zealand offer either a certificate or graduate degree in VRT, which can be combined with certification in LVT and/or O&M.

All university and certificate programs specify core competencies in the following areas, supplemented by specific methodology courses required by each discipline:

- Anatomy of the eye and functional implications of vision loss, including anatomy, diseases, and disorders; medical, surgical, and optical remediations; assessment and intervention of low vision; and instruction in a range of visual skills
- Knowledge of the blindness system
- Blind or visually impaired individuals with additional cognitive, physical, and mental disabilities
- Psychosocial adjustment to vision loss
- Teaching and learning strategies
- Professionalism, practice methods, and case management

Certification Process

While TVIs are certified through their appropriate state Departments of Education, the Academy for Certification of Vision Rehabilitation and Education Professionals (ACVREP) offers national certification in O&M, VRT, and LVT to qualified applicants. Some states also have state certification for O&M through Departments of Education. To receive the ACVREP credential, applicants must meet specific educational and clinical practice requirements and pass a national examination. TVIs, O&Ms, LVTs, and VRTs are governed by and adhere to a code of ethics specific to each discipline that delineates professional philosophy and ethical principles of practice.[9-11]

Vision Rehabilitation Services Network

Edwards, Duffy, and Ray[12] emphasize that individuals with vision impairment often require a broad range of comprehensive, holistic, and interdisciplinary vision-related rehabilitation services that may vary across the individual's life span, within individual rehabilitation programs, and within individual plans of instruction. In addition to TVIs, O&Ms, LVTs, and VRTs, there are a number of additional vision-related rehabilitation services that exist within the education and rehabilitation networks. These professionals and the services that they provide include communication specialists, OTs, physical therapists, speech and language therapists, rehabilitation counselors, job coaches, social workers, case managers, vocational evaluators, and special education teachers with additional knowledge in developmental and learning disabilities, hearing impairments, and physical impairments.

A critical choice that must be made either by or for clients or students who are blind or visually impaired is the selection of an appropriate medium (either braille or print) for reading and writing. For students, it is crucial that this decision be made as early as possible to ensure proficiency in the literacy medium of choice. The Learning Media Assessment, developed by Koenig and Holbrook,[13] is an assessment instrument that is used by TVIs and VRTs to assess and facilitate the choice of preferred literacy medium. It addresses the stability and prognosis of the eye condition, the tactual abilities of the client or student, the potential to become literate, and the ability to maintain literacy. In addition, the Learning Media Assessment considers the general environmental and related learning media to which an individual will habitually be exposed. For example, a child may use calendars, charts, figures, manipulatives, videos, computers and the Internet, or other related classroom materials, while adults may choose to use materials that are relevant to rehabilitation instruction or employment: mail, bills, package instructions, cookbooks, brochures, magazines, computers, and the Internet.

Environmental Assessment and Modification for Individuals With Low Vision

Before introducing adaptive instruction in activities of daily living, it is recommended that the OT and the appropriate vision rehabilitation professionals jointly perform a thorough, systematic assessment of an individual's work, home, leisure, and/or school environments. The purpose of such an assessment is to determine the modifications that may be required in order to meet the daily living, safety, mobility, and accessibility needs of the individual who is visually impaired.

Environmental assessment is the process of systematically analyzing the area and surroundings in which individuals with low vision will be living, walking/traveling, working, or attending school. This range of environments can be quite diverse and may include private homes and apartments/condominiums, classrooms, dormitories, offices and other work settings, long-term care and assisted-living facilities, clinics, and rehabilitation centers. To be effective, environmental assessment should encompass two broad areas: the individual's general environment and surroundings and specific tasks that the individual will be performing within those environments. *Environmental modification* describes the process of using information obtained from the systematic assessment to initiate concrete modifications in the physical environment that enhance the safety, accessibility, and functionality of those environments for individuals of all ages with visual impairments.[14,15]

Prior to commencing the environmental assessment process, it is essential that the appropriate vision professionals obtain the following information regarding the individual's visual status: diagnosis, prognosis, visual acuities, visual field measurements, prescription and low vision device requirements, lighting needs, preferred lighting conditions, and results of color perception and contrast sensitivity testing. These data provide a crucial foundation for the assessment process, which is highly individualized and requires knowledge of "the basics" in three essential areas: lighting, color, and contrast.

Lighting

This is the first and most crucial factor to consider in a systematic analysis of school, home, work, and recreational environments. Usually, it is possible to manage or control the quality and quantity of light in most of these settings. There are five different types of light that must be considered when evaluating the environment, each with its own distinct characteristics:

1. Sunlight/natural light: Contains all colors of light in the visible spectrum (red, orange, yellow, green, blue, and violet) in equal amounts; in other words, the sun is a full-spectrum light.

    Advantages: The best, most natural type of light; good for all outdoor and indoor visual tasks.

    Disadvantages: Brightness is not always constant or reliable; creates outdoor and indoor glare problems and shadows.[16]

2. Incandescent (lightbulb): Emphasizes the red/orange/yellow end of the visible light spectrum; however, full-spectrum incandescents are now available. Incandescent bulbs are available in a variety of wattages and are used primarily in table lamps, floor lamps, and ceiling fixtures.

    Advantages: Light is very concentrated; better for "spot" lighting on near tasks or close work, such as reading, sewing, and crafts; light is very stable and does not "flicker" like fluorescent light.

    Disadvantages: Not recommended for general room lighting; creates shadows and "pinpoint" glare spots; as wattage increases, heat also increases; therefore, incandescent light is not recommended for prolonged close work.[16]

3. Fluorescent: Emphasizes the green/blue/violet end of the visible light spectrum; however, full spectrum or "warm" fluorescents are now available. Fluorescent tubes come in several wattages and are used primarily in ceiling fixtures. Compact fluorescent bulbs fit into regular lamp sockets and provide illumination that is comparable to incandescent light (Figure 14-1).

    Advantages: Better for general room lighting; illuminates a wider area than incandescent light and does not create shadows; cooler than incandescent; uses less energy and is less expensive to operate.[16]

    Disadvantages: Light is not stable; it can flicker and produce a "stroboscopic" effect; cannot be dimmed as easily as incandescent light; compact fluorescent bulbs require approximately 30 seconds to 1 minute to reach full illumination.

4. Combination (incandescent and fluorescent): Incandescent light (red/orange/yellow) "fills in" gaps in the fluorescent (green/blue/violet) spectrum; this combination serves to create a fuller spectrum light. Lamps with combined fluorescent and incandescent bulbs (Figures 14-2 and 14-3) are available from lighting supply stores and specialized resources.

    Advantages: The most natural and comfortable type of artificial light; fluorescent light can be used for general room illumination, with supplementary incandescent light used for reading, sewing, or other near tasks.

    Disadvantages: May require the purchase of additional lamps and lighting fixtures or rearrangement of furniture; specialized lighting fixtures can be expensive to purchase and operate.

5. Halogen: More concentrated than regular incandescent light bulbs and are used in lamps, track lights, and recessed ceiling fixtures.

    Advantages: Brighter than incandescent light; gives more illumination and uses lower wattage; more energy efficient than regular incandescent light bulbs.

    Disadvantages: Light is hotter, more focused, and requires a shield; not recommended for prolonged close work; bulbs need to be replaced frequently and are more expensive than comparable incandescent lights.[16]

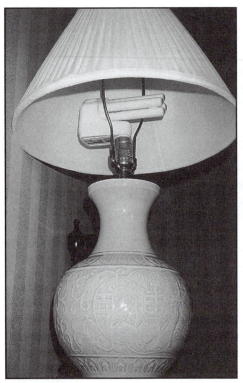

Figure 14-1. A compact fluorescent bulb used in a table lamp. (Reprinted with permission from Maureen A. Duffy, MS, CRVT.)

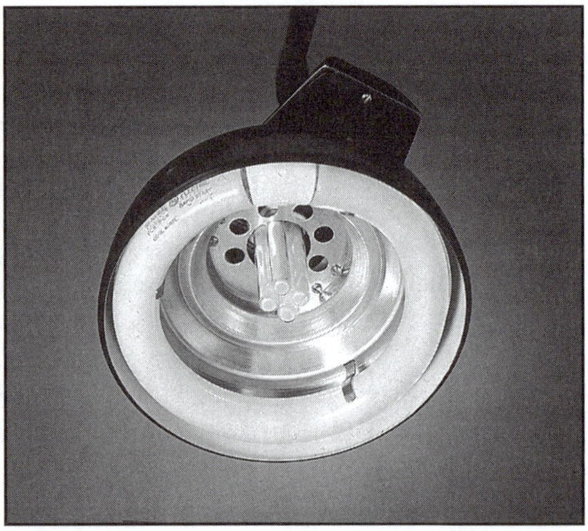

Figure 14-2. Lamp with combined incandescent and fluorescent bulbs. (Used with permission of Dazor Manufacturing Corp.)

Figure 14-3. Lamp with controls for separate and combined incandescent and fluorescent illumination. (Used with permission of Dazor Manufacturing Corp.)

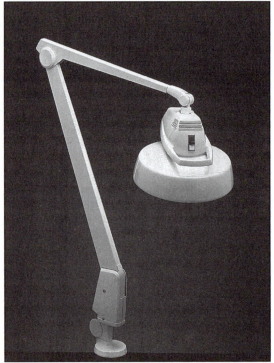

Note: When evaluating the various sources of light within the environment, it is also important to check for accompanying glare. *Glare* is defined as reflected or uncontrolled environmental light that shines directly into the eyes and causes either physical discomfort or a reduction in visual clarity.

Color

This is a key factor to consider when assessing and modifying the environment. Although many visually impaired individuals experience difficulty distinguishing between groups of colors, such as navy blue/brown/black, blue/green/purple, and pink/yellow/pale green, it is still possible to use color to enhance physical safety, accessibility, and independent participation in activities of daily living. There are several distinct characteristics of color that are relevant to the assessment process[15]:

- Hue: The particular color an object appears to have because it reflects or transmits specific wavelengths of light.
- Saturation: The intensity of a color or the amount of pure pigment that a color contains. For example, scarlet is more saturated than pink, which is composed of red combined with white.
- Brightness: How luminous or full of light the color appears.

Therefore, the following principles can be applied to the use of color in environments for individuals who are visually impaired:

- Bright colors are generally the easiest to see because of their ability to reflect light.
- Solid, bright colors such as red, orange, and yellow are usually more visible than pastels because they are more saturated.
- Lighting can influence the perception of color—dim light can "wash out" some colors; bright light can intensify others.
- Color can also provide important safety cues—an indicator of change in surface or level; a warning for potential hazards, such as steps or construction; a means of coding for location or identification; and a crucial factor in judging depth perception.

Contrast

Contrast sensitivity refers to the ability to detect differences between light and dark areas. Generally, increasing the contrast between an object and its background will make the object more visible. Enhancing contrast between elements of the environment is one of the simplest and most effective modifications to implement in most school, home, work, and recreational environments. There are several categories and principles of contrast that are relevant to the assessment process[14]:

- Contrast of hue: Compares two or more colors. Objects appear to have a particular hue or color because they reflect or transmit specific wavelengths of light.
- Light and dark contrast: Compares light colors to dark colors. Hues may be compared to white or black, with lighter hues being closer to white and darker hues being closer to black.
- Contrast of extension: Refers to the size of the surrounding contrasting areas. Generally, light colors on a dark background are more visible than equal-sized dark colors on a light background.

Therefore, the following principles can be used to implement contrast in environments for individuals who are visually impaired:

- White or bright yellow objects or print against a black background usually provide the strongest color contrast.

- Use solid colors as backgrounds to make objects "stand out." Avoid the use of patterns, prints, or stripes.
- Place light-colored objects against darker backgrounds. A white dinner plate is more visible against a brown or navy blue table covering.
- Place dark objects against lighter backgrounds. A dark handrail stands out against white or cream-colored walls. When combined appropriately with color, contrast can provide important cues for judging depth perception.

Environmental Modifications to Consider

- Miniblinds or vertical shades control direct sunlight and can be adjusted for variable lighting conditions according to the weather and time of day. They can also be used in combination with sheer window curtains or coverings.[16]
- Remember to control glare (Figure 14-4). If possible, switch to a nonglare floor wax, use matte floor tiles (either vinyl or ceramic), or use solid, nonpatterned carpeting. Position mirrors carefully to avoid "glare spots," especially in bathrooms. Counters and desks should have matte, nonglossy surfaces. Install dimmer switches on lamps and ceiling fixtures to control illumination levels and glare.
- Try to maintain continuous lighting levels throughout the building; install supplementary lighting along hallways to eliminate dim or excessively bright areas, especially in key safety locations (stairways, entrances, lobbies).
- Use additional sources of light, such as flexible "swing-arm" and "goose neck" lamps, for activities that require brighter, more concentrated light (reading, sewing, writing, crafts, dialing the telephone).[16]
- Whenever possible, use a combination of fluorescent and incandescent lighting. Install fluorescent ceiling fixtures for general room lighting supplemented with incandescent lighting in desk lamps, floor fixtures, and flexible "swing-arm" and "goose neck" lamps.
- Light switches, elevator buttons, call buttons, and other critical safety features can be painted in bright colors (red, orange) or outlined with fluorescent tape or paint to increase their visibility. Ensure that the color offers sufficient contrast with the wall, control panel, or other background.[16]
- Steps and staircases can be especially hazardous for visually impaired children and adults. Mark the leading edge of the first and last steps with bright paint or light-reflecting tape that contrasts with the background color of the flooring. If using tape, be sure to change it frequently and keep it in good repair. **Note:** In many instances, it is not necessary to adapt each step. Placing a mark on the first and last steps is sufficient to indicate where a staircase begins and ends.[16]
- Use solid, brightly colored hallway or stair runners (Figure 14-5) to clearly define traffic flow and walking spaces. Be sure to keep runners in good repair, because frayed or uneven edges can create a safety hazard.
- When designing printed reading material such as brochures, schedules, and menus, use black print (at least 18-point font size) on a nonglossy white background. Use plain, simple font styles (such as Arial), and avoid complicated formats.
- Signs, lettering, and clocks should be positioned at eye level whenever possible. Use large-print letters in simple fonts on a nonglossy, nonglare, contrasting background. Try to use either black letters on a white background or white letters on black.
- When towels, washcloths, and bath mats need replacement, purchase solid colors that contrast with the tub, floor, and wall tile. Wrap bathtub grab bars with brightly colored contrasting tape. Place a contrasting nonskid mat in the shower or tub to prevent falls and provide a cue for judging depth perception. Select a toothbrush with a dark handle that contrasts with the sink.

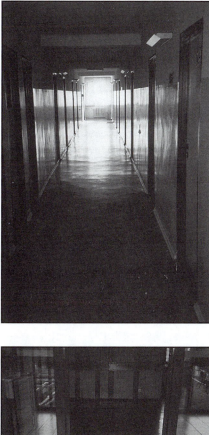

Figure 14-4. Note the glare in this hallway from an uncovered window and reflective floor and wall coverings. (Reprinted with permission from Maureen A. Duffy, MS, CRVT.)

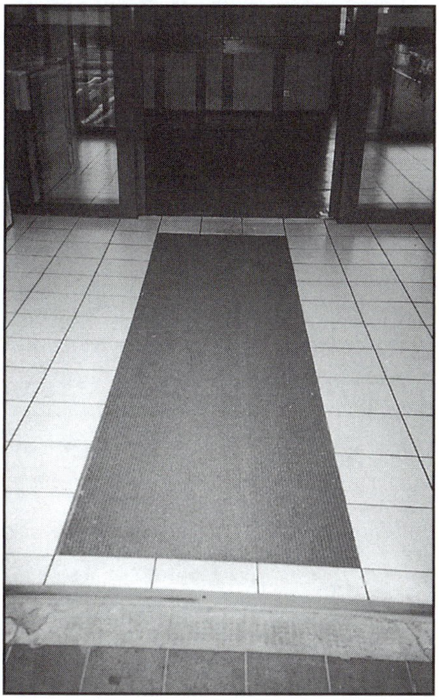

Figure 14-5. This contrasting floor runner helps define the entrance area. (Reprinted with permission from Maureen A. Duffy, MS, CRVT.)

Case Study: Activities of Daily Living

An Occupational Therapist/Vision Rehabilitation Therapist Collaboration

INTRODUCTION

Although several disciplines within the vision rehabilitation network have been discussed thus far, the authors have chosen to present an in-depth case study that focuses upon the cooperative disciplines of occupational therapy and VRT. Similar interdisciplinary collaborations between OT/TVI and OT/O&M are recommended for a variety of case management scenarios that may involve children, adolescents, working-age adults, and elderly people and can produce beneficial rehabilitation outcomes for students and clients.

The following case history represents a collaborative OT/VRT assessment and training effort in two specific areas of critical activities of daily living function: eating skills and handwriting, including signature and letter writing. The interdisciplinary vision-related OT/VRT collaboration is crucial in these areas because the subject exhibits multiple functional impairments in addition to low vision. This interdisciplinary collaboration represents the best synthesis of competencies that are germane to each discipline and culminates in a successful rehabilitation outcome for this individual.

BACKGROUND AND HISTORY

Marie is a widowed 72-year-old woman who lives alone in a fifth-floor apartment and employs a home attendant on a part-time basis. Her adult daughter lives nearby and visits several times a week. Marie has been an insulin-dependent diabetic for 23 years and experiences severe neuropathy in her right hand and both feet. She reports Paget's disease, hypertension, lupus, and rheumatoid arthritis in her spine and upper and lower extremities. In addition, she has a history of myocardial infarctions, angina, and kidney dysfunction. The following medications comprise her daily regimen: insulin, Isoptin (verapamil), Lasix (furosemide), Lidex (fluocinonide), Librium (chlordiazepoxide), nitroglycerin, Mylanta, and Tagamet (cimetidine); however, she experiences difficulty organizing and identifying most of these medications due to fluctuating vision and neuropathy. Her daughter premeasures her insulin dosage, and Marie self-injects twice a day. She uses a wheelchair to travel outside the home and wears a knee brace at all times. When walking indoors, she uses a support cane and wheelchair as needed. Her support network includes a diabetes education counselor, a visiting nurse, a rehabilitation counselor, Meals on Wheels, and volunteer high school students for chore and reading services. Her medical team includes a cardiologist, renal specialist, ophthalmologist, and endocrinologist.

Visual Acuity

Obtained during semi-annual ophthalmological examination—OD: FC; OS: 10/200; Fields: unable to test.

Ocular Status

- Proliferative diabetic retinopathy OU, with history of laser treatment OU.
- Paget's disease: Ocular implications include paralysis of extraocular muscles, diplopia, angioid streaks, hemorrhaging, retinal detachment, and macular scarring.
- During a prior low vision assessment, no optical devices were recommended.

POSSIBLE FUNCTIONAL VISUAL IMPLICATIONS

Fluctuating vision, photophobia, decreased color perception, increased sensitivity to glare, reduced detail vision, reduced contrast sensitivity, difficulty with depth perception.

Initial Assessment Results: Vision Rehabilitation Therapy

The initial assessment was conducted independently by the VRT and included the following component areas: general information; general health status; self-assessment of visual functioning; home management; medication management; clothing and personal management; communication abilities, including braille, computer skills, handwriting, reading, and recording; recreation and leisure activities; and indoor mobility. The results of this assessment facilitated the development of the following goals, adaptive equipment recommendations, environmental modifications, and instructional strategies:

Assessment. Difficulty locating food on plate and using utensils for scooping, piercing; difficulty using a knife and fork; unable to pour hot and cold liquids without spillage; unable to prepare simple meals independently or reheat Meals on Wheels.

Housekeeping Goals. Eating skills; pour hot and cold liquids; simple meal preparation.

Recommended Adaptive Equipment. Electronic liquid level indicator; toaster oven with asbestos mat; safety food turner; Hot Shot hot beverage maker; Dycem pads; tactile long-ring timer.

Environmental Modifications.

- Improve the lighting: See recommendations on page 312.

- Increase contrast: Use white dishes or plates on a dark tablecloth or dark plates on a white or light-colored cloth; avoid using clear glass cups and dishes.

- Implement color: Use fluorescent marking tape on handles of utensils; use brightly colored Dycem pads and trays for working surfaces.

Assessment. Unable to sign name independently on documents or greeting cards; unable to write shopping lists for her home attendant; unable to identify the time independently.

Communication Goals. Handwriting, including signature and list writing; time identification.

Recommended Adaptive Equipment. Signature guide; Marks Script Guide; envelope guide; 20/20 pen; talking clock; talking watch.

Environmental Modifications.

- Improve the lighting: See recommendations on page 312.

- Increase contrast: Place white paper on dark working surface; use dark-colored signature and envelope guides if possible; use 20/20 pen for maximum contrast and to decrease "bleed-through" on writing paper.

Assessment. Unable to independently identify coins and bills; unable to differentiate medications and administer them independently as appropriate.

Personal Management Goals. Money identification (coins and bills); medication identification.

Recommended Adaptive Equipment. Hi-Mark Tactile Pen or Spot 'n Line Pen for medication identification.

Environmental Modifications.

- Improve the lighting: See recommendations on page 312.

- Increase contrast: Place bills and coins on a light-colored, nonpatterned surface.

- Implement color: Use brightly colored tactual marking material on all medication containers.

Assessment. Unable to monitor blood glucose levels independently.

Health Management Goals. Test blood sugar levels at periodic intervals throughout the day and adjust insulin dosage as appropriate.

Recommended Adaptive Equipment. Talking blood glucose monitor.

Environmental Modifications.

- Improve the lighting: See recommendations below.

- Increase contrast: Place blood glucose monitor and blood glucose testing materials on a contrasting work surface or tray.

Lighting Recommendations for All Tasks. Adjustable swing-arm task lamps with combination fluorescent/incandescent bulbs; Chromalux and compact fluorescent bulbs for existing light fixtures; dimmer switches where appropriate.

Control Potential Sources of Glare. Assess for the presence of highly polished floors, shiny or reflective table tops and counters, chrome fixtures and mirrors in bathrooms, uncovered lightbulbs in lamps and ceiling fixtures, uncovered windows.

Additional Instructional Strategies. Slow the pace of instruction; incorporate frequent rest periods; emphasize sedentary tasks; minimize standing.

Additional Professional Referrals. To O&M for indoor and possible outdoor wheelchair mobility lessons; to social work for assistance with housing modifications and adaptations.

Assessment Results: Occupational Therapy

RATIONALE

After activities of daily living instruction was initiated, the VRT requested an interdisciplinary OT consultation in two specific training areas: eating skills and handwriting. It was apparent that the functional impact of Marie's combined visual and physical impairments created a significant barrier to the mastery of these specific activities of daily living skills through VRT intervention alone. The OT conducted the assessment in conjunction with a regularly scheduled VRT in-home training session and developed the following goals, adaptive equipment recommendations, and instructional strategies.

PHYSICAL FUNCTION EVALUATION

Marie experiences back and pelvic discomfort when seated for extended periods of time. Severe neuropathy in her right hand makes it difficult to grasp utensils and writing instruments, and she cannot detect elevated heat levels, such as those produced by a mug of hot water. She also experiences a loss of sensation in both lower extremities.

Wheelchair Evaluation. Repair current wheelchair, which is on loan. Recommend a replacement lightweight wheelchair with pneumatic tires and removable arms.

Recommended Adaptive Equipment. Wheelchair cushion (extra large) to stabilize trunk muscles; adapted orthopedic stool to minimize strain on lower back and extremities while engaged in kitchen and table activities.

Assessment. Difficulty executing safe, independent bathtub and toilet transfers.

Bathroom Self-Care Goals. Safe and effective bathtub and toilet transfers.

Recommended Adaptive Equipment. Bathtub chair with backrest, bathtub grab bars, elevated toilet seat, toilet grab bar.

Assessment. Difficulty grasping handles of utensils when scooping and piercing; difficulty using a knife and fork to cut, slice, and sever food items.

Housekeeping Goals. Adaptive eating skills.

Recommended Adaptive Equipment. Nonskid insulated mug, foam tubing, rocker knife, plate guard, round scoop dish.

Treatment Plan. Interdisciplinary OT/VRT collaboration to develop teaching/training sequence.

Assessment. Difficulty grasping 20/20 pen and applying appropriate downward pressure when writing; tendency to flatten the pen tip.

Communication Goals. Handwriting, including signature and list writing.

Recommended Adaptive Equipment. Foam gripper for 20/20 pen; possibly switch to a therapeutic retractable pen.

Treatment Plan. Interdisciplinary OT/VRT collaboration to develop teaching/training sequence.

COLLABORATIVE OCCUPATIONAL THERAPIST/VISION REHABILITATION THERAPIST TRAINING SEQUENCE

As a result of this collaborative consultation and assessment, both professionals jointly developed an individualized interdisciplinary training program that synthesized discrete competencies germane to OT and VRT. This interdisciplinary program of instruction in eating skills and handwriting used the following adaptive instructional strategies that addressed the combined functional effects of her physical and visual disabilities:

Goal 1: Instruction in Adaptive Eating Skills With the Addition of a Therapeutic Plate and Utensils

Functional Impact. Difficulty locating food on plate; grasping handles of utensils; using utensils for scooping and piercing; using a knife and fork to cut, slice, and sever food items.

Interdisciplinary Adaptive Instructional Strategies.

- Ensure that seating provides appropriate height and support.
- Check the quantity and quality of lighting on the task; use an adjustable swing-arm lamp with a 75-watt bulb to illuminate the plate and eating surface.
- Use a contrasting tray or placemat to facilitate orientation to the table setting; stabilize the plate with a brightly colored Dycem pad; when appropriate, use white dishes or plates on a dark tablecloth.
- Keep the head and face positioned over the plate to catch food items that may fall from utensils.
- Place foam tubing on utensils to facilitate effective manipulation and grasp.
- When appropriate, use a plate guard on the dinner plate or a round scoop dish for food items that are difficult to locate and pierce.
- Use the fork and knife to systematically explore contents of the plate.
- Use clock face orientation to describe the location of food items.
- When cutting foods with a knife and fork, use the index fingers to apply consistent downward pressure.
- Use the rocker knife when appropriate to apply consistent downward pressure to sever food items.
- Use the weight of food on the fork or spoon to indicate the relative portion size.

- Use the "buffer" technique with a knife, piece of bread, mashed potatoes, or the plate guard to push items onto the fork.
- Periodically check the location and arrangement of food on the plate; also check for dropped food items.

Goal 2: Instruction in Signature and Handwriting Skills With the Following Adaptations: Signature Guide; Marks Script Guide; Envelope Guide; 20/20 Pen With Foam Gripper; Therapeutic Retractable Pen

Functional Impact. Unable to sign name independently or write shopping lists; difficulty grasping the writing instrument and applying appropriate downward pressure when writing.

Interdisciplinary Adaptive Instructional Strategies.

- Ensure that seating provides appropriate height and support.
- Check the quantity and quality of lighting on the task; use an adjustable swing-arm lamp with a Chromalux bulb to illuminate the working surface.
- Examine the distance from the eye to the task and determine whether it can be adjusted; use the principle of relative distance magnification whenever possible.
- Place white paper on a dark working surface; use dark-colored signature and envelope guides for maximum contrast.
- Use 20/20 pen for maximum contrast and to decrease "bleed-through" on writing paper; place foam gripper on pen to facilitate effective manipulation and grasp.
- Alternatively, use the therapeutic retractable pen when appropriate to facilitate effective manipulation, grasp, and writing pressure.
- Practice letter formation without the guide (loops, points, circles).
- Use tactual methods to insert paper into the appropriate writing guide (Figures 14-6a through 14-6d).
- Introduce a method to determine the beginning of the writing line.
- Apply appropriate amount of downward pressure, and remain on the baseline when writing.
- Introduce a method for dotting i's and crossing t's.
- Use the nondominant index finger to maintain appropriate spacing between words.

Figure 14-6a. An assortment of adapted signature guides. (Reprinted with permission from Maureen A. Duffy, MS, CRVT.)

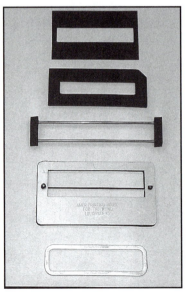

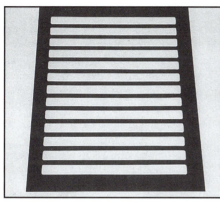

Figure 14-6b. An adapted handwriting guide. (Reprinted with permission from Maureen A. Duffy, MS, CRVT.)

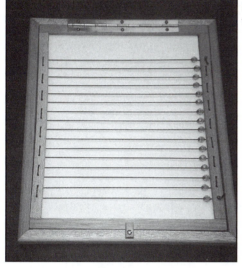

Figure 14-6c. An adapted handwriting guide. (Reprinted with permission from Maureen A. Duffy, MS, CRVT.)

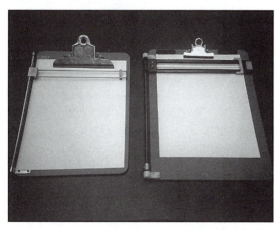

Figure 14-6d. An adapted handwriting guide. (Reprinted with permission from Maureen A. Duffy, MS, CRVT.)

Summary

This interdisciplinary collaboration represents the best synthesis of competencies that are germane to each discipline and culminates in a successful rehabilitation outcome for this individual. This case study demonstrates that OT or VRT intervention alone may not always be sufficient to teach specific daily living skills to blind or visually impaired adult consumers with additional functional physical impairments. The same is true when visually impaired children and adolescents have additional physical disabilities that require the knowledge and skills of an OT; thus, it is recommended that OTs and vision-related rehabilitation professionals continue to explore the benefits of such interdisciplinary collaborations within the rehabilitation process to produce more satisfactory outcomes for children and adults who are visually impaired.

Acknowledgments

The authors would like to acknowledge Nancy D. Miller, Executive Director, and the staff of VISIONS/Services for the Blind and Visually Impaired, New York, for their generous assistance in providing background material and the service delivery model that forms the basis for this composite case study.

References

1. Orr AL, Huebner KM. Toward a collaborative working relationship among vision rehabilitation and allied health professionals. *Journal of Visual Impairment and Blindness*. 2001;95(8):468-482.
2. Kern T, Miller NW. Occupational therapy and collaborative interventions for adults with low vision. In: Gentile M, ed. *Functional Visual Behavior*. Bethesda, MD: American Occupational Therapy Association; 1997.
3. Council for Exceptional Children. *What Every Special Educator Must Know: The International Standards for the Preparation and Licensure of Special Educators*. 3rd ed. Reston, VA: Council for Exceptional Children; 1998.
4. Hatlen P. The core curriculum for blind and visually impaired students, including those with additional disabilities. *RE:view*. 1996;28(1):25-32.
5. Corn AL, Hatlen P, Huebner KM, Ryan F, Siller MA. *The National Agenda for the Education of Children and Youths With Visual Impairments, Including Those With Multiple Disabilities*. New York, NY: AFB Press; 1995.
6. Huebner KM, Merk-Adam B, Stryker D, Wolffe K. *The National Agenda for the Education of Children and Youths With Visual Impairments, Including Those With Multiple Disabilities*. New York, NY: AFB Press; 2004.
7. Crews JE, Luxton L. Rehabilitation teaching for older adults. In: Orr AA, ed. *Vision and Aging: Crossroads for Service Delivery*. New York, NY: AFB Press; 1992:233-253.
8. Koenig AJ, Holbrook MC. Professional practice. In: Holbrook MC, Koenig AJ, eds. *Foundations of Education: History and Theory of Teaching Children and Youths With Visual Impairments*. 2nd ed. Vol 1. New York, NY: AFB Press; 2000:260-276.
9. Association for Education and Rehabilitation of the Blind and Visually Impaired. *Code of Ethics for Teachers of Students With Visual Impairments*. Alexandria, VA: Author; 1992.
10. Academy for Certification of Vision Rehabilitation and Education Professionals and Association for Education and Rehabilitation of the Blind and Visually Impaired. *Code of Ethics for Orientation and Mobility Specialists*. Tucson, AZ: Author; 1990.
11. Academy for Certification of Vision Rehabilitation and Education Professionals and Association for Education and Rehabilitation of the Blind and Visually Impaired. *Vision Rehabilitation Therapy Code of Ethics*. Tucson, AZ: Author; 2000.
12. Edwards LE, Duffy MA, Ray JS. The vision-related rehabilitation network. In: Brilliant RL, ed. *Essentials of Low Vision Practice*. Woburn, MA: Butterworth-Heinemann Publishers; 1998.
13. Koenig AJ, Holbrook MC. *Learning Media Assessment*. Austin, TX: Texas School for the Blind and Visually Impaired; 1993.
14. Duffy MA. Assessing and modifying the workplace environment for persons with visual impairments. In: Adamowicz-Hummel A, Yeadon A, eds. *Guidebook for Employers of Persons With Blindness and Visual Impairment*. Warsaw, Poland: The United States Embassy; 2000.
15. Duffy MA. *New Independence! Environmental Adaptations in Community Facilities for Adults With Vision Impairments*. Mohegan Lake, NY: Associates for World Action in Rehabilitation and Education (AWARE); 1997.
16. Duffy MA. *Making Life More Livable: Simple Adaptations for Living at Home After Vision Loss*. New York, NY: AFB Press; 2002.

Suggested Reading

Duffy MA, Beliveau-Tobey M, eds. *New Independence! For Older Persons With Vision Loss in Long-Term Care Facilities.* Mohegan Lake, NY: Associates for World Action in Rehabilitation and Education (AWARE); 1992.

Huebner KM, Prickett JG, Welch TR, Joffee EJ, eds. *Hand in Hand: Essentials of Communication and Orientation and Mobility for Your Students Who Are Deaf-Blind.* New York, NY: AFB Press; 1995.

Inkster W, Newman L, Weiss DS, Yeadon A. *Rehabilitation Teaching for Persons Experiencing Vision Loss.* 2nd ed. New York, NY: CIL Publications; 1997.

Mulholland ME, Welch TR, Huebner KM. *Hand in Hand: It Can Be Done. A Video With Discussion Guide.* New York, NY: AFB Press; 1995.

Ponchillia PE, Ponchillia SV. *Foundations of Rehabilitation Teaching With Persons Who Are Blind or Visually Impaired.* New York, NY: AFB Press; 1996.

Prickett JG, Joffee EJ, Welch TR, Huebner KM, eds. *Hand in Hand: Essentials of Communication and Orientation and Mobility for Your Students Who Are Deaf-Blind—A Trainer's Manual.* New York, NY: AFB Press; 1995.

Van S. *New Independence! Craft Adaptations for Adults With Vision Impairments.* Mohegan Lake, NY: Associates for World Action in Rehabilitation and Education (AWARE); 2007.

Weiner WR, Welsh RL, Blasch BB, eds. *Foundations of Orientation and Mobility. 3rd ed. Vol 1. History and Theory.* New York, NY: AFB Press; 2010.

Weiner WR, Welsh RL, Blasch BB, eds. *Foundations of Orientation and Mobility. 3rd ed. Vol 2. Instructional Strategies and Practical Applications.* New York, NY: AFB Press; 2010.

Wormsley DP, D'Andrea FM, eds. *Instructional Strategies for Braille Literacy.* New York, NY: AFB Press; 1997.

Related Web Sites

Academy for Certification of Vision Rehabilitation & Education Professionals
www.acvrep.org

American Foundation for the Blind
www.afb.org

American Foundation for the Blind Senior Site
www.afb.org/seniorsitehome.asp

Association for Education and Rehabilitation of the Blind and Visually Impaired
www.aerbvi.org

Journal of Visual Impairment & Blindness
www.jvib.org

VisionAWARE: The Self-Help Resource Center for Vision Loss
www.visionaware.org

Resources

Ableware/Maddak Inc
661 Route 23 S
Wayne, NJ 07470
Phone: 973-628-7600
Fax: 973-305-0841
Email: custservice@maddak.com
www.maddak.com

American Printing House for the Blind
1839 Frankfort Ave
PO Box 6085
Louisville, KY 40206-0085
Phone: 502-895-2405
Fax: 502-899-2274
Email: info@aph.org
www.aph.org

CIL Publication Series
500 Greenwich St, 3rd Floor
New York, NY 10013
Phone: 888-CIL-8333
Fax: 212-219-4078
Email: cilpubs@visionsvcb.org
www.cilpubs.com

Dazor Manufacturing Corp
2079 Congressional St
St. Louis, MO 63146
Phone: 800-345-9103 or 314-652-2400
Fax: 314-652-2069
Email: info@dazor.com
www.dazor.com

Independent Living Aids
200 Robbins Lane
Jericho, NY 11753
Phone: 800-537-2118
Fax: 516-937-3906
Email: orders@independentliving.com
www.independentliving.com

LS&S
145 River Rock Dr
Buffalo, NY 14207
Phone: 800-468-4789
TTY: 866-317-8533
Fax: 877-498-1482
www.lssgroup.com

Maxi-Aids
42 Executive Blvd
Farmingdale, NY 11735
Phone: 800-522-6294
TTY: 800-281-3555
Fax: 631-752-0689
Email: sales@maxiaids.com
www.maxiaids.com

VisionAWARE.org

Find Independent Living Products: www.visionaware.org/find_products

Find State and Local Vision Rehabilitation Services: www.visionaware.org/find_vision_rehabilitation_vision_services_in_your_state

Chapter Fifteen

Getting Involved in
Low Vision Rehabilitation

Maxine Scheiman, MEd, OTR/L, CLVT and
Mitchell Scheiman, OD, FCOVD, FAAO

The prevalence and incidence of low vision in the United States are high and experts predict a large increase over the next two decades because the prevalence of low vision increases sharply in persons older than 65 years. In the study by Congdon et al,[1] persons older than 80 years made up only 7.7% of the population but accounted for 69% of the severe visual impairment. It is this group that is the fastest-growing segment of the US population. Based on this information, the American Occupational Therapy Association (AOTA) has called low vision rehabilitation one of the top 10 emerging fields in occupational therapy. Occupational therapists working with the adult population will encounter many clients with low vision, even if this is not the primary reason the client has been referred for occupational therapy

It is our hope that if you have reached this section of the book you have a strong interest in becoming more involved in this new and exciting practice area of occupational therapy. If so, you are likely to be left with a number of important questions about educational requirements, certification, practice opportunities, billing, and reimbursement.

Some of the important questions that need to be addressed include:

- What are the educational requirements for an occupational therapist to provide low vision rehabilitation services?
- Is certification necessary to provide low vision rehabilitation services?
- How does the occupational therapist interact with other vision rehabilitation professionals?
- What practice opportunities are available?
- Are low vision rehabilitation services provided by occupational therapists covered by Medicare and other insurance?
- How do I properly bill insurance for low vision rehabilitation services?
- What equipment do I need to get started in the field of low vision rehabilitation?

This chapter is designed to provide answers to these critical questions.

Scheiman M
Understanding and Managing Vision Deficits: A Guide for
Occupational Therapists, Third Edition (pp 321-338)
© 2011 SLACK Incorporated

Didactic Education/Clinical Training

Although information about the visual system is certainly part of every occupational therapy curriculum, the information provided is generally basic and introductory. Few programs are designed to prepare the entry-level occupational therapist for the practice of low vision rehabilitation either from a didactic or clinical training perspective. Mary Warren states that "Although occupational therapists have been involved in the rehabilitation of persons with vision loss since the inception of the profession in 1917, we never played an extensive role in low vision rehabilitation."[2] Occupational therapists have indeed always played a role in low vision rehabilitation because nearly two-thirds of older adults with low vision have at least one other chronic medical condition that may interfere with activities of daily living and require occupational therapy.[3] Thus, in the context of providing care for other chronic conditions, occupational therapists must routinely manage issues related to low vision in their elderly clients.

Perhaps the entry-level occupational therapy program curricula need to be reconsidered, given the prevalence of low vision in the adult population. However, at the present time, most occupational therapy graduates, as well as experienced occupational therapists need to gain additional information and clinical experience to feel comfortable practicing low vision rehabilitation at a sophisticated level, much as hand therapists seek specialized training.

A wide range of educational opportunities are now available for occupational therapists to receive this additional educational experience. These opportunities include new low vision textbooks designed for occupational therapists, graduate-degree-level programs, multiple-day continuing education workshops (both on-site and online), presentations from companies that sell and produce optical aids, and home study courses.

While all registered/licensed occupational therapists are legally qualified and currently able to provide and bill for low vision rehabilitation services without any additional education or certification, most will need additional education and clinical experience to competently function as low vision therapists. The decision about how much additional educational experience and the nature of the educational experience is a personal one that each occupational therapist must make. Individuals vary in their preferred learning style. For an assertive, self-assured individual with strong independent learning skills, reading a book, taking a home-study course, and gaining some experience with optical aids from a manufacturer's workshop may be sufficient to develop the core knowledge base. Additional clinical practice supervised by an experienced low vision therapist is also recommended. For those preferring self-study, a useful guide to the knowledge base required to practice low vision therapy is provided by the Academy for Certification of Vision Rehabilitation & Education Professionals ([ACVREP] www.acvrep.org). Others may prefer to enroll in a formal graduate program in low vision rehabilitation that includes clinical training. The various opportunities are listed with contact information in Table 15-1. We have tried to make this listing as complete as possible. Of course, organizations come and go and new programs are being developed. Thus, it is important to use this table as a starting point and be aware that new programs and educational opportunities will certainly be available after publication of this book.

Low Vision Textbooks

There is only one low vision textbook written specifically for occupational therapists at this time. The book is entitled: *Low Vision Rehabilitation: A Guide for Occupational Therapists,* published by SLACK Incorporated.

In the Preface, the authors state: "This textbook is designed to provide a practical and clinically oriented guide to enable occupational therapists to begin this process of independent study and reading in order to seize this opportunity and the responsibility of joining the team of professionals that care for this population."[4] A unique aspect of this textbook is that it incorporates concepts from the AOTA's *Occupational Therapy Practice Framework: Domain and Process*.

Table 15-1	
Postgraduate Educational Opportunities for Education in Low Vision Rehabilitation	
Name of Organization/Web Site	*Type of Education*
Salus University www.salus.edu	Graduate level I All distance learning Certificate or master's in low vision rehabilitation Certificate or master's in rehabilitation teaching Certificate or master's in orientation and mobility
University of Alabama, Birmingham www.uab.edu/ot	Graduate level education Master's or certificate in low vision rehabilitation
Vision Education Seminars www.visionedseminars.com	2-day workshops on low vision presented across the United States
Lighthouse courses www.lighthouse.org	Workshops on low vision presented across the United States
Eschenbach Optik courses www.Eschenbach.com	2-day workshops on low vision presented across the United States
visABILITIES www.visabilities.com	2-day workshops on low vision presented across the United States
AOTA home study course www.aota.org	Home study course
AOTA/Jewish Guild for the Blind Online Study Course www.aota.org	Online course
The Hadley School for the Blind www.hadley-school.org/	Online course
Lions Vision Research and Rehabilitation Center at the Johns Hopkins Wilmer Eye Institute http://lowvisionproject.org/	Online course

Continuing Education Courses

It is common for occupational therapists to gain knowledge about new areas of practice through post-graduate, continuing education seminars and workshops. One- and 2-day workshops are offered periodically for low vision rehabilitation. Some of the companies offering such workshops are listed in Table 15-1. These workshops generally cover information about epidemiology of low vision, diseases causing low vision, basic optics, the occupational therapy evaluation and low vision rehabilitation, billing for services, and hands-on experience with optical aids. After completing one or two of these courses most occupational therapists would feel comfortable providing basic low vision rehabilitation services to clients presenting with low vision as a secondary diagnosis. Some self-assured occupational therapists might feel comfortable enough to initiate a low vision service in a hospital setting or provide home-based low vision rehabilitation services with clients presenting with a primary diagnosis of low vision.

Companies that produce and sell optical devices sometimes provide inexpensive continuing education for occupational therapists and these seminars offer an excellent opportunity to gain hands-on experience with microscopes, magnifiers, telescopes, closed-circuit televeisions, and other video display technology. For example, Eschenbach Optik of America (http://eschenbach. com/seminars.php) has been providing this service for many years and this company offers seminars in many cities around the country on an annual basis. The Eschenbach course is entitled "Low Vision Care...What's It All About?" This low vision care presentation for eye care and rehabilitation professionals is designed as an introduction into low vision care and optical devices.

The primary missing ingredient from short, continuing education courses, of course, is clinical experience with clients. Gaining meaningful clinical experience is the greatest challenge facing therapists who would like to be involved in low vision rehabilitation. Opportunities may exist in some communities for an interested occupational therapist to volunteer or find employment in a situation in which low vision rehabilitation is already being provided by another experienced therapist. In any case, finding a setting to acquire supervised clinical instruction is a challenge.

Home Study and Distance Education

In 1995, the AOTA devoted its entire October issue to the topic of low vision and in 1998 developed the AOTA *Occupational Therapy Practice Guidelines for Adults With Low Vision*. In 2000, Mary Warren edited a home study course entitled *Low Vision: Occupational Therapy Intervention With the Older Adult*, published by the AOTA.[5] This home study course has been revised in recent years. These documents provide a wonderful starting point for independent learning.

A recent trend in education is online or distance learning and many opportunities now exist for this type of education in the area of low vision rehabilitation. The Hadley School for the Blind (www.hadley-school.org/) currently offers a number of online courses for professionals including coursework in braille, low vision technology, introduction to low vision, self-esteem and adjusting with blindness, and macular degeneration. These courses are provided without any tuition charge.

The Lions Vision Research and Rehabilitation Center at the Johns Hopkins Wilmer Eye Institute offers some exceptional distance learning opportunities and outstanding up-to-date information about low vision rehabilitation on their Web site (http://lowvisionproject.org/). This site is also the gateway to the Low Vision Rehabilitation Network. This is a network of low vision providers and researchers and membership allows individuals to participate in a number of collaborative projects including:

- Free online continuing professional education courses
- Exchange ideas and views with colleagues in online forums
- Participate in live online low vision case conferences
- Participate in live online low vision research symposia
- Participate in an online "What's New in Low Vision" Web site
- Help plan the Low Vision Rehabilitation Outcomes Project

Membership in the Low Vision Rehabilitation Network is free and open to low vision rehabilitation practitioners, researchers, students, educators, administrators, policymakers, business people, and anyone else who is interested in advances in the field of low vision rehabilitation.

A course currently offered on this Web site is entitled "Understanding Visual Impairments and Functional Rehabilitation of Visually Impaired Patients." The course consists of 22 lectures and supplemental material that cover topics such as anatomy and physiology of vision, diseases of the visual system, optics and optical devices, functional and activities of daily living assessments, visual skills training, rehabilitation services and resources, and vision enhancement and adaptive technology.

An online course entitled "Low Vision in Older Adults: Foundations for Rehabilitation" is the result of collaboration between the AOTA and SightCare, a program of The Jewish Guild for the Blind. The course was written by low vision optometrist, a certified environmental design specialist, and an occupational therapist. It is made up if three lessons including:

1. An orientation to vision loss: Its causes, effects, and interventions

2. Vision enhancement with magnification: Theory and practice

3. Environmental considerations

Of course, textbooks, like this one, are available to assist occupational therapists in gaining information about low vision rehabilitation as independent learners.

University-Based Graduate Education

Some occupational therapists may prefer more formal, university-based, graduate education. Two excellent programs designed for occupational therapists are now available to meet this need and are listed in Table 15-1. Both programs offer a certificate or master's degree in low vision rehabilitation.

The College of Education and Rehabilitation at Salus University (www.salus.edu/cer/index. html) prepares a variety of professionals to work with people who are visually impaired. These programs include master's degree and certificate programs in:

- Low vision rehabilitation

- Orientation and mobility

- Education for teachers of children with visual and multiple disabilities

- Vision rehabilitation therapy

The program most likely to be of interest to occupational therapists is the Master of Science and Certificate in low vision rehabilitation. All of these programs, with the exception of the full-time master's degree in orientation and mobility, are now available through distance education.

The University of Alabama, Birmingham Department of Occupational Therapy, offers a graduate certificate program in low vision rehabilitation (http://main.uab.edu/Shrp/default. aspx?pid=76987). This program is designed for occupational therapists with bachelor's, master's, or doctorate degrees. It consists of 17 credit hours of specialized courses in low vision rehabilitation. Students take 11 credits of core courses designed to provide a foundation in providing low vision rehabilitation services, four credits of elective courses to address specific aspects of intervention in greater depth, and a two-credit course in advanced application. All of the courses are offered online through a Web-based curriculum. The curriculum is designed with the working occupational therapist in mind. Coursework emphasizes practical application of the information taught. Students can enroll in the certificate program or combine completion of the certificate program with a post-professional master's degree in occupational therapy. Students completing the certificate program need to complete an additional 10 credits of coursework and six credits of research to receive the post-professional master's degree. Coursework for the post-professional degree is also online.

Thus, many educational opportunities are available for an occupational therapist who would like to become involved in low vision education. It is simply a matter of deciding on one's learning style and researching some of the available options listed.

Certification

Certification in low vision therapy is not required at this time for occupational therapists. Any registered/licensed occupational therapist is able to provide low vision rehabilitation and bill for these services. In Chapter One, we discussed the various professionals involved in low vision rehabilitation of adult clients. These include occupational therapists, low vision therapists, vision rehabilitation therapists (formerly rehabilitation teachers), and orientation and mobility specialists. Of these four groups, only occupational therapists are licensed and function as independent service providers in the Medicare system and in some regions for other commercial insurance programs. Vision rehabilitation therapists, low vision therapists, and orientation and mobility specialists often work for state agencies, private organizations, and school systems. In 2009, the services of these professionals were not reimbursed by Medicare, Medicaid, or most private insurance.

Although occupational therapists do not require certification to practice low vision rehabilitation, it is a desirable goal for the following reasons:

- Certification demonstrates that the therapist has advanced skills low vision rehabilitation and in the future
- Certification may indeed be required by insurers for reimbursement even for occupational therapists

Academy for Certification of Vision Rehabilitation & Education Professionals

Currently there is only one active certification program for low vision therapy. This certification process is run by the ACVREP, which was established in January 2000. It is an independent and autonomous legal certification body governed by a volunteer board of directors. ACVREP's mission is to offer professional certification for vision rehabilitation and education professionals in order to improve service delivery to persons with vision impairments. As of January 2010, there were about 350 certified low vision therapists. Although ACVREP does not release data on how many occupational therapists are certified, it is likely that many of the 350 who are certified low vision therapists are occupational therapists.

The ACVREP certification program that is appropriate for occupational therapists is called the certified low vision therapist. To be eligible to take the written certification test candidates must meet the eligibility criteria listed in Table 15-2. Candidates passing a 100-item written examination receive certification that is valid for a 5-year period. Certified low vision therapists must go through a recertification process every 5 years. To be recertified an individual must demonstrate that he or she has maintained continuing professional competence in the field of vision rehabilitation and education much like the requirements for occupational therapy certification. Acceptable activities include continuing education, professional experience, publications and presentations, and professional service. Full details of all requirements can be obtained from the ACVREP Web site.

The advantages of ACVREP certification are:

- The guidelines for the examination and study program have been developed by experienced professionals in the field. The applicant must have his or her study program reviewed and a multiple-choice examination must be passed to ensure that the occupational therapist has the requisite knowledge base for competent practice.
- The organization will help applicants locate and arrange for clinical supervision. Although some direct supervision is necessary, most of the 350 hours of clinical practice may be supervised by a certified therapist off site.
- Certification allows the occupational therapist to join rather than compete with the professionals who have been providing low vision and blindness rehabilitation services long before the recent increase in occupational therapy practitioners in the field.

Table 15-2	

Criteria for Eligibility for Certification
Academy for Certification of Vision Rehabilitation &
Education Professionals

- Proof of a minimum of a bachelor's degree from an accredited college or university (or foreign equivalent, as verified through an independent credential evaluation company) in any field. In addition, the CLVT supervisor must verify that the applicant demonstrates basic competency in all core domain areas.

- Have completed 350 hours of "discipline specific, supervised practice that includes, but is not limited to, direct service hours, and related phone calls, meetings, observations, report writing, etc." The practice must be supervised by a CLVT and a physician (OD or MD) practicing in low vision. The CLVT practice supervisor may be off site. The applicant must meet the CLVT clinical competencies.

- Pass the LVT written exam demonstrating knowledge of low vision principles and their applications.

CLVT=certified low vision therapy/ist, LVT=low vision therapy.

American Occupational Therapy Association Certification

AOTA low vision specialty certification is based on a peer-reviewed reflective. Candidates identify the professional development activities they have engaged in that best demonstrate their knowledge, critical and ethical reasoning, and interpersonal and performance skills relative to identified competencies and criteria. How those activities helped them meet the criteria, supported their professional development, and influenced client outcomes is then described in a single brief narrative for each competency. Candidates for certification also must include a self-assessment that they use as a guide to establish five measurable goals that will be worked toward for the 5 years immediately following initial certification. Full details are available at www.aota.org/Practitioners/ProfDev/Certification.aspx.

Candidates must demonstrate the following:

- Professional or technical degree or equivalent in occupational therapy.

- Certified or licensed by and in good standing with an AOTA-recognized credentialing or regulatory body.

- Minimum of 2000 hours of experience as an occupational therapist or occupational therapy assistant.

- 600 hours of experience delivering occupational therapy services in the area of low vision rehabilitation to clients (individuals, groups, or populations) in the last 5 calendar years. Service delivery may be paid or voluntary.

Other Professions and Interprofessional Issues

It is important that occupational therapists have a firm understanding of the history of low vision in the United States.[4] Vision rehabilitation therapists and orientation and mobility specialists have been in low vision rehabilitation for many more years than occupational therapists. With the inclusion of low vision as a disability under Medicare guidelines in the early 1990s, occupational therapists suddenly became involved in low vision rehabilitation and this created controversy. The primary basis for this controversy is that the impetus for occupational therapy's entrance into the low vision arena was not a change in education and preparation of its practitioners, rather, it was purely based on reimbursement issues. Thus, other vision rehabilitation therapists have raised questions about occupational therapy's qualifications, education, and clinical experience in the area of low vision. For example, Lambert[6] raised the following concerns about occupational therapists:

- They may be unfamiliar with the various disciplines in the field, and thereby fail to appropriately refer clients for other needed services.

- They have inadequate knowledge or specialized training in low vision.

- Clinics may favor occupational therapy in the delivery of low vision services even though more disability-specific professionals may be the most appropriate provider.

Similar concerns were raised by Orr and Huebner[7] in 2001 when they expressed their unease about occupational therapists' lack of specialized knowledge base and skills needed to work with the low vision population.

Others have argued that there are a number of important reasons why occupational therapist should play a primary role in low vision rehabilitation[2,8]:

- Although the elderly comprise the majority of the low vision population, they are the most underserved by existing state, charitable, and private programs. Because of the lack of availability of services treatment through the blindness system, rehabilitation may be delayed and these individuals are likely to become socially isolated, depressed, and dependent. Involvement of occupational therapists through the health care system provides significantly greater access to low vision rehabilitation for the elderly.[8]

- Two-thirds of older persons have at least one other chronic condition in addition to low vision that limits their independent functioning. Occupational therapists are already primary providers for older clients with other chronic conditions.[2,8] Occupational therapists are trained in the physical, cognitive, sensory, and psychological aspects of disability and aging, and therefore, may be the natural choice of professionals to work with older persons whose limitations in daily living are a result of a combination of deficits.[2]

- Occupational therapists are more evenly distributed throughout the United States than orientation and mobility specialists and vision rehabilitation therapists who tend to be located in larger metropolitan areas. Low vision services can be more widely disseminated through the health care delivery system.[2]

Occupational therapy on a national level, as well as individual therapists, have reacted in a positive way to this debate. In the past 20 years, many occupational therapists have gained the knowledge base and clinical skills necessary to provide excellent care to clients requiring low vision rehabilitation. This has been accomplished though a variety of learning formats including independent study, continuing education courses, clinical internships, and university-based training. In addition, many occupational therapists have completed the certification process run by the ACVREP.

Occupational therapist active in low vision rehabilitation may work closely with vision rehabilitation therapists and orientation and mobility specialists in various clinical settings. As occupational therapists become involved it is critical to be aware of the history of low vision rehabilitation in the United States, the various professions involved, and some of the sensitivities and important political issues described above.

Practice Opportunities

There are many potential practice opportunities available for occupational therapists who wish to become involved in the field of low vision rehabilitation. These opportunities range from employment in hospitals (both inpatient and outpatient), nursing homes, assisted-living facilities, offices of ophthalmologists and optometrists, and independent home health care, as well as employment in home health agencies. The underlying essential ingredient to finding these opportunities is to know where to look for patients with low vision. Based on the information about prevalence and incidence of low vision we know this means looking for patients who are 65 years of age and older. These patients are found in nursing homes, assisted-living facilities, and hospital settings. The ophthalmologists most likely to see patients with low vision are the retinal, cataract, and glaucoma specialists. Optometrists with a specialty practice in low vision, of course, are also likely to be good resources for patients with low vision.

Home Health

A wonderful private practice opportunity for occupational therapists is providing low vision evaluations and rehabilitation in the client's home. To function in this capacity the occupational therapist must first enroll as a private practitioner in Medicare and obtain a Medicare provider number. Information about becoming a provider and an application are available at www.cms.gov. A list of Medicare carriers can be found at the Centers for Medicare and Medicaid Services (CMS) Web site: http://cms.hhs.gov/contacts/incardir.asp. After obtaining this provider number the therapist is able to perform both evaluation and treatment services and bill Medicare. In this mode of practice the occupational therapist is a private practitioner and must have an office address for billing while providing care in the client's home. The therapist must market him- or herself to other professionals who are likely to encounter elderly clients with low vision. Such professionals include ophthalmologists (primarily retinal, glaucoma, and cataract specialists), low vision optometrists, geriatricians, large eye hospitals, social workers, and rehabilitation therapists such as physical therapists, speech-language pathologists, other occupational therapists, and recreational therapists.

Nursing Home

Research has shown that a high percentage of nursing home residents are visually impaired. For example, Horowitz[9] conducted a study of a 250-bed, long-term facility and found that 23% were visually impaired. Vision loss among nursing home residents complicates many of the care-related tasks for which providers of nursing home services are responsible, and interferes with the clients' ability to engage in activities of daily living.[10] Thus, there is a significant need for occupational therapists who currently work in nursing homes to become involved in low vision rehabilitation in order to care for a large percentage of their clients.

Acute Care/Rehabilitation Hospital

We know that the two most common causes of low vision are macular degeneration and diabetic retinopathy. Older people with cardiovascular disease and diabetes make up a significant percentage of the patients in acute care and rehabilitation hospitals. These are the same people who are likely to have macular degeneration and low vision. In addition, many patients admitted to rehabilitation hospitals with cerebrovascular accident or traumatic brain injury may experience significant visual field loss, which also falls into the category of low vision impairment. Thus, occupational therapists working in this setting have an opportunity to establish a low vision service within such rehabilitation departments. Development of such a service helps to ensure that there are therapists with appropriate clinical ability and that clients receive appropriate and timely treatment. Occupational therapists may practice in outpatient and home-health services associated with rehabilitation hospitals enabling reimbursement from private insurers as well and Medicare and Medicaid.

Retirement/Assisted-Living Communities

Opportunities also exist in assisted-living communities because of the aging population that live in such facilities. The basic underlying theme when looking for the population that is likely to need low vision care is to find older adults. An occupational therapist can arrange to make educational presentations about low vision and low vision rehabilitation in assisted-living communities. Providing such education and helping people better understand what can be accomplished in spite of permanent vision loss can be quite important for people. Many individuals do not even seek care because they have simply been told by previous professionals that there is not much that can be done. The occupational therapist can develop a working relationship with an ophthalmologist and/or a low vision optometrist. People seeking more information or additional care for their visual impairment can be referred to an eye care professional for an evaluation. If low vision rehabilitation is required, the eye care professional can then refer the client to the occupational therapist for such care. This care would be provided by the occupational therapist as an independent provider.

Community-Based Agencies

Until the late 1990s, most of the low vision rehabilitation in the United States was provided within the service delivery system that has been called the "Blindness System."[4] This system is also sometimes referred to as the educational rehabilitation model, or the nonmedical vision rehabilitation system.[4,11] This system is a comprehensive nationwide network of services consisting of state, federal, and private agencies serving children and adults with blindness and low vision.[4,12] Because of limited public funds to support these services, however, only a limited percentage of people requiring low vision rehabilitation are able to receive these services in community-based, state, or federally funded agencies. This scarcity of resources has led some vision rehabilitation agencies to hire occupational therapists to provide services.[7] The advantage is that occupational therapists can be reimbursed by Medicare while vision rehabilitation therapists and orientation and mobility specialists cannot. Thus, there may be opportunities for occupational therapists in these agencies. Occupational therapists working in these agencies would generally be salaried employees.

Low Vision Optometrist

A nonconventional opportunity would be to become affiliated with a low vision optometrist. They design and prescribe low vision devices (eg, optical, non-optical, electronic) and make recommendations about lighting, contrast, and other environmental factors that influence vision. Although low vision optometrists should ideally work closely with low vision therapists, this may not always be the case. Some low vision optometrists are not fully aware of the capabilities of occupational therapists. Thus, once an occupational therapist identifies a low vision optometrist in the area, one challenge may be to educate this eye care professional about the role of occupational therapy in low vision rehabilitation.

A second challenge is trying to locate a qualified low vision optometrist. The profession of optometry does not recognize "specialties." Therefore, any optometrist can provide low vision services, regardless of his or her experience in this area. However, the American Academy of Optometry Low Vision Section has a Diplomate program for interested optometrists. To become a Diplomate in Low Vision, an optometrist must pass a written test, an oral examination, and a practical low vision examination. Currently, there are only about 45 practicing Low Vision Diplomates worldwide. A current list of optometrists who have successfully completed this process can be found on the American Academy of Optometry Web site (www.aaopt.org/).[13] The American Optometric Association also has a Vision Rehabilitation Section (www.aoa.org/x4786.xml). Although there is no testing program required to become a member of this section, optometrists who have joined are likely to have a strong interest in the area of low vision. Some low vision optometrists have completed a residency program, while others have chosen to specialize in this area and have acquired additional knowledge and clinical skills through continuing education and independent learning. Currently, there are about 38,000 optometrists in the United States and there are about 1000 members in the Vision Rehabilitation Section of the American Optometric Association.

There are two potential ways of working with the low vision optometrist. The first method would be as an employee. The low vision optometrist would refer patients to the occupational therapist working in his or her practice. The therapist would evaluate and provide treatment in the doctor's office. The office would bill and be reimbursed for the therapist's services and provide an hourly salary to the occupational therapist. Another scenario would be for the low vision optometrist to refer patients to an occupational therapist functioning as an independent provider. In this case, the therapist would not provide services in the doctor's office. Rather he or she would need an office and also could provide services in the client's home. In either case, the occupational therapist would require registration as an independent provider. In some states not all private insurers recognize occupational therapists as independent providers. In these situations occupational therapists may work for and bill through agencies or outpatient rehabilitation services.

Ophthalmologist

Perhaps the most effective way of finding clients who require low vision rehabilitation is to work with an ophthalmologist. Ophthalmologists are physicians who specialize in the diagnosis and treatment of eye disease by completing a residency in ophthalmology. Many ophthalmologists also complete a fellowship program to further specialize in an area of ophthalmology. A number of specialty areas exist including specialists in cataract, glaucoma, retina, cornea, pediatric ophthalmology, and neuro-ophthalmology. Ophthalmologists most likely to treat clients with low vision are the retinal, glaucoma, and cataract specialists. Since most patients who have low vision have retinal problems or loss of vision due to glaucoma, these are the types of specialists with whom the occupational therapist should develop relationships. Doctors in these offices examine a high percentage of patients with various retinopathies on a daily basis. A very high percentage of their patients require further care. Unfortunately, many ophthalmologists do not refer for low vision rehabilitation.[14] Occupational therapists can identify these ophthalmologists and arrange a visit at which the therapist can educate the physician about his or her capabilities and the potential advantages for the patients in the practice. There is no specific subspecialty of low vision in the profession of ophthalmology. There are currently about 16,000 practicing ophthalmologists in the United States.

The primary areas of interest and responsibility of ophthalmologists are the diagnosis and treatment of eye disease. Treatment modalities generally involve the use of medication and surgery. Thus, clients often see the ophthalmologist first because of a perceived significant change in vision. The ophthalmologist attempts to restore normal visual function by treating the eye disease. In some cases this fails; in other cases the vision can never be restored to normal and the client is now faced with permanent low vision. It is at this point that the ophthalmologist should refer the client with low vision to other professionals for further evaluation and rehabilitation.

The same working relationships described for the low vision optometrist apply to working with the ophthalmologist.

Eye Hospital

Some large metropolitan areas in the United States have free-standing eye hospitals. A high percentage of adult patients seen at these hospitals have low vision. Many of these institutions have a low vision optometrist on staff and some may already have established low vision rehabilitation programs. If not, eye hospitals represent a potential opportunity for occupational therapists. Occupational therapists working in such a setting would generally be employees.

Colleges of Optometry—Patient Care Clinics

There are 20 Colleges of Optometry in the United States and Puerto Rico. All of these colleges have large patient care clinics with a low vision service. These low vision services are used to train optometry students in all aspects of low vision care, including rehabilitation. The low vision departments are staffed by optometrists who have completed residencies in low vision and/or have many years of experience as low vision specialists. They are generally well-versed in the current trends in low vision care and research and should have an understanding of the important role that occupational therapists have begun to play in low vision rehabilitation. Some of these clinics may already employ rehabilitation therapists. Others, however, may not offer full-scope low vision care. Thus, this is a potential opportunity for an occupational therapist. The key contact person would be the Chief of the Low Vision Service at the College of Optometry. The occupational therapist would not have to convince this individual of the importance of low vision rehabilitation. Rather, the presentation would emphasize the unique contributions that occupational therapists could make in the low vision service.

Billing/Insurance/Medicare Issues

Reimbursement Sources

The impetus for occupational therapy's involvement in the area of low vision rehabilitation was the 1991 amendment by the Health Care Financing Administration that allowed Medicare coverage for the first time for licensed health care providers for low vision rehabilitation. Medicare is currently the main source of reimbursement for low vision rehabilitation for occupational therapists. Other potential reimbursement sources are HMOs (health maintenance organizations), private insurance companies, State agencies for the blind and visually impaired, and private paying clients.

Medicare and Low Vision Rehabilitation (Outpatient Settings)

The information we provide in this section was current when our manuscript was submitted to the publisher. However, it is important to understand that the CMS occasionally make policy changes and the reader should carefully review the CMS Web site and seek current information about billing for low vision rehabilitation services (www.cms.gov).

The current CMS policy on low vision rehabilitation in an outpatient setting (Medicare B) states that occupational therapy is a covered service if it meets the following criteria:

- Services must be prescribed by a physician and furnished under a physician-approved plan of care.
- Services must be performed by an occupational therapist or occupational therapy assistant under the supervision of an occupational therapist.
- Services must be reasonable and medically necessary for treatment of an individual's illness (must result in significant improvement in level of function within reasonable period of time). Medically necessary is defined by the diagnostic code and rehabilitation potential.

According to CMS, the purpose of vision rehabilitative therapy is to maximize the use of residual vision and provide patients with many practical adaptations for activities of daily living. In doing so, it builds the confidence that is necessary for ongoing creative problem solving. Rehabilitation appears to be more effective if it is started as soon as functional visual difficulties are identified.

There can be coverage variations among Medicare contractors, called fiscal intermediaries, which are allowed to establish local policies. Thus, it is important to check with your local Medicare fiscal intermediary before initiating any low vision rehabilitation with clients.

According to CMS, coverage of low vision rehabilitation services is considered reasonable and necessary only for patients with a clear medical need. To meet the criteria established by CMS you must demonstrate that:

- The patient has a moderate to severe visual impairment not correctable by conventional refractive means.

- The patient has a clear potential for significant improvement in function following rehabilitation over a reasonable period of time.

Before providing services the occupational therapist must develop a written evaluation and treatment plan. The treatment plan should include:

- An initial assessment that documents the level of visual impairment
- A plan of care identifying specific goals to be fulfilled during rehabilitation
- A definition of specific rehabilitative services to be provided during the course of rehabilitation
- A reasonable estimate of when the goals will be reached and the frequency at which the services will be provided

Periodic follow-up evaluations must be performed by the referring physician during the course of the rehabilitation.

Currently, CMS bases the maximum number of treatment sessions on the severity of the visual impairment, and the level of visual impairment is based on visual acuity with best correction and some forms of field loss. As of January 2010, individuals with central field loss, generalized field constriction, homonymous and heteronymous bilateral field deficits, or acuity loss of worse than 20/60 in the better eye are eligible for services.

Sessions are generally conducted over a 3-month period of time with intervals appropriate to the patient's rehabilitation needs. If additional sessions are necessary, medical record documentation must indicate the need for additional sessions.

Coding Guidelines

Vision rehabilitation therapy should be provided by an occupational therapist or a physician or incident to a physician's professional services when performed by nonphysician personnel under direct supervision. The incident to a physician rules apply to vision rehabilitation therapists and orientation and mobility specialists who are not licensed and are unable to perform these services independently. Occupational therapists can perform these services independently and do not require direct supervision by the physician.

Proper coding requires determination of the primary and secondary diagnoses and the use of ICD-9-CM (*International Classification of Diseases, Ninth Revision, Clinical Modification*) codes. The 369 codes reflect the level of visual impairment and this must always be the primary diagnosis. The secondary codes are the 362-377 codes and these reflect the actual eye disease causing the visual impairment. The eye disease must always be listed as the secondary diagnosis.

Table 15-3 is a convenient chart that can be used to determine the appropriate code to be used for a client based on the distance visual acuity measurement. To demonstrate the use of the chart, let us assume we have a client who has been referred to us for low vision rehabilitation. The referring eye doctor reports that the visual acuity in the right eye is 20/120 and the visual acuity in the left eye is 20/1500. The first step is to determine the level of impairment that each visual acuity represents. Looking at Table 15-3, one can determine that 20/120 falls into the category of "moderate impairment" (left-hand column of table) and 20/1500 falls into the category of "near total impairment" (left-hand column of table). The next step is to locate the category of "moderate impairment" on the left hand column of the chart and move across that row until it intersects with the column with the heading of "near total impairment." The code found at the intersection of these the row and column is the primary diagnosis used for Medicare billing. In this case the code would be 369.17. A second example is a client with a visual acuity of 20/200 in the right eye and 20/300 in the left eye. Use the approach suggested above. In this case both acuities fall in the category of "severe impairment." Locate "severe impairment" in the left-hand column and move across this row until it intersects with "severe impairment" on the top column. The diagnostic code is 369.22.

Table 15-3

ICD-9-CM Codes for Visual Impairment—Primary Diagnosis

	Normal Vision	Near Normal Vision	Moderate Impairment	Severe Impairment	Profound Impairment	Near Total Impairment	Total Impairment
Normal vision 20/20 to 20/25			369.76	369.73	369.69	369.66	369.63
Near normal vision 20/30 to 20/60			369.75	369.72	369.68	369.65	369.62
Moderate impairment 20/80 to 20/160	369.76	369.75	369.25	369.24	369.18	369.17	369.16
Severe impairment 20/200 to 20/400 or VF ≤20 degrees	369.73	369.72	369.24	369.22	369.14	369.13	369.12
Profound impairment 20/500 to 20/1000 or VF ≤10 degrees	369.69	369.68	369.18	369.14	369.08	369.07	369.06
Near total impairment 20/1250 to 20/2500 or VF ≤5 degrees	369.68	369.65	369.17	369.13	369.07	369.04	369.03
Total impairment No light perception (NLP)	369.63	369.62	369.16	369.12	369.06	369.03	369.01
Visual field defects		368.41 Scotoma involving central area		368.45 Visual field defects, generalized contraction or constriction		368.46 Homonymous bilateral field defects	368.47 Heteronymous bilateral field defects

Adapted from Hart AC. *The Professional ICD-9-CM Code Book.* Reston, VA: St. Anthony Publishing; 2000.

Table 15-4

Common ICD-9-CM Billing Codes for Secondary Diagnosis

362.01	Diabetic retinopathy, background
362.02	Diabetic retinopathy, proliferate
362.35	Central retinal vein occlusion
362.51	Macular degeneration, dry
362.52	Macular degeneration, wet
362.74	Retinitis pigmentosa
365.10	Glaucoma, open-angle, unspecified
365.20	Glaucoma, primary, angle-closure, unspecified
366.10	Cataract, senile, unspecified
368.46	Field deficit homonymous, bilateral
377.10	Optic nerve atrophy
377.41	Optic neuritis

Table 15-5

Physical Medicine and Rehabilitation Codes Used for Low Vision Rehabilitation

Evaluations

97003	Occupational therapy evaluation
97004	Occupational therapy re-evaluation

Therapeutic Procedures

97110	Therapeutic procedure, one or more areas, each 15 minutes; therapeutic exercises to develop strength and endurance, range of motion, and flexibility.
97112	Neuromuscular re-education of movement, balance, coordination, kinesthetic sense, posture, and proprioception.
97530	Therapeutic activities, direct (one-on-one) patient contact by the provider (use of dynamic activities to improve functional performance), one-on-one treatment each 15 minutes.
97533	Sensory integrative techniques to enhance sensory processing and promote adaptive responses to environmental demands, direct (one-on-one) patient contact by provider, each 15 minutes.
97535	Self-care/home management training (eg, activities of daily living and compensatory training, meal preparation, safety procedures, and instructions in use of adaptive equipment), direct one-on-one contact by provider, each 15 minutes.
97537	Community/reintegration training (eg, shopping, transportation, money management, avocational activities and/or work environment/modification analysis, work task analysis), direct one-on-one contact by provider, each 15 minutes.

The secondary diagnosis must be determined by the referring eye doctor. Table 15-4 lists some of the more common diagnoses of low vision clients.

The treatment codes for low vision rehabilitation are the traditional PM&R codes used by occupational therapists and are listed in Table 15-5.

Referrals for Low Vision Rehabilitation

Medicare requires that an occupational therapist receive a referral from a physician before initiating an evaluation or low vision rehabilitation. Initially, this referral could only be issued by an ophthalmologist or other medical doctor. However, the Balanced Budget Refinements Act (P.L. 106-113) signed into law November 29, 1999, includes a technical amendment that recognizes optometrists as "physicians" for purposes of certifying a Medicare beneficiary's need for occupational therapy services under Medicare Part B. This new Federal law does not, however, supercede State law. Currently, optometrists can provide a referral to an occupational therapists in 37 of the 50 states. To determine the regulation in your state it is important to check with your state occupational therapy association. You can check your state law using the "Licensure Area" on the AOTA Web site at www.aota.org to access the State Occupational Therapy Law Database.

Current Reimbursement Rates for Vision Rehabilitation Services

Information about Medicare reimbursement rates can easily be accessed for any location in the United States at the CMS Web site (www.cms.gov/physicians/mpfsapp/step0.asp).

Summary

In this chapter we tried to provide answers about many of the critical questions and issues that occupational therapists encounter when they begin to provide low vision rehabilitation services. We have included information about low vision education, certification, interaction with other vision rehabilitation professionals, practice opportunities, reimbursement and coding, and Medicare requirements. It is our hope that many readers will use the information in this book to help meet the growing demand for low vision rehabilitation services in the adult client.

References

1. Congdon N, O'Colmain B, Klaver CC, et al. Causes and prevalence of visual impairment among adults in the United States. *Arch Ophthalmol.* 2004;122(4):477-485.
2. Warren M. Including occupational therapy in low vision rehabilitation. *Am J Occup Ther.* 1995;49(9):857-860.
3. Elliott DB, Trukolo-Ilic M, Strong JG, Pace R, Plotkin A, Bevers P. Demographic characteristics of the vision-disabled elderly. *Invest Ophthalmol Vis Sci.* 1997;38:2566-2575.
4. Scheiman M, Scheiman M, Whittaker S. *Low Vision Rehabilitation: A Practical Guide for Occupational Therapists.* Thorofare, NJ: SLACK Incorporated; 2007.
5. Warren M. *Low Vision: Occupational Therapy Intervention With the Older Adult.* Bethesda, MD: American Occupational Therapy Association; 2000.
6. Lambert J. Occupational therapists, orientation and mobility specialists and rehabilitation teachers. *J Vis Imp Blind.* 1994;88:297-298.
7. Orr AL, Huebner K. Toward a collaborative working relationship among vision rehabilitation and allied health professionals. *J Vis Imp Blind.* 2001;95(8):468-482.
8. McGinty Bachelder J, Harkins D. Do occupational therapists have a primary role in low vision rehabilitation? *Am J Occup Ther.* 1995;49(9):927-930.
9. Horowitz A. Vision impairment and functional disability among nursing home residents. *The Gerontologist.* 1994;34:316-323.
10. Horowitz A, Balistreri E, Stuen R, Fangmeier R. Visual impairment and rehabilitation needs of nursing home residents. *J Vis Imp Blind.* 1995;88:7-15.
11. Mogk L, Goodrich G. The history and future of low vision services in the United States. *J Vis Imp Blind.* 2004;Oct:585-600.
12. Ponchillia PE, Ponchillia SV. *Foundations of Rehabilitation Teaching With Persons Who Are Blind or Visually Impaired.* New York, NY: American Foundation for the Blind; 1966:3-21.
13. American Academy of Optometry. *American Academy of Optometry Low Vision Section List of Low Vision Diplomates.* 2010.
14. Pankow L, Luchins D. Geriatric low vision referrals by ophthalmologists in a senior health center. *J Vis Imp Blind.* 1998;92(11):748-753.

Resources

Academy for Certification of Vision Rehabilitation & Education Professionals
www.acvrep.org/

Chapter Sixteen

The Inter-Relationship Model

Mitchell Scheiman, OD, FCOVD, FAAO and
Maxine Scheiman, MEd, OTR/L, CLVT

Overview

The objective of this chapter is to describe an inter-relationship model for occupational therapists, optometrists, and other professions involved with vision rehabilitation. Pediatric occupational therapists care for children with a wide variety of problems including cerebral palsy, Down syndrome, other types of mental retardation, spina bifida, low birth weight syndrome, pervasive developmental delay, sensory integrative dysfunction, and child abuse and neglect. The most common conditions found in these children include optical problems such as hyperopia, myopia, astigmatism, strabismus, amblyopia, nystagmus, optic atrophy, and visual information processing problems.

For occupational therapists working with adults, the most common patients seen are those who have experienced cerebrovascular accident, traumatic brain injury, and spinal cord injury. Studies demonstrate that nearly half of the patients admitted to a long-term rehabilitation facility after brain injury have visual system deficits, primarily in the areas of binocular vision, accommodation, eye movement disorders, visual field deficits and neglect, strabismus, reduced visual acuity, and decreased contrast sensitivity. In recent years, occupational therapists have also become more involved in low vision rehabilitation and, in many settings, are now part of the low vision rehabilitation team.[1-3]

Whether working with children or adults, occupational therapists often manage patients who have vision disorders. Hopefully, we have demonstrated that optometry, as a result of its expansive model of vision and concern about function and performance, is the profession of choice to help occupational therapists manage patients with vision disorders.

In previous chapters, we included case reports of various patients co-managed by optometrists and occupational therapists and other visual rehabilitation professionals. These cases are representative of the type of inter-relationship we feel is appropriate. The model we propose is one in which occupational therapists, optometrists, vision rehabilitation therapists (formerly rehabilitation teachers), orientation and mobility specialists, and teachers of children who are visually impaired recognize that certain patients require close interaction between the various professions to achieve maximum benefit.

Of course, the need for co-management works both ways. There are certainly patients who optometrists evaluate who should be co-managed with occupational therapists and other vision rehabilitation specialists. A good example is the learning disabled child with visual information processing problems. Many of these children have difficulty with visual motor integration that interferes with handwriting and copying skills. Some optometrists may design vision therapy programs to treat these children without consultation with occupational therapists. In our experience, some of these children also have fine motor and gross motor problems that could be interfering with handwriting skills, and they would benefit from an occupational therapy evaluation to evaluate these areas. Occupational therapists certainly have much broader clinical training in these areas. We believe that optometrists should seek consultation with occupational therapists in these cases. If gross and fine motor problems are present, optometrists should co-manage these patients with occupational therapists.

Inter-Relationship Model

We suggest a four-step model that can be applied to most patients seen by occupational therapists. We expect that this model will lead to the most successful management possible for learning disabled children, developmentally delayed children, and children with brain injury, cerebrovascular accident, and visual impairment.

Step One: Rule Out Vision Problems

Our first recommendation is that occupational therapists rule out vision problems in all patients before developing a treatment approach. This can be accomplished in one of two ways. Some therapists may choose to screen all patients using the screening battery presented in Chapter Six. If a patient fails any portion of this screening battery, a referral should be made to an optometrist with the education, experience, and philosophy suggested in this book. As discussed in Chapter Six, the screening battery cannot be used with all patients. Infants, preverbal children, and adults with severe perceptual, cognitive, and attention problems will be very difficult to evaluate. In such cases, a referral for a comprehensive vision examination should be made. Alternatively, some occupational therapists may make the decision to simply refer all patients for a comprehensive vision examination before initiating a therapy program.

There will certainly be many patients who return to the occupational therapist with a report that all three areas of visual function—acuity and eye health, visual efficiency, and visual information processing—are normal. This is critical information and allows the occupational therapist to confidently plan a treatment approach having eliminated vision as an issue. In this text, we have shown, however, that a large percentage of patients will have vision deficits that need to be addressed. The case studies presented in Chapters Eight, Ten, Eleven, Twelve, and Fourteen are characteristic of the types of patients occupational therapists treat on a daily basis. If you review these cases, you will appreciate the wide variety of visual deficits that can occur and the importance of early identification.

In Chapter Eight, two cases of learning disabled children were presented. The first child was evaluated by a school occupational therapist and had a visual efficiency problem and only required optometric intervention. The second child was considerably more complicated and had binocular vision, ocular motility, and visual information processing problems along with problems with bilateral integration, strength, upper limb coordination, fine motor control, postural instability, and low muscle tone. The occupational therapist and optometrist worked together to prioritize the treatment program for the various problems identified. Eyeglasses were prescribed immediately, and the child had one vision therapy and one occupational therapy visit per week. The occupational therapist worked on fine motor skills, handwriting, and low muscle tone while the optometrist simultaneously treated the binocular vision and ocular motor problems with vision therapy.

In Chapter Ten, Dr. Hellerstein discussed five case studies involving patients with brain injury. All five cases demonstrated the importance of early identification and treatment of vision disorders. In the first case, a patient required optometric intervention 2½ years after the original injury because she was still suffering from headaches, double vision, blurred vision, and attention and concentration deficits. These problems interfered with almost every aspect of her life, and she was unable to perform everyday tasks such as cooking, shopping, writing, and driving. Visual efficiency problems were found, and the optometrist prescribed two pairs of glasses and vision therapy. This treatment led to significant improvement in activities of daily living. This case is particularly supportive of the first step in our model, which is referral for a vision examination. This patient would have undoubtedly progressed more quickly in her various rehabilitative programs had the vision problems been identified and treated initially.

The second case demonstrated the importance of ocular motor therapy after cerebrovascular accident and the benefit of vision therapy for subsequent occupational therapy to improve walking and mobility skills. In the third case, prescription of eyeglasses and recommendations for ocular motor therapy by the occupational therapist under optometric supervision were helpful in teaching the patient to compensate for a lower visual field deficit. This case is important because it demonstrates that in some clinical settings it may be more appropriate for the occupational therapist to carry out vision therapy under the supervision of an optometrist than for the optometrist to perform the vision therapy him- or herself. The final two cases demonstrated how simply prescribing glasses for refractive error is important and how attention to the type of lens used (single vision lens compared to bifocal) can be instrumental in helping overcome certain problems.

In Chapter Eleven, Drs. Appel and Ciner presented an important case study of a 7-year-old developmentally disabled girl with a history of head trauma who had been undergoing a vision stimulation program in her educational setting that involved eye movement activities. The child's mother reported that she was very frustrated during these activities, and the vision teacher was frustrated by the girl's lack of cooperation, especially during vertical tracking activities. Optometric testing revealed a marked vertical gaze palsy that prevented the girl from initiating and maintaining vertical gaze movements. She had been asked to perform an activity that was impossible for her to successfully accomplish. Therapy goals were re-established to teach her to compensate for the problem rather than try to remediate it.

Another interesting case was presented about a 10-year-old girl with a history of clumsiness. This resulted in many bumps and bruises incurred during mobility-related activities. The optometric evaluation revealed a constriction in the upper visual field area to approximately 5 degrees above fixation. The cause for the clumsiness was actually an upper visual field impairment. A referral was made for orientation and mobility services, and protective eyewear was prescribed.

Step Two: Occupational Therapy Evaluation

After consultation with an optometrist, the occupational therapist can develop an appropriate evaluation to assess strengths and weaknesses of the patient. Knowing that the visual system has been adequately examined allows the therapist to select appropriate evaluation tools and more confidently interpret the results of his or her testing. This point has been emphasized by several authors.[4-6] They stress that normal visual information processing or visual perceptual function is dependent on normal visual acuity and visual efficiency. Scheiman and Rouse,[4] Warren,[5] and Bouska et al[6] have all developed evaluation models that have emphasized this point. They discuss the importance of detecting and treating ocular motor, accommodative, and binocular vision disorders before the management of visual processing disorders.

Table 16-1

Conditions That Require Vision Therapy Treatment in an Optometric Office

- Amblyopia
- Strabismus
- Intermittent strabismus
- Nonstrabismic binocular vision disorders
- Accommodative disorders
- Ocular motility disorders associated with accommodative and binocular vision disorders

---

Table 16-2

Circumstances That Suggest Vision Therapy in an Occupational Therapy Setting Under Optometric Supervision

- Preschool children with other impairments and delays, very limited attention and concentration
- Older children with mental retardation and multiple impairments
- Traumatic brain injury and cerebrovascular accident patients undergoing rehabilitation in a rehabilitation hospital

---

In the area of low vision rehabilitation, it is recommended that the occupational therapist and appropriate vision-related rehabilitation professional jointly perform a thorough, systematic assessment of an individual's work, home, and/or school environments. The purpose of such an assessment is to determine the modifications that may be required in order to meet the daily living, safety, and accessibility needs of the individual who is visually impaired.

Step Three: Consultation

After both evaluations have been completed, the various professionals should discuss their respective test findings and conclusions. This consultation would most likely occur over the phone. The objectives of this phone consultation are to develop a complete list of deficits, to prioritize the significance of these disorders in terms of the urgency for treatment, and, finally, to develop a treatment program in which all professionals contribute when appropriate.

If vision therapy is appropriate, a decision will have to be made about who will provide the vision therapy. We have suggested in this book that in some cases vision therapy must be implemented in an optometric office and at other times vision therapy may be performed by an occupational therapist with direct supervision by the optometrist. The determining factors are the type of disorder (Table 16-1) and the developmental age or level of functioning of the patient (Table 16-2).

Generally, patients must be functioning at about a 6-year-old level to benefit from vision therapy in an optometric office. The sessions usually last about 45 minutes and require a certain level of attention and concentration. We have found that for preschool and for developmentally delayed children, certain vision conditions can be effectively treated by an occupational therapist with optometric supervision. Tracking and visual information processing problems and saccadic and pursuit disorders are included in this category. In our experience, occupational therapists are very effective with these populations and can incorporate vision therapy for these conditions into the overall occupational therapy treatment plan.

The cases discussed in Chapter Twelve are examples of this approach. In all three cases, significant visual deficits were present. Glasses were prescribed for two of the children and a low vision aid for the third. In all three cases, the optometrist helped develop a vision therapy program that could be administered by the occupational therapist. The vision conditions treated included visual information processing problems and tracking disorders. The optometrists provided ongoing consultation and follow-up during the course of treatment.

If low vision rehabilitation is necessary, the occupational therapist will often have to work along with the vision rehabilitation therapist and/or orientation and mobility specialist. For example, in Chapter Fourteen, a case is presented in which the vision rehabilitation therapist performed an evaluation of home management; medication management; clothing and personal management; communication abilities, including braille, computer skills, handwriting, reading, and recording; recreation and leisure activities; and indoor mobility. Based on these results, she developed goals for adaptive equipment, environmental modifications, and instructional strategies. The vision rehabilitation therapist requested an occupational therapy consultation in two specific training areas: Eating skills and handwriting. It was apparent that the functional impact of the patient's combined visual and physical impairments created a significant barrier to the mastery of these specific activities of daily living skills through rehabilitation therapy intervention alone. The occupational therapist conducted the assessment in conjunction with a regularly scheduled rehabilitation therapy in-home training session and developed goals for adaptive equipment recommendations and instructional strategies.

Step Four: Periodic Phone Consultation

When various professionals are providing treatment for the patient, periodic phone consultation is important to discuss progress and re-evaluation findings. In other cases, the decision may have been made initially about how to prioritize the various treatments that may be necessary. In such cases, periodic phone consultation is necessary.

Summary

Occupational therapists, whether working with children or adults, often manage patients who have vision disorders. If the four-step inter-relationship model presented in this chapter is followed, we believe that patients served by both professions will achieve maximum benefit.

References

1. American Occupational Therapy Association. *Vision Services and Occupational Therapy*. Bethesda, MD: Author; 2000.
2. Warren M. *Occupational Therapy Practice Guidelines for Adults With Low Vision*. Bethesda, MD: American Occupational Therapy Association; 1998.
3. Kern T, Miller N. Occupational therapy and collaborative interventions for adults with low vision. In: Gentile M, ed. *A Therapist's Guide to the Evaluation and Treatment of Low Vision*. Bethesda, MD: American Occupational Therapy Association; 493-536.
4. Scheiman M, Rouse MW. *Optometric Management of Learning Related Vision Problems*. 2nd ed. St. Louis, MO: CV Mosby; 2006.
5. Warren M. Identification of visual scanning deficits in adults after cerebrovascular accident. *Am J Occup Ther*. 1990;44:391-399.
6. Bouska MJ, Kauffman NA, Marcus SE. Disorders of the visual perceptual system. In: Umphred DA, Jewell MJ, eds. *Neurological Rehabilitation*. St. Louis, MO: CV Mosby; 1985:552-585.

Chapter Seventeen

Theory and Guidelines for Visual Task Analysis and Synthesis

Kathleen Tsurumi, OTR and Valorie Todd, OTR

Introduction

Task analysis and synthesis are primary tools of occupational therapy. They form the basis for eliciting behaviors along a function/dysfunction continuum in both evaluation and intervention.[1] Task analysis is the process of examining an activity to distinguish its component parts. Task synthesis is the process of combining component parts of the human and nonhuman environment so as to design an activity suitable for evaluation or intervention.[1] In this chapter, we propose theory and guidelines for a task analysis and synthesis of visual activities that can be used to incorporate many of the concepts discussed earlier in this book into occupational therapy practice.

If an occupational therapist plans to use a standardized test in evaluation, it is analyzed into its component parts so that the score at the end can be interpreted meaningfully. For example, how much visual precision is required to score well on the Bruininks-Oseretsky Test of Motor Proficiency? We know that there are differences in the requirements for motor speed, dexterity, and precision among the subtests of the Bruininks. We need to ask, are there differences in the visual requirements also? In a similar fashion, we need to analyze each standardized test we use. How much does success on the Test of Visual Perceptual Skills (TVPS) depend on attention? How much does success on this test depend on efficient eye movement? How much does it depend on the cognitive ability to detect similarities and differences?

If an occupational therapist prepares a task for intervention, it is synthesized to meet the needs of the particular client. For example, if a client has a peripheral field loss, what modifications must be made in the task so that it is within his or her capability? The design of a specific activity for a specific client is central to a basic assumption of all frames of reference in occupational therapy (ie, that the change process is initiated in that stage of function at which the client is currently able and then proceeds sequentially to more advanced stages of function).[1-3]

Our conceptual framework for visual task analysis and synthesis is consistent with the hierarchical model of vision presented in Chapters Three through Five. It is based on the assumption that two processes are at work when visual function is intact. First, the visual stimulus is seen with

Scheiman M
Understanding and Managing Vision Deficits: A Guide for Occupational Therapists, Third Edition (pp 345-364)
© 2011 SLACK Incorporated

clarity, comfort, and efficiency. Second, the information carried in the visual stimulus is analyzed in a way that meets the needs of the client for the functional demands of daily life. The first process—clarity, comfort, and efficiency of vision—has been addressed in the preceding chapters. This chapter will incorporate this information into an analysis of how visual information processing develops.

Definition of Terms and Organization

We use the term *visual information processing* (or *visual information analysis*) as Dr. Scheiman has defined it in Chapter Five.

Visual information processing refers to a group of cognitive skills used for extracting and organizing visual information from the environment and integrating this information with other sensory modalities, previous experiences, and higher cognitive functions.

As Dr. Scheiman points out, other terms such as *visual perception*, *visual perceptual motor*, and *visual processing* have been used to describe this skill. When we use the terms *perceive* or *perception* in this chapter, we will use them in their narrowest definition: "to become aware of directly through the senses" and "the process of perceiving; becoming aware of directly through the senses."[4] The literature in applied sciences, including occupational therapy, frequently uses the term perception in its broader definition: "any insight, intuition, or knowledge gained by perceiving."[4] Because there seem to be as many meanings of the term perception as there are authors, we will use the terms visual information processing or visual information analysis as defined above rather than the term visual perception when the broader meaning is intended.

Because of the nature of occupational therapy, the range of activities that an occupational therapist uses in evaluation and treatment settings is more extensive than those used in optometry. An occupational therapist can conceivably use any visual activity as a therapeutic medium, ranging from self-care to mobility to recreation to work-related and academic activities. Thus, a conceptual framework for visual task analysis and synthesis for occupational therapy must include all sources of visual stimulation.

We have chosen to use Eleanor Gibson's[5] classification of types of visual stimulation and will organize this chapter around these classifications. The first five sections will cover, in turn, the development of visual information analysis skill in each of Gibson's five categories of visual stimulation. Each section will initially emphasize the process of normal visual information analysis skill. From this, we will extract postulates regarding intervention and draw an application to occupational therapy. Postulates regarding intervention are principles derived from the theory base that can guide the therapist in designing activities for evaluation or intervention. We will give selected examples of how these postulates can translate into occupational therapy practice with adults and children who have dysfunctions in vision or visual information analysis. Section one, which covers the visual information analysis of objects, is divided into three parts and is lengthier than subsequent sections because it introduces concepts that recur in other sections. In the sixth and last section, a quick reference gives in outline form the factors that can be manipulated in the analysis and synthesis of visual tasks for evaluation and for intervention.

Sources of Visual Stimuli

Eleanor Gibson writes that she developed a classification of types of visual stimuli by choosing a classification that would be useful, natural, and functional.[5] This useful, natural, and functional approach suits the occupational therapist very well. Gibson's categories of sources of visual stimuli add clarity to dealing with the sheer volume of possible visual stimuli. Gibson's five categories are:
1. Objects
2. Space

3. Events
4. Representations of objects, space, and events
5. Symbols

Every source of visual stimulation in an activity used by an occupational therapist will fall into one of these five categories.

The occupational therapist will discover in reading this chapter that most of the literature on visual perception has focused on Gibson's fourth category of visual stimulation—representations. This focus has been too limiting for a field as inclusive as occupational therapy. Our activity analysis and synthesis must have a broader base, and Gibson's work gives us this base.

OBJECTS

Objects are three-dimensional forms. A human face is an object that attracts intense visual regard by the infant in the first months of life. The world is full of objects, and the young child attends to them and learns over time to recognize them. How does the child learn to distinguish one object from another visually? How does the adult learn to interpret minute differences between objects that appear to have similar physical characteristics? These questions are important for the therapist who wishes to facilitate learning of visual object discrimination in a child or relearning in an adult who has suffered a loss of function.

As noted earlier, the development of visual discrimination of objects will be discussed in detail. Three crucial processes will be covered separately:
1. An object is differentiated from its background.
2. The salient features that distinguish one object from another are abstracted.
3. Invariant properties and relationships are abstracted.

Together, these active processes support the development of visual recognition, matching, and categorization.[5] Each of these functions requires visual attention and visual memory. For the sake of brevity, attention and memory will be acknowledged, but the reader is referred to texts dedicated to the analysis of these skills for a more complete discussion.[6,7]

Differentiation of an Object From Its Background

To perceive objects, or forms, it is necessary to isolate one aspect of the visual array while "ignoring" other aspects. The initial isolation of one object from a background occurs through the physiological effect of light on the retina.[8] An inhibitory interaction between neighboring retinal cells—lateral inhibition—heightens the contrast at borders, contours, and edges of an object. Other contrast phenomena based on retinal stimulation also create and support form perception. For example, the measure of acuity called contrast sensitivity function, discussed in Chapter Three, is fundamental to form perception under degraded lighting conditions.

In addition to physiological retinal processes, a set of organizing principles have been identified that govern the detection of a figure in a background. These are the Gestalt grouping principles. The Gestalt grouping principles are a set of fundamental, unlearned tendencies to organize the visual field on the basis of the arrangement and relative location of elements.[9] Because they stimulate object detection, these principles can have a direct application to how visual materials might be presented in a treatment or evaluation setting:

- The principle of nearness or proximity. Elements that are closer together tend to be organized or grouped together.
- The principle of similarity. Elements that are similar in physical attributes tend to be grouped together.
- The principle of good continuation. Elements that appear to follow in a uniform direction encourage the continuation of a figure once movement or direction is established.
- The principle of common fate. If a number of elements are in movement, those that appear to be moving in parallel lines tend to be grouped together.

- The principle of closure. Even if elements are fragmentary, grouping occurs in a way that favors the perception of an enclosed figure or a complete figure.

- The principle of symmetry. More balanced and symmetrical forms tend to be given priority over asymmetrical ones.

The factors discussed thus far—lateral inhibition, contrast sensitivity, Gestalt grouping principles, plus other factors related to light energy and retinal structure—influence initial differentiation of an object from its background. These factors are considered to be innate, unlearned, and, therefore, available for use by any client who has normal visual and ocular motor function. Subsequent differentiation of forms is considered to be a learned process based on attention, memory, and cognitive analysis abilities.

Postulates Regarding Intervention in Relation to Visual Information Analysis: General Postulates

1. Visual information processing is enhanced by an intact visual and ocular motor system.

2. If remediation of the visual system is not possible, then compensation strategies must be employed.

These general postulates will apply to all subsequent categories of visual stimulation.

Postulates Regarding Intervention in Relation to the Visual Analysis of Objects: Detection

1. Differentiation of a form from the background is enhanced by adequate lighting conditions, good contrast, and the absence of glare.

2. Differentiation of a form from the background is enhanced when elements in a visual array are organized according to the Gestalt grouping principles of proximity, similarity, good continuation, common fate, closure, and symmetry.

Examples of Occupational Therapy Intervention: Detection of Objects

For the initial detection of an object (ie, the visual isolation of a form from its background), some conditions are within the control of the occupational therapist and some are not. Whether or not the client has an intact retina with normal acuity, optics, peripheral vision, contrast sensitivity, eye movements, and binocular vision and accommodation will obviously affect his or her object detection. Remediation and compensation strategies for deficits in these areas are described in previous chapters.

The environment surrounding the object, which is often accessible to modification, also affects object detection. For example, an occupational therapist attempting to facilitate a client in differentiating a form from the background would monitor the client's environment for appropriate and adequate lighting. Natural, fluorescent, incandescent, and halogen lighting have varying effects on brightness and glare. Fluorescent lights produce a great deal of glare but are commonly used in public environments including schools, hospitals, and offices. The judicious use of supplementary incandescent light, natural light, or even a visor can reduce glare for clients in these environments.

Occupational therapists who make home visits to low vision clients or post-trauma clients can make suggestions for environmental modifications to increase the possibility of adequate object detection for food preparation, self-care, and safe mobility. These suggestions include increasing the brightness of lightbulbs, adding lamps to portions of the home where they were not previously needed, changing floor coverings to add contrast, and providing enlarged or contrasting stove indicators.[10,11]

In schools, occupational therapists can work with teachers to identify and modify the many factors in a classroom that produce glare, such as glossy paper, Formica desks, and sunlight on chalkboards. The occupational therapist can also monitor and modify factors in classrooms that produce poor contrast, such as poorly reproduced worksheets and poor contrast between chalk and chalkboard.[12]

In schools and rehabilitation clinics, Gestalt grouping principles can be applied to enhance the environment for easier detection of objects. Therapists and teachers can work together to modify classroom worksheets so that the child's eye is directed to attend to the appropriate information. Math problems can be separated into distinct units by using grids or color coding. The many elements on a language worksheet can be grouped into similar units by judicious use of spacing and symmetry.

In an occupational therapy clinic, labels for various materials that clients use should be visually clear, consistent, and designed for easy detection. Following Gestalt principles, for example, a set of cabinets containing kitchen supplies in a therapy clinic would have labels that are similar rather than random and that are placed symmetrically rather than in disarray. This organization would facilitate detection of the appropriate label by the client.

Abstraction of the Distinctive Feature

The world is full of objects, and once the young child has isolated the object from its background, he or she must learn over time to distinguish that object from other objects. He or she learns this by identifying salient or distinctive features, in other words, by the minimal set of features that will serve to distinguish the object from other objects that it is not. A cat, for example, is small, it moves in a certain way, and it is furry. This abstraction of distinctive features is at first rather general and becomes more and more specific with experience: my cat has a specific pattern of coloration, and Joey's cat has a different pattern of coloration. In infancy, high-contrast edges, vertices, spots, and moving parts attract attention and form the basis for early discrimination.[13] Attention in the infant is, in fact, stimulus bound or "obligatory attention." This gradually gives way to selective attention and voluntary extended vigilance.[5] By adulthood, the visual discrimination of objects reaches a highly refined state and, with training, can be the basis for earning a livelihood. For example, a horticulturist, trained through education and experience, has far more ability than the average person to achieve the seemingly instantaneous perception of the salient features that distinguish one plant from another, a healthy plant from an at-risk plant, and an edible plant from an inedible plant.

Abstraction of the salient feature or bundle of salient features that distinguish one object from another has been researched extensively.[5] In order to identify the distinctive feature, it is necessary to filter out the irrelevant features and attend to the relevant features. Thus, selective attention is basic to object discrimination. Selective attention is supported by exploratory visual activity. Scanning the visual field, fixation, head turning to direct vision to another location, and re-fixation are all aimed at exposing the feature that will hold the key to identification. Factors that have been found to facilitate identification of the salient feature include exaggeration of the distinctive feature, even to the point of caricature, and elimination or reduction of features that do not carry salient information.[5,8,14] Memory supports the recognition of a distinctive feature if it is encountered again. Recognition is used here to mean an awareness that something perceived has been perceived before (to recognize a face) or an identification of something from past experience or knowledge (to recognize a red-winged blackbird).[4]

Exploration and experience through other sensory systems influences the process of visual analysis. As a child develops more and more independent movement, input from the tactile, proprioceptive, vestibular, and auditory systems adds to the initial identification of salient features and reinforces the visual analysis.[5,15]

Postulates Regarding Intervention in Relation to the Visual Analysis of Objects: Recognition

1. Selective attention to detail is supported by efficient visual exploration.

2. Object identification is facilitated by selective attention and extraction of distinctive or salient features.

3. Identification of distinctive or salient features is facilitated by exaggeration or caricature of the feature and elimination or reduction of nonsalient features.

4. Identification of distinctive or salient features is facilitated by input from other sensory systems that reinforces the visual input.

5. Attention to distinctive or salient features requires ignoring nonsalient features.

6. Object recognition is facilitated by familiarity of visual stimuli.

Examples of Occupational Therapy Intervention: Recognition of Objects

The identification of an object and its subsequent recognition begins with visual attention. It is supported by the sensory and motor abilities of the eye to engage in exploratory activity. It culminates in the extraction of a distinctive feature or bundle of features.

Once again, we see that the efficiency of the ocular motor and visual system is a basic requirement for visual information analysis. This system must be addressed in treatment or in compensation before object discrimination and recognition develop comfortably.

Warren has demonstrated that deficits in visual scanning are present in post-cerebrovascular accident patients and can result in incomplete and erroneous acquisition of visual information about the environment, adversely affecting the performance of daily living skills.[16] Her treatment approach includes measuring visual scanning performance, making the client aware of deficient visual scanning performance, and providing a systematic means of overcoming the deficit with "intellectual override" and/or with intensive, structured training using a scan board.[16]

When visual exploration ability is intact but attention is the interfering factor, object recognition can be facilitated by modifications in the environment. For a low arousal client, a highly stimulating visual target can be designed using primary or neon colors, movement, and auditory embellishments. For a hypervigilant client, providing a secluded, distraction-free environment through such techniques as use of a study carrel or use of headphones to reduce auditory distractions can focus attention. For academic tasks, the density and detail in visual materials can be controlled. A bookmark under the line to be read can focus attention by masking the part of the page that is to be ignored.

The fact that identification and recognition of objects is facilitated by exaggeration can be applied to the design of communication boards for communication handicapped children and adults. If the symbols on these boards are caricatures that exaggerate salient details rather than complex reality-based pictures or photographs, quick visual recognition will be facilitated.

Distinctive features such as shape, contour, weight, and texture are discovered and reinforced through sensory manipulation of objects. Occupational therapists can provide exploratory activities that combine sound, touch, proprioception, and kinesthesia paired with vision. Activities incorporating mouthing, banging, stroking, turning, lifting, dropping, and tracing can contribute to future visual recognition of objects.

Because familiarity of visual stimuli facilitates object recognition, occupational therapists may choose familiar environments or tasks for therapy sessions. The client's own kitchen or bathroom may be the environment of choice for learning daily living tasks. Habituation resulting from familiarity also allows attention to be reallocated to more novel visual stimuli, so that new demands can be added to an intervention.

Abstraction of Invariant Properties and Relationships

An invariant is the relation or property that remains constant over change. One example of this is size, shape, and lightness constancy. Constancy means that the same object can be viewed from different distances, at different angles, and in different lighting conditions and still be perceived as retaining a constant, stable size, shape, and brightness. When we watch a person walk away from us, the image of the person shrinks on our retina, but we perceive the person as retaining true size. When we see a red hat in a dim light, we perceive true red although it may in fact be received on our retina as a darker shade. We see a plate from an angle, and the image on our retina is an ellipse, but we perceive a circular plate. Is this the result of learning, or is it yet another effect of the structure of light and the structure of the retina?

Research has shown that size constancy is almost completely dependent on distance cues that originate in the structure of the retina. The size of the image cast on our retina by light energy is inversely proportional to the distance of the object from us. In addition, all objects in the visual array are subject to this same effect. If a person at a distance appears smaller, all the other objects in the visual array at that distance are relatively smaller as well, in the same inverse proportion.[8]

In shape constancy, an object appears to possess the same shape even when the angle from which it is viewed changes radically. Shape constancy results from and depends on visual cues from the context in which an object is seen. For example, when we look at an open door, we see both the door and the opening. The actual image of the door on the retina may be a parallelogram, but we register the door as a rectangle, because the gap made by the open door is rectangular. Shape constancy therefore depends on visual cues from the environment.

Lightness constancy also depends on environmental cues. When the absolute level of illumination is reduced, objects in the environment are seen as keeping the same relative lightness in relation to one another.[8]

These invariants of size, shape, and lightness are recognized very early in life through retinal cues. Other invariant properties and relationships are learned through experience: the child sees that when milk spills, it flows and takes on many shapes; when the plastic bottle falls, it may bounce but it remains solid and does not change its shape. The recognition of these invariant properties, combined with experience, produces greater and more refined object discrimination. Classes of objects can be formed: some are liquid, some are solid, and some are elastic. Objects can be categorized in a higher order structure. Concept formation based on visual information analysis becomes possible.

Invariant properties are also discovered through other sensory systems. The tactile system registers solidity, liquidity, and elasticity, as does the proprioceptive system. As exploration increases, identification of invariant properties increases.[5,15]

The ability to name objects and concepts leads to a faster identification when a similar visual stimulus is encountered in the future: Is it a hat? A coat? Is it blue? Large? Square? Language facilitates identification and supports progression to finding the most economical set of distinctive features: It's a blue hat with interlocking letters N and Y. Memory facilitates further identification: It's a New York Yankees baseball hat.[5]

Postulates Regarding Intervention in Relation to the Visual Analysis of Objects: Matching and Categorization

1. Constancy of size, shape, and lightness arises from retinal cues.

2. The ability to form concepts is facilitated by abstraction of invariant properties in the visual stimulus.

3. The development of skill in matching objects is facilitated by concept formation based on visual analysis.

4. The development of skill in categorizing objects is facilitated by concept formation based on visual analysis.

5. Progressive differentiation toward the most informative distinctive features is facilitated by language, experience, and memory.

Examples of Occupational Therapy Intervention: Matching and Categorization of Objects

Occupational therapists who work with children will have seen children move through the stages of visual analysis. A 2-year-old child will match colors and shapes to a model but will not be able to take a collection of circles, squares, triangles, and rectangles and order them into separate categories as a 5-year-old child would do. Parents, teachers, and therapists will almost instinctively speak to young children with language that emphasizes the development of visual matching and categorization: "Look, it's a red one." "Oh, this one is the same." Therapists who work with adults with visual information processing dysfunction train themselves to speak to another adult with the same economy and selection in language.

Tasks that encourage awareness of similarities and differences for the development of matching skills can be graded from simple to complex in several ways:

- By type of visual stimulus: From familiar and concrete to unfamiliar and abstract.
- By degree of difference: From gross differences to subtle differences.
- By amount of stimuli: From few visual targets to many visual targets.
- By presentation: From highly organized to less organized.
- By ocular motor requirements: From vertical to horizontal to diagonal placement of visual targets.[12]

Categorization tasks can also be designed on a graded continuum:

- By grouping identical objects into categories (objects that are identical in size, color, internal detail, general configuration).
- By grouping nonidentical objects into categories (objects that differ in internal detail but are alike in general configuration, eg, all the cups, regardless of floral pattern and color; all of the flowers, regardless of type).[17]

Language facilitates concept development. Occupational therapists can follow the developmental pattern in language acquisition in order to apply this principle to task analysis and synthesis. Development of labeling usually begins with identification of objects (nouns) and moves toward identification of other distinctive features such as color and shape (adjectives) and then progresses to action words (verbs).

SPACE

Objects exist in three-dimensional space. The object is a figure on a spatial background. To move toward an object or around an obstacle, the continuity of the surface on which it rests must be appreciated, and gaps in that surface must be recognized. Gaps in a horizontal surface present possible danger of falling. Gaps in a vertical surface present possible opportunity for passing through. Depth and distance judgments are crucial for safety and productivity. In activity analysis and synthesis, the occupational therapist will need to be aware of three aspects of space as a visual stimulus: How the eye perceives space, how movement through space is refined, and how measures of space are learned.

Many theorists have held in the past that a child learns to perceive where objects, obstacles, and gaps are in space by sensory motor learning (eg, by having reached for an object many times, walked toward objects over and over, stumbled over obstacles, and fallen into gaps in the spatial surface). Piaget has been a very strong influence in this direction through his theory of acquisition of schemata as the fundamental process of perceptual learning. He emphasizes the role of exploratory motor activity and repetition of sensory motor situations as essential for schema formation.[17]

More recent research has shown that the awareness of distance and depth, particularly as a basis for locomotion, is inborn, automatic, and unconscious, and can be demonstrated in human infants by at least 6 months of age. The awareness of depth and distance is generated by binocular and monocular cues arising from the optic flow across the retina.[8,18] This optic flow produces motion parallax, binocular disparity, and pictorial cues. These in turn produce invariant relationships that form the basis for the discrimination of real spatial features, just as invariant relationships and properties form the basis for the discrimination of objects.

Motion parallax is the relative apparent movement of elements in the visual array as the observer moves the head or changes the fixation point. One effect of motion parallax is that near objects move across the visual field more rapidly than distant objects. Another effect of motion parallax is that the apparent movement of objects in the visual array will change direction depending on the fixation point. These are monocular cues that both animals and humans use to recognize depth and distance. Research on humans and on many species of animals has shown that this depth perception is an unlearned, innate capability, and that it is present by the age of locomotion. In animals capable of locomotion at birth, depth perception is present at birth. In humans, depth perception can be demonstrated by the age of first locomotion (by the age of crawling).[5,18]

The cues that we use to detect depth and distance in near space, within 16 inches of our eyes, come from binocular parallax. Because the two eyes are set 2 to 3 inches apart in the human, the two slightly different retinal images received by the eyes are fused, creating stereopsis in near space.

Additional information on depth and distance comes from pictorial cues, so named because they are the effects of the interaction of light with the retina that are imitated in paintings. These monocular cues are linear perspective, texture gradient, elevation, interposition, and shading and lighting.

Most theorists now believe that these retinal cues contain the basic information that enables the perception of depth and distance and that refined movement through space is developed using these cues in combination with practice in movement.[8] A ballet dancer leaps to an exact spot by combining retinal cues with the motor control achieved in years of practice. A basketball player scores a basket by combining retinal cues with finely honed reflexes and physical skill. A child sees a distant target at age 2 but has the rotation movements required to throw a ball that far only at age 5. An inexperienced teenage driver has the same retinal cues as an adult to indicate how wide the garage door is, but must learn through practice exactly what degree of attention and motor precision is required to park the car in the garage safely.

Spatial features are identified, recognized, and categorized in the same way that objects are identified, recognized, and categorized: By focused attention to the space, extraction of distinctive features of the space, and extraction of invariant properties and relationships.[5] Language and memory support the process. The young child on a tricycle judges the distance he or she has traveled from home by retinal cues for distance, remembers his or her experience of being that far away once before, and decides whether to continue down the sidewalk or to turn around. The adult skier uses retinal cues to assess the trail before him or her: The degree of slope, the width, the depth of the drop at the edge of the cliff. He or she "names" the trail using the international symbols for degree of difficulty using green circle for easy, blue rectangle for intermediate, black diamond for difficult. He or she remembers his or her past experience with a similar trail and decides whether or not to descend by that route.

We judge distance and depth using retinal cues. We learn to name that distance and depth using the language symbols of our culture: Inches, feet, miles, centimeters, meters. These are two separate skills, one innate and related to whether or not we have intact vision, the other learned and therefore related to memory, attention, and practice. Refinement of "metric space," the sense of judgment of a certain quantity or measure of distance, is considered to be a learned skill, one that probably develops from both sensory motor activity and from education in culturally based symbols of measurement.

Postulates Regarding Intervention in Relation to the Visual Analysis of Space
1. Awareness of depth and distance is generated by binocular and monocular cues arising from the optic flow across the retina.
2. Awareness of depth and distance in near space is generated by binocular cues arising from binocular parallax.
3. Awareness of depth and distance is facilitated by selective attention.
4. Refined movement through space is developed by using retinal cues to depth and distance in combination with practice in movement.

5. Detection, recognition, and categorization of the features of real space are facilitated by identification of the salient features of a space and the invariant relationships and properties within a space.

6. Progressive differentiation toward the most informative and reliable judgment of space is facilitated by language and memory.

7. Naming measures of distance and depth using culturally appropriate symbols is facilitated by education and experience in measuring.

Examples of Occupational Therapy Intervention: Visual Analysis of Space

The occupational therapist is often called upon to determine whether a client can move safely through a particular environment. In these cases, each of the factors that affect the visual analysis of space and movement through space must be considered separately:

*   Is the visual system intact?
*   Are other sensory systems intact?
*   Is attention adequate?
*   Is the ability to identify and categorize intact?
*   Is memory of previous encounters with similar space reliable?
*   Is motor control sufficient?

It is crucial for the occupational therapist to consider that even if the question to be addressed is whether or not a client can ambulate or drive, run, or skip through an environment safely, the first factor to be evaluated is not gross motor control but vision. Before any movement takes place, reliable judgments about space must be made.

These judgments are largely dependent on retinal cues and on the complex balance of muscle alignment, accommodation, and refractive condition that allows for clear and comfortable vision, as described in Chapters Three and Four. If clarity and consistency of vision is present, and if the client is in an appropriate state of alertness, then the spatial features of gaps, obstacles, drop-offs, elevations, depressions, and passages can be detected.

Applying the theory and postulates presented here, the occupational therapist will also understand that a stable, consistent, and complete image from a single eye can support most activities of daily living because most of the retinal cues for depth and distance are monocular. Binocular vision is needed for depth perception in near space only, within 16 to 20 inches from the eyes, because stereopsis depends on input from two eyes. The effects of binocular vision disorder on activities of daily living are listed in Chapter Four.

Events

Events are happenings over time. Watching an object come toward one's self or recede from one's self requires an awareness of a continuity over time. Objects and space are continuously seen in a different perspective as they move or as we move. To watch a ball roll across a floor or to watch words appear on a video screen is to watch an event in real time, a happening "before our eyes." To run after the ball or to write words across the page is to participate in the event. For success in participation, the eye must maintain fixation on the visual target no matter what direction, position, or velocity the observer or the visual target assume. Ocular pursuit movements maintain continuing fixation when the target is moving. Saccadic movements refixate the eyes precisely from one target to another. Vergence movements bring the eyes into position for binocular fixation at any distance. Lens accommodation changes the thickness of the lens to maintain focus as distance from the visual target changes. Vestibular ocular reflexes stabilize the image on the retina when the head is moving or when the head is not upright in relation to gravity. In addition, intact acuity and visual fields contribute to a clear and complete view of the target.

Research has shown that participation in events (ie, self-generated movement) when coupled with consistent visual input, produces visual-motor adaptation. Passive movement coupled with consistent visual input also produces visual-motor adaptation, but less effectively and less efficiently.[8,19,20]

Observing events and participating in events provide a foundation for the development of concepts of object permanence and causality. Continuous transformations in apparent size, shape, and lightness of objects occur over time through movement of the object, the viewer, or both, but the salient features and invariant properties can still be detected.[5,17] Recognizing these features and properties leads to the establishment of object permanence.

Most of the treatment and evaluation activities used by occupational therapists are events, simply because much of the visual stimulation of daily life is from events and involves the interplay of people with objects and space over time. The movement of objects in our environment creates events. Our own movements as we work or play create events. When the occupational therapist and the client work on activities of daily living such as dressing, eating, and driving, these activities are in the visual stimulation category of events.

Obviously, all events do not involve linear movement, but for those that do, we have devised cultural measures of movement over time. When stated in language, these measures are stated as velocity and are learned through education. However, accurate judgments of velocity and motion can be made from retinal cues and have been demonstrated to be well developed in children by 4 years of age, long before the language label for measures of speed can be attached.[5] When vision is impaired, however, the retinal cues for velocity and motion may not be reliable, and judgments may be affected.

Postulates Regarding Intervention in Relation to the Visual Analysis of and Participation in Events

1. Observation of or participation in an event is facilitated by an intact ocular motor and visual system.

2. Visual motor integration is facilitated by self-generated movement coupled with consistent visual input.

3. Visual motor integration is facilitated by passive movement coupled with consistent visual input.

4. The development of concepts of object permanence and causality is supported by observation of and experience with the movement of objects through space over time.

Examples of Occupational Therapy Intervention: Visual Analysis of and Participation in Events

Consistent visual input is a necessary requirement for the development of visual motor integration. The 7-year-old child who presents with illegible handwriting and who has no history of deficits in attention, memory, or motor development is likely to be found to have an intermittent visual dysfunction upon examination. If vision is clear sometimes and blurred or double at other times, salient visual feedback is not consistently available. Without consistent visual feedback, a precise visually guided spatial activity, such as handwriting, cannot develop even in the presence of adequate fine motor potential.

On the other hand, therapists encounter some children who have never ambulated independently and who have severely limited self-generated movement because of congenital myotonia or because of the effects of some dystrophies and find that these children can learn very quickly to maneuver a motorized wheelchair with a skill in spatial judgment and speed control that any adult automobile driver would envy. This results from the fact that these children have had consistent visual input throughout their lives, and they have learned to visually analyze space by making observations while being carried or while being pushed in manual wheelchairs. Thus, when equipped with a motorized chair, they can successfully integrate accurate spatial judgments with their limited motor ability.

Occupational therapists who work with a vision-impaired population often train clients in the use of prisms.[11] Prisms distort the visual environment, but the distortion is consistent. Repeated practice of movement through space while viewing a consistently distorted world of objects and spatial features produces adaptation in visual motor integration.[20]

Conditions that create inconsistent visual input are discussed in detail in Chapters Two and Four. Many of the clients typically seen by occupational therapists will suffer from inconsistent visual input related to cerebrovascular accident, head trauma, developmental delay, and other causes. Once the visual dysfunction has been addressed through a remediation plan or a compensation plan, the occupational therapist is in a position to develop therapy activities that incorporate events involving movement through space and manipulation of objects in space.

Therapists are familiar with the many possibilities for grading such movement:

- By position: Supine, prone, sitting, all fours, tall kneel, half kneel, standing on a stable surface, standing on a moving surface, standing on one foot, etc.

- By mobility: Walking, running, on a scooter board, on a bicycle, in a wheelchair, in a car, etc.

- By complexity of the environment: With or without obstacles, in a narrow or wide space, at slow or fast speed, etc.[3]

Occupational therapists continually design activities graded to match the capacity of the client for self-generated movement in a meaningful and purposeful undertaking. This is indeed the "stock in trade" of the occupational therapist. Earlier chapters of this text contain detailed information for monitoring and managing the visual capacity of the client when designing treatment "events."

REPRESENTATIONS OF OBJECTS, SPACE, AND EVENTS

Representations are surrogates for three-dimensional reality. Two-dimensional drawings or photographs are representations of objects and space. Motion pictures and video are representations of events. Representations of familiar objects and events are recognized and identified easily by a person who has already learned to recognize and identify the real-life object, space, or event that it represents. Even an infant will recognize a picture of a dog or an apple if he or she has learned to recognize a dog or an apple in real life. Unfamiliar objects seen in representational form are subject to discrimination in the same way that unfamiliar objects seen in real life are subject to discrimination. A person notices distinctive features and identifies invariant properties and relationships, for example.

All of the information presented earlier in this chapter on visual information analysis as it applies to objects can be applied to the analysis of representations.

Postulates Regarding Intervention in Relation to the Visual Analysis of Representations

The postulates that apply to the visual analysis of objects apply equally to the visual analysis of representations.

Examples of Occupational Therapy Intervention: Visual Analysis of Representations

Much of the research on visual perception has been done using representations rather than real objects and real space. In addition, much of the published literature on visual perception fails to acknowledge the role of vision in any way. The unfortunate, if not tragic, result of this is that, in applied fields like education, occupational therapy, and clinical psychology, the visual information analysis of real objects, space, and events is sometimes overlooked, and the efficiency of the visual system is sometimes assumed to merit no particular attention.

Good visual perception is often understood to correlate with the ability to achieve a passing score on tests that use two-dimensional representations of invented forms as the stimulus material. Examples are the TVPS (Test of Visual Perceptual Skills) by Gardner[21] and the Motor Free

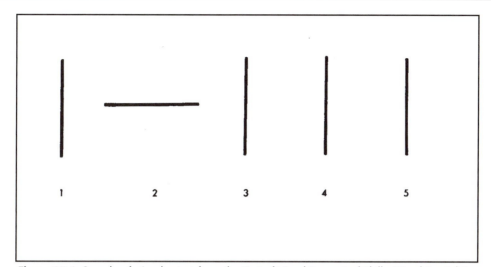

Figure 17-1. Sample of stimulus test from the Test of Visual Perceptual Skills: Visual Spatial Relationships Subtest. (Reprinted with permission from Psychological and Educational Publications Inc.)

Test of Visual Perception by Collarusso and Hammill.[22] Lending to the confusion is the fact that the names of the subsections of these tests imply that they test three-dimensional functioning rather than the interpretation of two-dimensional representations. The subsections named Spatial Relationships bear no relationship to the physiological process of perceiving three-dimensional depth and distance. The subsections named Figure Ground Discrimination bear no relationship to the physiological process of isolating a previously unidentified form from a background. The subsections named Form Constancy bear no relationship to the physiological process of experiencing the constancy of a real object as change occurs in the retinal image of that object. It is very important for the occupational therapist to be aware of the fact that scores achieved on these and similar tests tell us very little, if anything, about a client's ability to see the three-dimensional world, analyze it, and act in it.

Three items from the TVPS will be examined in the spirit of activity analysis in order to demonstrate how these tests might be interpreted and used by an occupational therapist.

Figure 17-1 is an illustration of one of the items from the section of the TVPS called Visual Spatial Relationships. When space is represented on paper, as it is here in two dimensions, it becomes a representation—a picture. It becomes a two-dimensional stimulus. It will be necessary to think of it as such when trying to analyze what the client can and cannot do with this particular task.

The directions are: "Here are some forms that are the same, but one form is going a different way or part of one of the forms is going a different way." The client is to indicate by pointing or by saying the number of the form that is going a different way. If the client gets the correct answer on this item, what do we know about his or her ability? We know that he or she can find the salient features, the set of relationships that make four of the forms the same and one of them different. He or she can put the forms that are the same in one category in his or her mind and put the form that is different in another category in his or her mind. This is an important cognitive skill. This test item, therefore, might more accurately be named after the cognitive analysis ability of categorization. This section of the TVPS, although named Visual Spatial Relationships, does not require processing space as depth and distance.

When an occupational therapist interprets the functional implications of a low score on this test, the implication is not that the person will have difficulty moving through space or acting in space. A low score on this test might imply that the person would have difficulty with matching

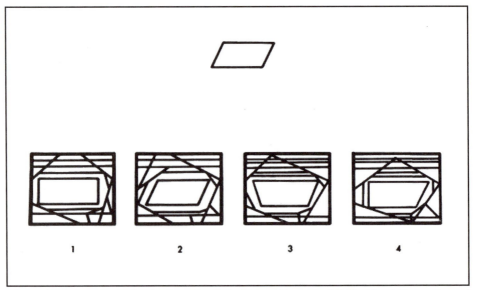

Figure 17-2. Sample of stimulus from the Test of Visual Perceptual Skills: Visual Figure Ground Subtest. (Reprinted with permission from Psychological and Educational Publications Inc.)

and categorization and with finding likenesses and differences in unfamiliar representational material. As noted in the earlier discussion of the visual information processing of objects, the crucial factors here, and in the next samples from the TVPS, are selective attention, efficient visual exploration, memory, ability to extract the distinctive feature or bundle of features, and ability to ignore irrelevant features.

Figure 17-2 illustrates an item from the section of the TVPS that is called Visual Figure Ground. In this test item, a specific two-dimensional stimulus figure is given at the top of the page, while another similar figure is hidden in one of several two-dimensional drawings at the bottom of the page. The client is required to scan the page and find a match for the stimulus figure. This task requires attention, visual search, and comparison of salient features. This is a matching task. This test item would more accurately be named after the cognitive analysis ability of matching. It tests an important cognitive analysis skill, but it is unrelated to physiological figure ground discrimination.

In daily life, with three-dimensional objects in three-dimensional space, figure ground discrimination is the tendency to perceive an object as set apart from the background, to experience the emergence of certain parts of a visual field as distinct from other parts, to perceive a previously unidentified form as being dominant in a visual array.

Figure 17-3 illustrates an item from the section of the TVPS that is called Visual Form Constancy. In this section, the client is directed to look at the stimulus form and find the form among five other given forms, even though it might be smaller, bigger, darker, turned, or upside down.

In the three-dimensional world of daily life, constancy means that the same object can be viewed from different distances, at different angles, and in different lighting conditions and still be perceived as retaining a constant, stable size, shape, or brightness. The correct answer to this test plate, number five, does not depict the same exact shape, but rather the same shape drawn smaller. This is also a matching task. The client must recognize the distinctive features and invariant properties of this shape and indicate the presence of the same shaped but different size.

Tests of visual perception that are presented in the form of two-dimensional representations are useful as measures of certain cognitive analysis skills, but scores on these tests should not be correlated with ability to perceive the three-dimensional world of objects and space. They should

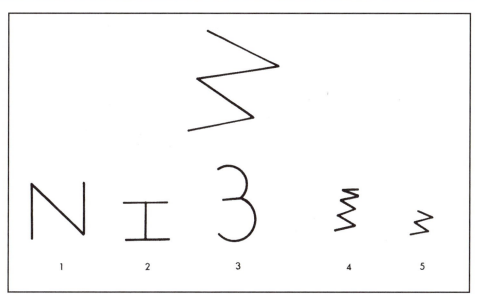

Figure 17-3. Sample of stimulus from the Test of Visual Perceptual Skills: Visual Form Constancy Subtest. (Reprinted with permission from Psychological and Educational Publications Inc.)

certainly not be assumed to correlate with the ability to move through and act in the three-dimensional world of objects and space.

SYMBOLS

Finally, a major source of visual stimulation comes in the form of symbols or codes. A primary example of a coded visual symbol system is written language. Speech is a coded auditory symbol system. Other examples of coded symbol systems are musical notation, mathematical notation, Morse code, and sign language.

Written words are symbols and, like representations, are man-made and "stand in place of" objects, space, and events. But symbols differ from representations in that they require a mental process of association. A drawing or photo of an apple, for example, corresponds to an actual apple, and the representation conveys to the eye the same visual information as the actual apple. The written symbol "apple" does not convey to the eye the same visual information as an actual apple. The meaning of the written word must be known and must be associated with the memory of the object to which it corresponds.[5]

Symbols differ from representations in another important way. The information given by symbols is almost always given in a sequence. Visual information from real objects, space, and events as well as from representations of objects, space, and events is simultaneously present to the eye. The eye registers visual information from a symbol system in a sequence. In the case of written language, the sequence itself has a particular structure and particular rules. In English, for example, spaces separate words from one another, and sentences begin with a capital letter and end with a punctuation mark; paragraphs mark units of thought. During reading, the eyes move to informative areas of the text based on cues from peripheral vision. Many of these cues are derived from the physical structure of the language on the page.[23] Structural elements are an integral part of the symbol system. For example, Withoutinterwordspaces,Englishisverydifficulttoread.

As indicated by the sentence above, without interword spaces, English is very difficult to read. Interword spaces are as critical a part of our language symbol system as are the letters of the alphabet. The structure as well as the content of a symbol system must be detected, recognized, and remembered.

Although symbols differ from other categories of visual stimulation in that they require mental association and sequencing, they are similar to objects, space, events, and representations in that the symbols themselves must be detected, recognized, and discriminated one from another. Just as a toddler learns to recognize a doll by its particular distinctive features and invariant properties, the kindergartner must learn to recognize the letter "w" by its distinctive features and learn to distinguish it from "m" or "v" by its differences. The adult linguist must learn to distinguish the written forms of other language systems before he or she can decode and read that language.

But a man-made symbol presents a new problem to a developing child. In his or her previous experience, retinal cues for constancy of shape have indicated to him or her that a positional difference did not change the essential identification of an object, even when the positional difference created a different image on the retina. The doll remained the doll when viewed from behind or when held upside down. In the alphabet, positional difference becomes a distinctive feature of the letter and actually changes the identification of the letter. New readers are prone to confuse "b" and "d" and other "reversible" pairs of letters until they learn that, in a symbol system, position is indeed a salient distinguishing feature. Rotation and reversal change "u" to "n" and "b" to "d."[24]

Postulates Regarding Intervention in Relation to the Visual Analysis of Symbols

The postulates that apply to the visual information analysis of objects apply equally to the visual information analysis of symbols. In addition, the following postulates apply:

1. Analysis of visual symbols or symbol systems is facilitated by the mental process of association with memory of the reality to which they correspond.

2. Analysis of the visual symbol system of written language is facilitated by recognition of the rules of sequence and structure in the language.

3. Discrimination of symbols is facilitated when position, particularly reversal and rotation, is understood to be a salient feature in identification.

Examples of Occupational Therapy Intervention: Visual Analysis of Symbols

Symbols are similar to objects, space, events, and representations in this way: They must be seen clearly by the eye before the information they contain can be analyzed. For example, if words on a page are blurred because of binocular dysfunction, or only partially seen because of a field cut, a correct association is compromised. "Fight" might be read as "Eight." If words on a page are read out of order because of a problem with saccadic eye movements, correct sequencing for meaning is compromised. The occupational therapist has a responsibility to screen for ocular motor or vision deficits when a client presents with problems in using symbol systems and to suggest a vision evaluation by a vision professional.

Sequencing becomes a particularly important skill in schools or in any work activity that deals primarily with words and numbers or other symbol systems. An evaluation of a client who must function in such a setting should include an evaluation of ability to attend to detail and ability to remember a sequence.

When a client has difficulty learning to discriminate letters and numbers because of a lack of understanding that reversals and rotation change the identity of symbols, the occupational therapist can provide recognition and matching activities that reinforce or exaggerate the importance of position as a distinguishing feature. Tactile cues, tracing, verbal cues, and mnemonics using concrete associations are helpful. Self-evaluation and self-correction techniques can be introduced, using alphabet and number strips for self-reference. In educational settings, the role of the occupational therapist is frequently one of consultation to the educator. An understanding of the types of visual stimuli and the differences between other visual stimuli and symbol systems can be communicated to the educator. This will add clarity and efficiency to the consultation meetings.

Visual Task Analysis and Synthesis: An Outline

This section is offered as a quick reference to the factors that can be considered or manipulated in visual task analysis and synthesis. It is divided into two sections:

1. Factors related to clarity of sight and ocular motor skill.
2. Factors related to visual information analysis.

In each section, these factors are separated into those that characterize the task, the client, and the environment.

Also, in a general sense, the factors are listed in a continuum from easier to more difficult. For example, stationary targets, a stationary client, and a stationary environment present an easier ocular motor task than a moving target, moving client, and moving environment. As an example, think of the relative ease of reading an acuity chart while seated versus playing a game of ice hockey. Similarly, detecting a familiar object in a familiar, relatively simple environment is an easier visual information processing task than categorizing unfamiliar symbols in an unfamiliar, complex environment. Think of these examples: Finding one's own coat in one's own closet versus finding the correct subway line in an unfamiliar city terminal.

Characteristics of the Task That Relate to Clarity of Sight and Ocular Motor Skill

Factors Related to the Task

- Stationary targets
- Moving targets
- Near point targets
- Far point targets
- Converging or diverging targets

Factors Related to the Client

- Stationary client
- Moving client
- Client upright or not relative to gravity
- Specific impairments of client (such as focal vision, peripheral vision, acuity, and binocularity)

Factors Related to the Environment

- Stationary environment
- Moving environment
- Relative brightness and contrast level (degraded lighting conditions)
- Gestalt grouping principles:
  - Nearness
  - Similarity
  - Continuity
  - Parallel movement
  - Closure
  - Symmetry

Characteristics of the Task That Relate to Visual Information Analysis

FACTORS RELATED TO THE TASK

Sources of Visual Stimuli

- Objects
- Space
- Events
- Representations of objects, space, and events
- Symbols

Degrees of Complexity

- Degree of familiarity
- Amount of stimuli
- Degree of organization
- Degree of abstraction required

FACTORS RELATED TO THE CLIENT

Capable of Abstraction

- Detection
- Recognition
- Matching
- Categorization

Capable of Attention

- Arousal/alertness level
- Selectivity
- Vigilance

Capable of Memory

- Short-term memory
- Long-term memory

Past Experience With the Task

- Education
- Practice

FACTORS RELATED TO THE ENVIRONMENT

- Degree of familiarity
- Amount of stimuli
- Degree of organization
- Number and type of cues
- Feedback and reinforcement

Summary

In his introductory chapter, Dr. Scheiman discusses the growing realization among optometrists and occupational therapists that, in some instances, optimal care for clients requires a joint effort between the two professions. Subsequent chapters in this book describe visual function in normal development and visual dysfunction as it affects the populations typically served by occupational therapists. Of particular interest to occupational therapists is information throughout these chapters on how the optometrist manages vision problems and uses the tools of the optometry profession: Lenses, prisms, and vision therapy.

In this chapter, we have focused on one of the primary tools of occupational therapy: Task analysis and synthesis. We have presented a conceptual and practical basis for the analysis and synthesis of activities that have a visual and visual information processing component. It is our hope that this framework will be helpful not only to occupational therapists but also to optometrists who are interested in learning how occupational therapists formulate their intervention plans when a client has a problem with vision or with visual information analysis.

Our presentation differs from much of the previously published literature on visual perception that has been directed to an occupational therapy audience in that we have included all sources of visual stimulation rather than limiting our discussion to two-dimensional representations.

By using Gibson's five categories of visual stimulation—objects, space, events, representations, and symbols—we believe that we reflect the inclusive and comprehensive nature of occupational therapy.

We hope that this inclusive approach, coupled with the extensive overview of visual function and visual dysfunction contained in the preceding chapters, can contribute to the knowledge base of occupational therapists so that we can become more expert in three endeavors:

1. Recognizing visual dysfunction in our clients, particularly if it has not been previously identified.

2. Referring clients to appropriate vision professionals.

3. Incorporating an understanding of vision and visual information processing into the activities that we analyze and synthesize for our evaluations and interventions.

References

1. Mosey AC. *Occupational Therapy: Configuration of a Profession*. New York, NY: Raven Press; 1981.

2. Mosey AC. *Three Frames of Reference for Mental Health*. Thorofare, NJ: SLACK Incorporated; 1970.

3. Kramer P, Hinojosa J. *Frames of Reference for Pediatric Occupational Therapy*. Baltimore, MD: Williams and Wilkins; 1993.

4. Morris W, ed. *The American Heritage Dictionary of the English Language*. Boston, MA: Houghton Mifflin Co; 1979.

5. Gibson EJ. *Principles of Perceptual Learning and Development*. New York, NY: Appleton-Century-Crofts; 1969.

6. Posner MI, Rafal RD. Cognitive theories of attention and the rehabilitation of attentional deficits. In: Meier MJ, Benton AL, Diller L, eds. *Neuropsychological Rehabilitation*. New York, NY: Guilford Press; 1987.

7. Levine M. *Developmental Variation and Learning Disorders*. Cambridge, MA: Educators Publishing Service; 1987.

8. Shiffman HR. *Sensation and Perception: An Integrated Approach*. New York, NY: John Wiley & Sons Inc; 1990.

9. Wertheimer M. Principles of perceptual organization. In: Beardslee DC, Wertheimer M, eds. *Readings in Perception*. New York, NY: Van Nostrand; 1958.

10. Lampert J, Lapolice DJ. Functional considerations in evaluation and treatment of the client with low vision. *Am J Occup Ther*. 1995;49:877-883.

11. Warren M. Providing low vision rehabilitation services with occupational therapy and ophthalmology: a program description. *Am J Occup Ther*. 1995;49:877-883.

12. Todd VR. Visual perceptual frame of reference: an information processing approach. In: Kramer P, Hinojosa J, eds. *Frames of Reference for Pediatric Occupational Therapy*. Baltimore, MD: Williams and Wilkins; 1993.

13. Frantz RL. The origin of form perception. *Sci Am*. 1961;204:66-72.

14. Ryan TA, Schwartz CB. Speed of perception as a function of mode of representations. *Am J Psychol.* 1956;69:60-69.

15. Kimball JG. Sensory integrative frame of reference. In: Kramer P, Hinojosa J, eds. *Frames of Reference for Pediatric Occupational Therapy.* Baltimore, MD: Williams and Wilkins; 1993.

16. Warren M. Identification of visual scanning deficits in adults after cerebrovascular accident. *Am J Occup Ther.* 1990;44:391-398.

17. Ginsburg H, Opper S. *Piaget's Theory of Intellectual Development: An Introduction.* Englewood Cliffs, NJ: Prentice-Hall Inc; 1969.

18. Walk RD. Depth perception and experience. In: Walk RD, Pick HL, eds. *Perception and Experience.* New York, NY: Plenum; 1978.

19. Howard IP. *Human Visual Orientation.* New York, NY: John Wiley; 1982.

20. Kohler I. Experiments with goggles. *Sci Am.* 1962;206:62-86.

21. Gardner MF. *Test of Visual Perceptual Skills.* San Francisco, CA: Health Pub Co; 1988.

22. Collarusso R, Hammill D. *The Motor Free Test of Visual Perception.* Novato, CA: Academic Therapy Publications; 1972.

23. Lane KA. *Developing Your Child for Success.* Lewisville, TX: Learning Potentials Pub Inc; 1993.

24. Gibson EJ, Gibson JJ, Smith OW, Osser HA. A developmental study of the discrimination of letter-like forms. *Journal of Comparative Physiological Psychology.* 1962;55:897-906.

Glossary of Key Terms

accommodation: The ability to change the focus of the eye so that objects at different distances can be seen clearly.

accommodative excess: A condition in which the amplitude of accommodation is normal but the ciliary muscle has a tendency to spasm. Typically the problem is intermittent and variable. The individual reports that after reading for a period of time, he or she experiences blurred vision when looking at a distant object.

accommodative infacility: A condition in which the amplitude of accommodation is normal, but the speed of the response is reduced. The most common complaint associated with accommodative facility is blurred vision when looking from near to far or far to near.

accommodative insufficiency: A condition in which the amount of accommodation available (amplitude of accommodation) is less than expected for the individual's age.

ambient processing mode: Concerned with the "where" or the location of objects. Information about movement and position of objects is transmitted to the posterior parietal cortex, which provides a reference of where objects are located in space. The ambient mode is important in posture, motion, and spatial orientation.

amblyopia: A condition in which the visual acuity is less than 20/20 and this loss of visual acuity cannot be attributed to refractive error or observable eye disease. Most people are familiar with amblyopia, which is commonly called "lazy eye" by the public. The term *lazy eye* is a misnomer and does not really describe the condition well. The eye is not lazy; it simply has not received proper stimulation.

anisometropia: A condition in which there is a significant difference in the magnitude of the refractive error between the two eyes.

anisometropic amblyopia: A condition in which the prescription in one eye is considerably stronger than the prescription in the fellow eye.

anomalous correspondence: A condition associated with strabismus in which the visual system adapts to the misalignment of the eye by altering the neurophysiology of the visual system. This adaptation eliminates double vision.

Scheiman M
Understanding and Managing Vision Deficits: A Guide for Occupational Therapists, Third Edition (pp 365-370)
© 2011 SLACK Incorporated

aqueous humor: A clear, watery fluid produced in the posterior chamber that fills the anterior chamber of the eye.

astigmatism: A condition in which vision is blurred and distorted at both distance and near. An astigmatic eye is not spherical. Rather, it has an oval shape and this causes the light rays entering the eye to focus at two different points.

Best's vitelliform macular degeneration: Juvenile form of macular degeneration typically inherited as an autosomal dominant trait. Onset is typically during the first decade of life. Vision loss may be mild or progress to more significant central vision loss.

congenital ocular motor apraxia: Abnormality in voluntary horizontal eye movements with reflex horizontal movements remaining intact. May be due to brain malformation or lesions.

contrast sensitivity: Contrast sensitivity tells us about the quality of the available vision. Problems associated with mobility and reduced ability to recognize faces and objects that are common after brain injury have been found to be associated with contrast sensitivity problems.

convergence excess: A condition in which the eyes have a tendency to turn inward rather than outward. Convergence excess has been found to be slightly more prevalent than convergence insufficiency in a clinical population.

convergence insufficiency: A condition in which the eyes have a tendency to drift outward when being used for near work such as reading, while at a far distance the eyes work well together. This is one of the leading causes of eyestrain and discomfort.

cornea: The anterior one-sixth of the outer coat of the eye is the transparent structure called the cornea. The cornea is an extremely important structure of the eye because it is the key optical component responsible for refraction of light that enters the eye. It is an unusual tissue because it is clear and has no blood vessels.

Crouzon syndrome: A syndrome associated with a forward pointed skull, beak-shaped nose, underdeveloped upper jaw, widely spaced eyes (hypertelorism), protruding eyes (exophthalmos), and exotropia. Inheritance is typically autosomal dominant.

directionality: The ability of the individual to interpret right and left directions in three separate components of external space.

divergence excess: A condition in which the eyes drift outward when looking at a distance and function normally when looking at near objects.

Down syndrome: A syndrome arising from a chromosomal abnormality involving an extra chromosome 21 (trisomy 21). Associated systemic findings include developmental disability, congenital heart disease, and large protruding tongue. Ocular findings typically include a mongoloid slant of the eyes, yellowish flecks on the iris (Brushfield's spots), myopia, keratoconus, and cataracts.

eccentric fixation: Fixation with a nonfoveal point under monocular conditions. This condition is common in strabismus.

emmetropia: The term used to describe the condition in which there is an absence of refractive error.

esophoria: A condition in which the eyes have a tendency to turn in but the person is able to control this tendency.

esotropia: A condition in which the eyes turn in and the person is unable to control this tendency.

exophoria: A condition in which the eyes have a tendency to turn out but the person is able to control this tendency.

exotropia: A condition in which the eyes turn out and the person is unable to control this tendency.

focal processing mode: Made up of the foveal, parafoveal, and primary visual cortex inputs. The focal mode contributes to the "what" of vision (object recognition and identification). The focal mode is attention oriented and centers on detail in small areas of space.

fovea: The fovea is the part of the eye that contains the area of most acute vision. Whenever we look at an object we must aim the eye so that the image of the object is focused on the fovea. Smooth eye movements called pursuits and jump eye movements called saccades are both designed to allow the individual to always use the fovea.

Hallermann-Streiff syndrome: A developmental disability associated with a parrot-like facial appearance (craniofacial dysplasia), skin atrophy, and hair loss with sparse or absent eyebrows. Ocular findings may include microphthalmos and congenital glaucoma.

hemianopsia: Blindness in one-half of the visual field of one or both eyes.

holoprosencephaly: An underdeveloped prosencephalon associated with developmental disabilities and facial abnormalities including cleft lip and palate. Ocular findings may include microphthalmos, coloboma, and optic atrophy.

hyperopia: A condition in which light rays entering the eye focus behind the retina and the individual must accommodate to see clearly. This need to accommodate requires the use of muscular effort. The amount of effort necessary is greater when the individual looks at near.

isometropic amblyopia: A condition in which there is a very high refractive error in both eyes.

keratoconus: A bulging of the central cornea associated with a thinning of that region. Typically associated with significant astigmatism.

keratoglobus: An enlarged protruding cornea with thinning of the periphery of the cornea.

laterality: The ability to be internally aware of and identify right and left on one's self.

Laurence-Moon syndrome: A syndrome associated with an autosomal recessive inheritance pattern, obesity, extra digits, developmental disability, underdeveloped sexual organs, and retinitis pigmentosa.

lens: A transparent, flexible structure that is held in position by zonular fibers. It is located posterior to the iris and anterior to the vitreous humor. Like the cornea, the lens is both transparent and avascular and is another key part of the refractive system of the eye.

macrencephaly: Enlarged brain with a thickened highly convoluted cortex, associated with optic atrophy, developmental disabilities, and seizures.

Marfan syndrome: A congenital connective tissue disorder associated with a tall stature, postural abnormalities, increased length of fingers and toes, joint hyperextension, cardiovascular disease, and aneurysm of the ascending aorta. Ocular findings may include displacement (subluxation) of the lenses, cataracts, strabismus, nystagmus, myopia, and megalocornea.

microcornea: A cornea that is smaller than 10 mm in diameter. Microcornea is typically associated with myopia.

microphthalmos: A developmental abnormality resulting in a smaller than normal eye. Microphthalmos may be associated with colobomas, glaucoma, and cataracts. Refractive error is typically hyperopia.

myopia: A condition in which the light rays entering the eye focus in front of the retina. In myopia the vision is blurred at distance but clear at near.

near point of convergence: The point at which the eyes are in the position of maximum convergence. This should occur about 2 to 4 inches from the eyes.

nystagmus: A condition in which there are involuntary, rhythmic oscillations of one or both eyes.

Pierre Robin syndrome: Syndrome associated with neonatal respiratory distress, swallowing difficulties, jaw abnormalities, and low set ears. Ocular findings may include microphthalmos, glaucoma, cataracts, myopia, and strabismus.

presbyopia: A condition in which near visual acuity is decreased because of an age-related decline in accommodative ability.

pursuit dysfunction: A condition in which the individual is unable to accurately follow a moving object.

refraction: The term used to describe the evaluation of the optical system of the eye. When the optometrist performs the "refraction," he or she determines whether the individual is emmetropic, myopic, hyperopic, or astigmatic.

retina: The most internal coat of the eye. It is a thin, delicate membrane composed of two layers: An outer pigment cell layer and an internal neural layer.

retinoscope: An instrument used for determining the refractive power of the eye.

saccadic dysfunction: A condition in which the accuracy and speed of saccadic eye movements are reduced relative to expected findings for the individual's age.

sclera: The white, external coat of the eye that covers the posterior five-sixths of the eye.

scotoma: An isolated area of absent vision or depressed sensitivity in the visual field, surrounded by an area of normal vision.

septo-optic dysplasia (de Morsier's syndrome): Brain malformation (septum pellucidum) associated with midline facial deformities such as cleft lip and palate and growth retardation. Ocular findings may include optic atrophy, optic nerve hypoplasia (underdevelopment), coloboma, and microphthalmos.

Stargardt's maculopathy: Juvenile form of macular degeneration typically inherited as an autosomal recessive trait. Onset is typically between the ages of 8 and 16. Vision loss progresses to between 20/200 and 20/400. Peripheral vision is preserved.

stereopsis: Binocular visual perception of three-dimensional space.

Stickler syndrome: Syndrome associated with joint and hip abnormalities, progressive myopia, retinal detachment, and glaucoma.

strabismic amblyopia: Amblyopia secondary to the presence of a strabismus. The strabismus must occur early in life, involve only one eye, and be present all of the time to cause amblyopia.

strabismus: A condition in which the eyes are misaligned all or part of the time. Many types of strabismus are possible, including esotropia (eyes turn in), exotropia (eyes turn out), and hypertropia (one eye turns up).

strabismus, comitant: A strabismus that is the same magnitude in the nine diagnostic positions of gaze.

suppression: A condition usually associated with strabismus and amblyopia in which the visual system ignores the input from one eye.

Treacher Collins syndrome (Franceschetti syndrome): Syndrome associated with facial deformity, malformation of the ears associated with deafness, downward slanting eyes, segmental absence of lashes, and lid deformities.

Turner syndrome: Syndrome associated with the presence of only one X chromosome or a severe deformity of the second X chromosome in a female. Associated systemic findings include immature sexual development, pulmonary stenosis, vascular disease, and autoimmune disease. Ocular findings may include ptosis (incomplete opening of the lids), strabismus, and cataracts.

vision therapy: Also known as orthoptics, vision training, visual training, and eye training. Vision therapy is an organized therapeutic regimen utilized to treat a number of neuromuscular, neurophysiological, and neurosensory conditions that interfere with visual function. Vision therapy encompasses a wide variety of procedures to improve a diagnosed neuromuscular or neurophysiological visual dysfunction.

visual acuity: A measure of the resolving power of the eye. An individual with 20/20 acuity is considered to have normal ability to see small detail at the distance tested.

visual analysis skills: These skills contribute to the individual's ability to analyze and discriminate visually presented information, to determine the whole without seeing all of the parts, to identify more important features and ignore extraneous detail, and to use visual imagery to recall past visual information. It includes the ability of the child to be aware of the distinctive features of visual forms including shape, size, color, and orientation.

visual efficiency: Refers to the effectiveness of the visual system to clearly, efficiently, and comfortably allow an individual to gather visual information at school, work, or play. The various component skills that are important in this process are called visual efficiency skills and include the subcategories of accommodation, binocular vision, and ocular motility.

visual field: The extent of physical space visible to an eye in a given position. Its average extent is approximately 65 degrees upward, 75 degrees downward, 60 degrees inward, and 95 degrees outward.

visual motor skills: These skills are related to the individual's ability to integrate visual information processing skills with fine motor movement. Another term for visual motor integration is *eye-hand coordination.*

visual spatial skills: These skills allow the individual to develop normal internal and external spatial concepts and are used to interact with and organize the environment. They allow the individual to make judgments about location of objects in visual space in reference to other objects and to the individual's own body.

vitreous body: A colorless, transparent gel that consists of 99% water and forms four-fifths of the eyeball. In addition to transmitting light, it holds the retina in place and provides support for the lens.

yoked prisms: Yoked prisms are used to alter a patient's spatial awareness, to modify a patient's midline perception, or to change weight shifting.

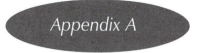

Resources

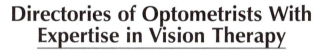

Directories of Optometrists With Expertise in Vision Therapy

American Academy of Optometry
6110 Executive Blvd, Suite 506
Rockville, MD 20852
Phone: 301-984-1441
www.aaopt.org

College of Optometrists in Vision Development
215 W Garfield Rd, Suite 200
Aurora, OH 44202
Phone: 888-268-3770 or 330-995-0718
www.covd.org

Optometric Extension Program Foundation
1921 E Carnegie Ave, Suite 3-L
Santa Ana, CA 92705-5510
Phone: 949-250-8070
www.oepf.org

Equipment

Avanti Educational Programs
Attn: Ms. Patricia Wilbarger
10 S Kearney St
Denver, CO 80224
303-782-5117

Scheiman M
*Understanding and Managing Vision Deficits: A Guide for
Occupational Therapists, Third Edition* (pp 371-374)
© 2011 SLACK Incorporated

Bangerter Foil Occlusion/Fresnel Prism & Lens Co
6824 Washington Ave S
Eden Prairie, MN 55344
Phone: 800-544-4760
www.fresnel-prism.com

Finger Fitness
451 Emerson Ave
Hamilton, OH 45013
Phone: 888-868-HAND (4263)
www.handhealth.com/

Hoyle Products Inc
937 A St
Fillmore, CA 93018
Phone: 805-524-1211

National Library Service for the Blind and Physically Handicapped
Library of Congress
Washington, DC 20542
Phone: 888-NLS-READ or 202-707-5100

Visual Information Processing Evaluation Tests

Source	Name of Test
Bernell Corp 4016 N Home St Mishawaka, IN 46545 Phone: 800-348-2225 www.bernell.com	Developmental Eye Movement Test
Lafayette Instrument Co PO Box 5729 Lafayette, IN 47903 Phone: 800-428-7545 or 765-423-1505 www.lafayetteinstrument.com/	Grooved Pegboard
Optometric Extension Program Foundation 1921 E Carnegie Ave, Suite 3-L Santa Ana, CA 92705 Phone: 949-250-8070 www.oepf.org	Developmental Test of Visual Motor Integration Gardner Reversal Frequency Test Wold Sentence Copy Test
Psychological and Educational Publications Inc PO Box 520 Hydesville, CA 95547 Phone: 800-523-5775	Test of Visual Perceptual Skills (TVPS)

Testing Equipment

Company	Equipment
Bernell Corp 4016 N Home St Mishawaka, IN 46545 Phone: 800-348-2225 www.bernell.com	Eye patch (Black Elastic Eye Patch SF3ES) Snellen Eye Chart (BC11931) Red Maddox Rod (BC1200R) Near Visual Acuity Chart (ODNVC) Disposable penlight (WC70206, Pkg of 6) Developmental Eye Movement Test (DEM) Viewer-Free Random Dot Tests (SY98) Pen-Pal Fixators (PENPALS)
Gulden Ophthalmics 225 Cadwalader Ave Elkins Park, PA 19027 Phone: 215-884-8105 www.guldenindustries.com	CPAC Visual Acuity Test Fixation Sticks
Optometric Extension Program Foundation 1921 E Carnegie Ave, Suite 3-L Santa Ana, CA 92705 Phone: 949-250-8070	Developmental Test of Visual Motor Integration
Psychological and Educational Publications Inc PO Box 520 Hydesville, CA 95547 Phone: 800-523-5775	Test of Visual Perceptual Skills (TVPS)
Vision Associates 295 NW Commons Loop, Suite 115-312 Lake City, FL 32055 Phone: 407-352-1200 www.visionkits.com	3-D Lea Symbols Set (#2516) Lea Symbols Chart Lea Symbols Near Vision Card

Vision Therapy Equipment

Company	Item
Bernell Corp 4016 N Home St Mishawaka, IN 46545 Phone: 800-348-2225 www.bernell.com	DEM Symbol Tracking (AADSB) Letter Tracking (AALTB) Hart Chart Tracing Patterns
Learning Potentials Publishers Inc 230 W Main St Lewisville, TX 75057 Phone: 972-221-2564	Developing Your Child for Success by Kenneth Lane, OD
Optometric Extension Program Foundation 1921 E Carnegie Ave, Suite 3L Santa Ana, CA 92705 Phone: 949-250-8070 www.oepf.org	Visual Tracing Workbook (2) Visual Fine Motor Workbook (2) Rotating Pegboard Helping Children Overcome Learning Difficulties—Jerome Rosner

Continuing Education

American Occupational Therapy Association offers a self-paced clinical course entitled "Low Vision: Occupational Therapy Intervention With the Older Adult."
Phone: 301-652-2682
www.aota.org

Association for Education and Rehabilitation of the Blind and Visually Impaired provides national and regional conferences and teleseminars.
Phone: 877-492-2708 or 703-671-4500
www.aerbvi.org

Lighthouse International offers courses, seminars, hands-on workshops, newsletters, and publications, including a workshop specifically for occupational therapists.
Phone: 800-829-0500
www.lighthouse.org

visABILITIES Rehab Services Inc provides continuing education seminars and educational materials for the treatment of visual impairment in adults and children.
Phone: 888-752-4364
www.visabilities.com

Vision Education Seminars sponsors continuing education courses for occupational therapists, physical therapists, speech pathologists, and educators of the visually impaired.
Phone: 610-664-5270
www.visionedseminars.com

Vision Screening Report Form

Name _____ DOB ___ / ___ / ___ Age _____

Wears glasses/contact lenses: No _____ Yes _____ Full-time _____

Distance only _____ Near only _____

Test	Performance	Referral Indicated If:
Symptom Questionnaire	_____ Significant symptoms _____ No significant symptoms	Significant symptoms are present
Visual Acuity Testing (distance) Distance _____ feet _____ with glasses _____ without glasses	Right eye 20/ _____ Left eye 20/ _____	20/40 visual acuity or worse in either eye A two line difference in acuity between the two eyes
Visual Acuity Testing (near) _____ with glasses _____ without glasses	Right eye 20/ _____ Left eye 20/ _____	20/30 visual acuity or worse in either eye A two line difference in acuity between the two eyes
Eye Alignment (distance)	_____ exophoria _____ esophoria _____ vertical phoria _____ suppression	6 exophoria or greater 4 esophoria or greater Any vertical phoria Suppression
Eye Alignment (near)	_____ exophoria _____ esophoria _____ vertical phoria _____ suppression	8 exophoria or greater 4 esophoria or greater Any vertical phoria Suppression

Scheiman M
Understanding and Managing Vision Deficits: A Guide for Occupational Therapists, Third Edition (pp 375-376)
© 2011 SLACK Incorporated

Test	Performance	Referral Indicated If:
Convergence	Break: _____ inches Recovery: _____ inches	A break greater than 4 inches A recovery greater than 6 inches
Stereopsis	_____ Identified all three symbols _____ Cannot identify all three symbols	Inability to identify all three symbols
Accommodative Amplitude	Right eye _____ diopters Left eye _____ diopters	2 diopters below age expected (18 minus one-third the patient's age)
Saccades: Direct Observation		See chart below
Pursuits: Direct Observation		See chart below
Saccades: Visual-Verbal Format (DEM)	Errors _____ percentile Ratio _____ percentile	A score below the 15th percentile for either errors or ratio
Visual Fields: Right Eye		Any field loss
Visual Fields: Left Eye		Any field loss
Gardner Reversal Frequency Test: Recognition Subtest	Raw score _____ Percentile _____	A score below the 15th percentile
TVPS: Form Constancy	Raw score _____ Percentile _____	A score below the 15th percentile
Developmental Test of Visual Motor Integration	Raw score _____ Percentile _____	A score below the 15th percentile

Northeastern State University College of Optometry
Saccade Test Referral Criteria by Age and Sex

Sex	Ability	Accuracy	Head Movement
Boys	Less than 5	Less than 3	5 to 6 years: less than 2 All other ages: less than 3
Girls	Less than 5	Less than 3	5 years: less than 2 6 to 9 years: less than 3 All other ages: less than 4

Northeastern State University College of Optometry
Pursuit Test Referral Criteria by Age and Sex

Sex	Ability	Accuracy	Head Movement
Boys	Less than 5	5 to 6 years: less than 2 7 to 9 years: less than 3 10 years and older: less than 4	5 to 6 years: less than 2 7 to 9 years: less than 3 10 years and older: less than 4
Girls	Less than 5	5 to 8 years: less than 3 9 years and older: less than 4	5 to 9 years: less than 3 All other ages: less than 4

Advanced-Degree Programs

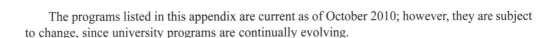

The programs listed in this appendix are current as of October 2010; however, they are subject to change, since university programs are continually evolving.

Orientation and Mobility

- California State University, Los Angeles, California
- Flinders University, Adelaide, South Australia
- Florida State University, Tallahassee, Florida
- Hunter College of the City University of New York, New York
- Massey University, Palmerston North, New Zealand
- Missouri State University, Springfield, Missouri
- Mohawk College, Brantford, Ontario, Canada
- New Mexico State University, Las Cruces, New Mexico
- North Carolina Central University, Durham, North Carolina
- Northern Illinois University, DeKalb, Illinois
- Salus University, Elkins Park, Pennsylvania
- San Francisco State University, San Francisco, California
- South Carolina State University, Orangeburg, South Carolina
- Stephen F. Austin State University, Nacogdoches, Texas
- Texas Tech University , Lubbock, Texas
- University of Arizona, Tucson, Arizona
- University of Arkansas at Little Rock, Little Rock, Arkansas
- University of Louisville, Louisville, Kentucky
- University of Massachusetts, Boston, Massachusetts

Scheiman M
Understanding and Managing Vision Deficits: A Guide for Occupational Therapists, Third Edition (pp 377-378)
© 2011 SLACK Incorporated

- University of Northern Colorado, Greeley, Colorado
- University of Pittsburgh, Pittsburgh, Pennsylvania
- Western Michigan University, Kalamazoo, Michigan

Low Vision Rehabilitation

- Salus University, Elkins Park, Pennsylvania

Vision Rehabilitation Therapy

- Academy for Special Education, Warsaw, Poland
- Hunter College of the City University of New York, New York
- Massey University, Palmerston North, New Zealand
- Mohawk College, Brantford, Ontario, Canada
- North Carolina Central University, Durham, North Carolina
- Northern Illinois University, DeKalb, Illinois
- Salus University, Elkins Park, Pennsylvania
- University of Massachusetts, Boston, Massachusetts
- University of Montréal, Montréal, Quebec, Canada
- Western Michigan University, Kalamazoo, Michigan

Organizations

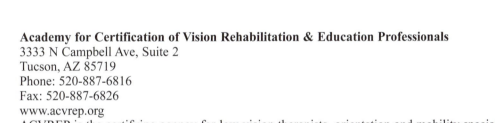

Academy for Certification of Vision Rehabilitation & Education Professionals
3333 N Campbell Ave, Suite 2
Tucson, AZ 85719
Phone: 520-887-6816
Fax: 520-887-6826
www.acvrep.org
ACVREP is the certifying agency for low vision therapists, orientation and mobility specialists, and rehabilitation teachers.

American Occupational Therapy Association
4720 Montgomery La
PO Box 31220
Bethesda, MD 20824-1220
Phone: 301-652-2682
Fax: 301-652-7711
www.aota.org
The AOTA is the nationally recognized professional association for more than 50,000 occupational therapists and occupational therapy assistants.

Association for Education and Rehabilitation of the Blind and Visually Impaired
1703 N Beauregard St, Suite 440
Alexandria, VA 22311
Phone: 877-492-2708 or 703-671-4500
Fax: 703-671-6391
www.aerbvi.org
The AER is an international membership organization dedicated to supporting and assisting the professionals who work in all phases of education and rehabilitation of blind and visually impaired children and adults.

Lighthouse International
111 E 59th St
New York, NY 10022-1202
Phone: 800-829-0500
www.lighthouse.org

Lighthouse International is a leading resource worldwide on vision impairment and vision rehabilitation. Through its pioneering work in vision rehabilitation services, education, research, and advocacy, Lighthouse International enables people of all ages who are blind or partially sighted to lead independent and productive lives.

Low Vision Supplies and Equipment

American Printing House for the Blind Inc
Phone: 800-223-1839
www.aph.org/index.html
- Adult life products catalog
- General products catalog
- Catalog of accessible books for people who are visually impaired or blind

Ann Morris
Phone: 800-537-2118
www.annmorris.com
- Online consumer products catalog

Eschenbach Optik of America Inc
Phone: 800-396-3886
www.Eschenbach.com
- Optical devices catalog

HumanWare Inc
Phone: 800-722-3393
www.humanware.com
- Assistive technology catalog

Independent Living Aids Inc
Phone: 800-537-2118
www.independentliving.com
- Consumer products catalog

Lighthouse International

Phone: 800-829-0500

www.lighthouse.org

- Professional products catalog—optical and nonoptical
- Publications and resources catalog
- Consumer product catalog

LS&S

Phone: 800-468-4789

www.lssproducts.com

- Consumer and professional products catalog

Maxi Aids

Phone: 800-522-6294

www.maxiaids.com

- Consumer and professional products catalog

NoIR Medical Technologies

Phone: 800-521-9746

www.Noir-medical.com

- Catalog of protective eyewear (sun lenses, absorptive lenses)

TeleSensory

Phone: 800-804-8004

www.telesensory.com

- Online catalog of closed-circuit televisions

Financial Disclosures

Dr. Sarah D. Appel has no financial or proprietary interest in the materials presented herein.

Dr. Elise B. Ciner has no financial or proprietary interest in the materials presented herein.

Ms. Maureen A. Duffy has no financial or proprietary interest in the materials presented herein.

Ms. Beth I. Fishman has no financial or proprietary interest in the materials presented herein.

Dr. Lynn Fishman Hellerstein has no financial or proprietary interest in the materials presented herein.

Dr. Paul B. Freeman has no financial or proprietary interest in the materials presented herein.

Ms. Marcy Graboyes has no financial or proprietary interest in the materials presented herein.

Dr. Kathleen Mary Huebner has no financial or proprietary interest in the materials presented herein.

Ms. Maxine Scheiman has financial interest in the Tracking and Perceptual Skills for Occupational Therapists software.

Dr. Mitchell Scheiman has financial interest in the Tracking and Perceptual Skills for Occupational Therapists software.

Ms. Valorie Todd has no financial or proprietary interest in the materials presented herein.

Ms. Kathleen Tsurumi has no financial or proprietary interest in the materials presented herein.

Dr. Stephen G. Whittaker has not disclosed any relevant financial relationships.

Dr. Diane P. Wormsley has no financial or proprietary interest in the materials presented herein.

Index

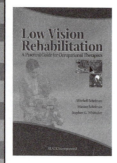
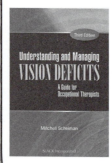

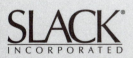